Placebo Tal

Placebo Talks
Modern perspectives on placebos in society

Edited by

Amir Raz and Cory S. Harris

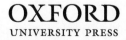

OXFORD
UNIVERSITY PRESS

OXFORD

UNIVERSITY PRESS

Great Clarendon Street, Oxford, OX2 6DP,
United Kingdom

Oxford University Press is a department of the University of Oxford.
It furthers the University's objective of excellence in research, scholarship,
and education by publishing worldwide. Oxford is a registered trade mark of
Oxford University Press in the UK and in certain other countries

First Edition published in 2016
Impression: 1

Published in the United States of America by Oxford University Press
198 Madison Avenue, New York, NY 10016, United States of America

British Library Cataloguing in Publication Data
Data available

Library of Congress Control Number: 2015939607

ISBN 978-0-19-968070-2

Printed and bound by
CPI Group (UK) Ltd, Croydon, CR0 4YY

*To Anyu's first grandchild, to Benci's berye, to my first Kook,
and to the four chickens.*
Amir Raz

To Mac, mes belles filles, and their ever-empowering hugs.
Cory S. Harris

Foreword

Anne Harrington

After decades of suspect status, the placebo effect seems finally to have become scientifically respectable. Recent high-profile brain imaging studies (looking at pain, Parkinson's disease, and depression) promise to cast direct light on at least some of the neurological mechanisms involved in the effect. Harvard University now supports an entire research center dedicated to the placebo effect and the doctor–patient relationship. While one meta-analysis of several decades of past clinical trials proposed that the placebo effect was more hype than reality (Hróbjartsson and Gøtzsche 2001), its criticisms have not stuck; indeed, the backlash against that article has instead had the effect of clarifying "best practice" methods of statistical analysis for the future. Meanwhile, television, radio, the internet, and the print media—interested in the potential practical implications of all of this scientific work—have put the placebo effect in the public eye as never before.

It is an astonishing—and also astonishingly rapid—turnaround for a phenomenon that, for so long, had been so marginalized. Back in our grandparents' day, placebos were understood to provide a kind of cheap psychotherapy in pill form. They belonged, in this sense, to the art rather than the science of medicine; they were a bit of benevolent deception played on patients by doctors who believed that there was nothing seriously wrong or that the symptoms were really "just in the mind." All of their effects—including the relief of anxiety and the disappearance of one or another psychosomatic symptom—were also believed to happen "in the mind."

By the 1950s, it is true, people like Harvard medical professor Henry Beecher had begun to argue that the placebo effect was actually so "powerful" in many patients that methods needed to be developed to protect clinicians seeking to test the efficacy of new drugs from being misled by it (Beecher 1955). The randomized, placebo-controlled clinical trial is a partial response to concerns like these. In such trials, patients in both the experimental and the control group often claim to feel better, and sometimes even show objective signs of improvement. The assumption remained, though, that whatever happened in the placebo group—however striking—was noise in the system, some kind of bodily theatrics rather than true physiological change with clinical interest in its own right.

Then, in the 1970s, two events happened that began to change things. The first of these was an outgrowth of the discovery of endorphins. The word "endorphin" is an abbreviation of "endogenous morphine-like substance." Endorphins were understood to be substances in the brain that are stereochemically similar to morphine, and function as the brain's own natural "painkillers." In 1978, it was reported that giving an experimental subject a placebo version of morphine or some other alleged painkiller—creating a situation in which the patient believed that he or she was going to experience pain relief—actually had the effect of stimulating the release of endorphins (Levine et al. 1978). In other words, the subject created the biochemical conditions that allowed his or her expectation to come true. This was confirmed by showing that administration of naloxone, an opioid receptor blocker, abolished the placebo pain relief. This result implied that placebo pain relief works through known bodily biochemistry. There was flesh and substance to the whole thing after all!

The second thing that began to change the fortunes of the placebo effect was an experiment that also helped to catalyze a new field of research known as psychoneuroimmunology. In 1975, University of Rochester psychologist Robert Ader put a powerful immune-suppressing drug, cyclophosphamide, in saccharine water and fed it to rats. (His goal was to create a state of nausea in the rats and condition them to associate it with the sweet taste of the water; at the outset, he had not realized that the drug also suppressed the immune system.) When his rats grew ill and began to die, he stopped offering them the tainted water and just fed them plain saccharine water. Nevertheless, the rats continued to grow ill and die. In the end, Ader concluded that the rats had been conditioned; that is, the experimental treatment had created an association between the taste of the saccharine water and the biochemical action of cyclophosphamide. As a result, on switching from cyclophosphamide-tainted saccharine water to "placebo" saccharine water, the rats' immune systems continued to act "as if" they were still being suppressed by the drug. In effect, Ader concluded, he had unwittingly demonstrated the potency of placebos, even in non-human experimental subjects (Ader and Cohen 1975).

These two findings appeared to demonstrate that the placebo effect might, after all, be "real." However, at first, no one really paid much attention. The 1970s was a time of new medical consumerism and interest in "holistic treatments," both in the United States and in Europe. These movements were aimed at empowering patients in the face of what was perceived to be a patronizing medical establishment; and in this context, the long-standing association of placebos with deception and paternalism made them seem part of the "bad old past" rather than the "bright new future" (Bok 1974). Holistic medicine was fascinated in other ways by the potential of the so-called mind–body connection, but placebos were not part of its original toolbox.

It was not until the 1990s, and against a backdrop of new questions and new concerns (ranging from the decay of the doctor–patient relationship under managed care to the dominance of big pharma) that people began to take a renewed interest in the power of the placebo. Returning to the suggestive work that had been done in the 1970s, some proposed that the doctor–patient relationship is a more important factor in the clinical equation than people had thought; or that our bodies have their "internal medicine cabinet," or innate capacity for healing that implies we should take fewer drugs and seek ways to cultivate that ability naturally. Helping all of these new conversations along in the 1990s were innovative brain imaging technologies that allowed scientists to create bold, colorful images of the living brain in action. In fact, nothing has helped to make the placebo effect feel real and relevant more than the technologies we now have that appear to let us watch the effect in action inside people's brains (Petrovic et al. 2002).

If we are now taking the placebo effect seriously, what sorts of conversations are we having about it? Here lies the interest and importance of this volume, *Placebo Talks*. This is one of the first books on the placebo effect in which the focus is no longer on making the case for taking the placebo effect seriously: that argument has now been won. Instead, the editors have reached out to scholars and researchers who collectively give us a sense of how we might begin to leverage what we know about the placebo effect in order to make progress on other important topics and questions. The placebo effect appears in this volume less as a cool phenomenon, the reality of which we can capture in brain scans and probe in experimental studies, and more as a lens that we can train onto phenomena as apparently diverse as the nature of false memory, the psychology and culture of dietetics, and what should be included in effective medical education.

Particularly welcome is the degree to which *Placebo Talks* aims to provide knowledge and perspectives that will be useful to people. The placebo effect that emerges in the majority of chapters in this volume is not the abstraction that exists only in the airy realm of philosophy. Nor is it even the carefully controlled phenomenon found only in the laboratory. It is instead a phenomenon grounded in the rich world of human collective experiences, cultural norms, and social institutions. This too strikes me as highly significant. No longer needing to justify our interest in the placebo effect, we find ourselves liberated to begin to identify a whole new set of questions and opportunities for new kinds of scholarly inquiry. In this sense, *Placebo Talks* represents an important milestone in this process of the placebo's coming of age.

References

Ader, R. and Cohen, N. (1975). Behaviorally conditioned immunosuppression. *Psycho-somatic Medicine*, **37**(4), 333–340.

Beecher, H. K. (1955). The powerful placebo. *Journal of the American Medical Association*, **159**, 1602–1606.

Bok, S. (1974). The ethics of giving placebo. *Scientific American*, **231**, 17–23.

Hróbjartsson, A. and Gøtzsche, P. C. (2001). Is the placebo powerless? An analysis of clinical trials comparing placebo with no treatment. *New England Journal of Medicine*, **344**(21), 1594–1602.

Levine, J. D., Gordon, N. C., and Fields, H. L. (1978). The mechanism of placebo analgesia. *The Lancet*, **312**(8091), 654–657.

Petrovic, P., et al. (2002). Placebo and opioid analgesia—imaging a shared neuronal network. *Science*, **295**, 1737–1740.

Contents

Part 4 **The placebo lens**

Part 5 **Concluding remarks**

Contributors

Natasha K. J. Campbell
Montreal Neurological Institute and
Hospital, Clinical Research Unit,
Canada

Bennett Foddy
Tisch School of the Arts Game
Center, New York University,
USA

Ian Gold
Department of Philosophy,
McGill University, Canada

Anne Harrington
Department of the History of
Science at Harvard University,
USA

Cory S. Harris
Department of Biology,
University of Ottawa,
Canada

Timothy Johns
Centre for Indigenous Peoples'
Nutrition and Environment,
School of Dietetics and Human
Nutrition, McGill University,
Canada

Veronica de Jong
Department of Psychiatry,
McGill University,
Canada

Stewart Justman
The Liberal Studies Program,
University of Montana,
USA

Laurence J. Kirmayer
Division of Social and Transcultural
Psychiatry, Department of
Psychiatry, McGill
University,
Canada

Irving Kirsch
Program in Placebo Studies,
Harvard Medical School,
USA

Elizabeth F. Loftus
Department of Psychology and
Social Behavior, Criminology,
Law and Society, and Cognitive
Sciences, University of
California, Irvine,
USA

Daniel E. Moerman
Department of Behavioral Sciences,
University of Michigan-Dearborn,
USA

Michael Orsini
School of Political Studies,
University of Ottawa,
Canada

Marie Prévost
Grenoble Applied Economics
Laboratory (GAEL-INRA),
Laboratory of Psychology and
Neurocognition (LPNC), Université
Pierre-Mendès-France, France

Amir Raz
Departments of Psychiatry,
Neurology and Neurosurgery, and
Psychology, McGill University,
Canada; Lady Davis Institute for
Medical Research at the Jewish
General Hospital of Montreal,
Canada

Paul Saurette
School of Political Studies,
University of Ottawa, Canada

Edward Shorter
Jason A. Hannah Professor
of the History of Medicine /
Professor of Psychiatry, Faculty
of Medicine, University of Toronto,
Canada

Steve Silberman
Investigative reporter (*Wired, PLoS*)
and author

Melanie K. T. Takarangi
School of Psychology,
Flinders University, Adelaide,
Australia

Anna Zuckerman
McGill University, Montreal,
Canada

Part 1

Introduction

Chapter 1

Introduction: placebos in modern society

Veronica de Jong and Cory S. Harris

More than ever, people around the world are talking about placebos. The term has entered our popular vocabulary and the concept, our popular culture. Whether in clinics or universities, boardrooms or courthouses, newspapers or internet forums, the subject of placebos is topical and intriguing and never fails to bring heated debate.

No longer simply the sugar pill given to clinical trial participants who do not get the "good stuff" or the fake prescription given to patients whose symptoms are "all in the head," contemporary concepts of placebos encapsulate much more. Appearing in many guises and in many contexts, placebos and placebo effects are rampant in society, not only in medicine and research but also in our everyday lives.

Why are placebos so intriguing and why are they garnering so much attention, confusion, and debate? At the surface, we find the paradox of *something* from *nothing* and the alluring yet mysterious potential of the mind. Digging deeper to the heart of much of this "placebo talk," we find topics at the fringe of modern medicine but central to human health and well-being. Personal rapport, expectation, empathy, hope, conditioning, symbolic thinking, and suggestion are highly relatable human experiences that lie at the root of placebo effects. Their influence on health and disease, however, is incongruent with our reigning medical paradigm and creates friction that, depending on your point of view, may be exciting, unsettling, or a bit of both.

1.1 Placebos in the twenty-first century

Placebo research has made impressive strides over recent years, most notably in the neurobiology of placebo effects and particularly in placebo analgesia but increasingly in other domains (as so eloquently described by Anne Harrington in the foreword). The existence of placebo effects (also referred to as context effects, meaning effects, care effects, etc.) (Di Blasi and Kleijnen 2003; Louhiala and Puustinen 2008; Moerman 2002), while still debated, is now well supported by convergent and interdisciplinary scientific evidence.

Survey studies confirm that physicians around the world use placebos routinely in clinical practice and consider them to be of legitimate therapeutic value. Not all placebos are equal, however, as the prescriptions for "pure" or "inert" placebos such as sugar pills or saline injections are far less common than those for "impure" or "active" placebos such as unwarranted vitamins or antibiotics (Fassler et al. 2010; Harris and Raz 2012). Clinical research demonstrates that placebo treatments can perform comparably with well-established drugs (e.g., antidepressants) (Kirsch et al. 2008; Temple and Ellenberg 2000) and procedures (e.g., arthroscopic knee surgery) (Moseley et al. 2002; Sihvonen et al. 2013) and better than standard care for conditions such as chronic pain and aggressive behavior (Haake et al. 2007; Tyrer et al. 2008). Clinical data reveal that different types of placebos can be more effective than others in different settings with, for example, sham acupuncture tending to outperform other physical placebos like surgery, which tend to outperform pharmacological placebos like injections and pills (Linde et al. 2010). We now also have evidence that placebos can work even if the nature of the treatment is openly disclosed to patients (Kaptchuk et al. 2010). Neurobiology, moreover, shows that placebo administration can activate the brain in numerous ways to mediate symptom relief, including through the activation of the opioid and endocannabinoid systems in pain relief and of dopamine release in parkinsonian patients (Benedetti 2014).

Despite this progress, however, many questions remain. Neither clinical trials nor neurobiology, for example, has managed to explain how and why red placebos stimulate whereas blue ones calm, four placebos work better than two, or sham interventions can perform on par with successful drugs and operations. Unfortunately, the tectonic nature of placebo science as a field of study complicates the consolidation and synthesis of relevant interdisciplinary research. At the same time, the place for placebos in clinical medicine continues to evade consensus; from the American Medical Association's restrictive position to the German Medical Association's permissive stance, policies regulating the use of placebos are nascent and contentious, if not entirely absent.

Offering a malleable paradigm with "blank" or even deceptive properties, placebos present a unique opportunity to investigate healing beyond the narrow range of variables typically attributed to medical interventions. As described briefly here and in more depth throughout this volume, the blossoming field of placebo science continues to surprise researchers, practitioners, and the public by highlighting both the shortfalls of clinical medicine and the riches of psychosocial influences on health and healing.

The existence of placebos and placebo effects—as well as the power of placebo science—is not limited, however, to medicine or healing. Analogies of placebo abound across cultures and societies, in the past, present, and foreseeable future. Such placebo-like situations similarly offer a unique paradigm through which to study non-medical phenomena that manifest through psychosocial influences on physiology or behaviors. For instance, placebos appear metaphorically as a developmental tool for the transition between dependence and independence, amateur and professional, or apprentice and teacher. When teaching a child to ride a bike, a caregiver initially supports the child's seat but, later, may only say they are doing so in leading the unsuspecting child to ride independently. The bestowal of a supposedly lucky or storied piece of equipment like a baseball bat (or, in the case of Harry Potter and Ron Weasley, a potion—Rowling 2005), can similarly help the recipient perform more confidently in sport. A photographer may similarly leave the camera empty during the first rounds of a photo shoot with new (and unaware) models to help them relax and gain confidence before starting the real shoot.

Some professionals, including entertainers, performers, and magicians, draw on placebo-like principles to build their reputation, mystique, and career. With certain other practices, elements of placebo arise in ways that are less agreeable, even though we accept them as part of the social fabric. In an attempt to influence consumer experience, for example, brand imaging seeks to construct symbolic associations and consumer expectations to enhance the cultural value of a product or service. As an extension, the production and sale of replica or counterfeit products capitalizes on the value created through branding while providing consumers with an inferior product, with or without their knowledge. Although none of these examples are particularly shocking, their implications are varied and far reaching. Like their medical counterparts, everyday placebos, their effects and their consequences, require more than a single lens to be appreciated and understood.

In order to capture the diverse roles that placebos play in modern society—including within medicine—we must take a fundamentally interdisciplinary approach. *Placebo talks* meets this challenge by presenting readers, for the first time, with a comprehensive, multifaceted view of placebos, seldom captured by either academic or popular sources alone.

1.2 **An interdisciplinary look at placebo use in society**

Combining perspectives from medicine, the social sciences, and beyond, we invite you to explore the diverse aspects and impacts of placebos in the twenty-first century. This volume does not attempt to prove the placebo effect but starts from the premise that it exists. The contributing authors build on a broad yet cohesive body of evidence to examine placebos and placebo effects as they exist not only in clinical practice and research but also in education, government, industry, media, culture, and everyday life. We also do not attempt to implement a standard definition. Instead, we leave it up to the individual authors to use their best definition for placebos and related terminologies. In fact, the volume will likely expose most readers to new definitions and interpretations, which we welcome given our intent to demonstrate the plurality of placebos. In the process, we transition from looking at medical placebos through the lens of science to looking at medicine, health, and social interactions through the lens of placebo science. The book moves beyond pain as the central model for exploring placebo effects to entertain the equally germane but less explored paradigm of depression (not to mention diet, politics, or sex). Through the voices and expertise of many of the field's most prominent scholars, this volume talks through the negative connotations and misconceptions embedded in placebo terminology, reconstituting placebos as a promising therapeutic tool, a bourgeoning field of study, and a rich framework for interdisciplinary investigation.

This volume is based, in part, on conversations and presentations from a two-day workshop held at the Jewish General Hospital, Montreal, in July 2010 under the sponsorship of the Social Sciences and Humanities Research Council. A number of chapters have been adapted from a subsequent special edition of the *Journal of Mind–Body Regulation* (June and October 2011) and others have since been added.

The book comprises three main sections, each looking at placebo use through a different lens—the practitioner lens, the cultural lens, and the placebo lens.

1.2.1 The practitioner lens

The "practitioner lens" section of the book addresses the use of placebos in contemporary medicine. Whereas some may think that modern practitioners have mostly done away with placebos, current practices provide ample opportunity for practical and conceptual explorations of placebo use. We begin in the context of clinical trials, where placebo research found its popular beginnings (see Anne Harrington's foreword for a historical account of placebos in medicine and research). We also introduce depression as a model for examining placebos and one that unifies much of the discussion throughout the book. From there, we explore how physicians currently use placebos in the clinic to examine some important ethical and philosophical considerations central to the doctor–patient relationship. Finally, we take a practical look at where placebos fit into today's medical education curricula.

In the opening contribution, clinical and experimental psychologist Irving Kirsch presents his astounding and controversial research on the relative effectiveness of antidepressants and placebos in randomized controlled trials (RCTs). Kirsch and colleagues' meta-analyses of placebo-controlled antidepressant trials expose a particularly disturbing reality of the pharmaceutical industry's influence on the apparent efficacy of antidepressants. Their findings, replicated by independent researchers (Fournier et al. 2010; Khan et al. 2002; Rief et al. 2009), reveal hardly any clinical benefit of antidepressants compared to placebos and raise pressing and provocative questions concerning the standard of care for the millions of patients suffering from mild-to-moderate depression worldwide.

Controversy in the literature surrounding treatments that fare no better than placebo demands investigation of how practitioners who rely on such treatments receive and apply this information. In the next chapter, placebo researchers Veronica de Jong and Amir Raz dig further into the use of a particular type of active placebo—sub-therapeutic doses—in the context of antidepressant therapy for depression. Attempting to elucidate the clinical rationales for such prescriptions, de Jong and Raz survey psychiatrist attitudes and opinions on the practice through one-on-one interviews. Do sub-therapeutic doses provide an outlet for clinicians wishing to harness the placebo effect and avoid handing out inert pills? Does their use sidestep the bad clinical form associated with placebo prescriptions, especially due to the deception presumably involved?

With all diagnoses and treatments, the context of the associated clinical encounter is ripe with potential placebo-like elements. Communication between the physician and the patient is a key component of some of the typical arguments for, but also against, placebos in the clinic. On the one hand, good communication is vital to the patient–physician relationship and an aspect of care known to induce positive therapeutic outcomes on its own (Thomas 1987). On the other hand, the use of a physical placebo may necessitate deceptive communication—a clinical faux pas with the potential of undermining the patient–physician relationship and compromising patient autonomy (Miller and Colloca 2009). However, philosopher and bioethicist Bennett Foddy makes a bold and carefully crafted argument against these common notions in his chapter, "Justifying deceptive placebos." Foddy breaks down deception, exposing its multifaceted nature, some of its forms being commonplace and permissible in the everyday. From Foddy's perspective, deceptive use of placebos is, in some circumstances, both ethically permissible and achievable without serious harm to the doctor–patient relationship, which in itself is central to fostering placebo effects and healing more broadly.

The fourth chapter within the practitioner lens section, "Trust and placebos," delves into the often mentioned but rarely explored aspect of trust within the patient–physician relationship. Philosophers of medicine Ian Gold, Marie Prévost, and Anna Zuckerman probe the contribution of a trusting relationship, versus a reliant one, to placebo outcomes and to medical treatment in general. Drawing on a non-medical example, they outline how one can rely on a computer to do something—but not trust it—to illustrate the point that a doctor may prescribe out of routine, without any trust-forming goodwill as motivation. However, while this trust may impact on placebo effects engendered by the patient–physician relationship, few empirical studied have explored the individual elements of this relationship. The authors call for direct investigation into the role of trust in placebo effects—a call echoed frequently with respect to other sociocultural factors in subsequent chapters.

Although many empirical questions remain concerning placebo effects in clinical care, placebo research has made substantial advances, especially in light of the complexity and chameleon-like appearance of placebo effects across medical domains. One might suspect that placebo effects—given their history, prevalence, and therapeutic potential—would be prioritized as a subject for medical students. In their chapter about placebos in medical education, Natasha Campbell and Amir Raz tell of a very different reality. Through their exploration of the current state of placebo teaching in medical schools across North America and Europe, placebo is apparently not a common utterance in the halls of the biomedical breeding grounds, at least not in terms of formal curricula and evaluation. Whereas in-depth knowledge of seventeenth-century physics is a prerequisite to entering medical school, many graduates are left to witness and comprehend placebo effects only once in the field, if ever.

Looking through the practitioner's lens raises many questions. How much of the doctor's role is writing prescriptions compared to talking to patients? Do we expect or want computer-like doctors processing available data to find the statistically favorable course of action, or trustworthy caregivers gauging their words and actions to best suit the needs of their individual patients? Should doctors continue to prescribe drugs or sub-therapeutic doses but not placebos—particularly not deceptive placebos—if evidence shows their efficacies are therapeutically comparable?

1.2.2 The cultural lens

The paradoxical nature of placebos and their effects presents a practical and conceptual obstacle for practitioners, researchers, and policy makers alike. In the "cultural lens" section of the book, Dan Moerman, Laurence Kirmayer, Stewart Justman, and Steve Silberman apply their distinct sociocultural lenses to help understand placebo effects in health and society and shed light on some resounding questions.

According to Moerman, a renowned cultural anthropologist, the paradox of placebo is based in terminology and easily rectified by changing focus from inert placebos to meaningful symbols, words, actions, and settings. Reviewing a spectacular diversity of research ranging from meta-analyses to qualitative psychology, he provides a personalized and updated review of his previous work on the meaning response, a tenor that continues to influence modern conceptualizations of placebo. He describes how elements such as language, visual cues, expectations, and beliefs impact on human physiology or patient outcomes for better or worse, highlighting recent studies where the power of meaning is both surprising and impressive. From this viewpoint, the variability of placebo effects between and within individuals and across diseases, time, and cultures begins to make sense.

In the next chapter, Kirmayer, a noted transcultural psychiatrist, takes the placebo concept outside the bounds of biomedicine. With a focus on mental illness and depression-like conditions, his chapter draws on indigenous healing systems as well as their associated cultural, social, and spiritual foundations in formulating an ethnographic model of placebo effects. Kirmayer discusses symbolic and ritual healing together with their real, potential, and believed-in efficacy. The paramount roles given to social interaction, community support, and collective belief in these settings are strikingly absent from modern treatment protocols, even for conditions like depression, where these elements directly contribute to diagnosis and morbidity.

Complementing Kirmayer's emphasis on social interactions in health and healing, Justman argues, in the next chapter, that placebo effects are about more than the relationship and context of the clinical encounter. Placebo effects have broader social roots through word of mouth, advertising, and popular culture. Considering examples from popular literature and comparing today's antidepressant hype to historical trends such as Mesmerism, Justman positions placebo effects as social forces brought by the public sphere to the medical arena. In this way, placebo effects can potentially manifest in various forms and aspects of our lives—a concept we explore more thoroughly throughout this section of the book.

Closing off the cultural lens section, Silberman takes the reader on an armchair tour of placebos in popular culture as only a journalist of his caliber can. Articulating in his chapter the process and aftermath of writing his popular 2009 *WIRED* article on placebos and the pharmaceutical industry (Silberman 2009), he juxtaposes the public appetite for controversial themes in health and healing against the largely superficial and inadequate coverage of science and medicine in the mainstream media. In doing so, Silberman not only highlights connections between placebo and healing, complementary and alternative medicine (CAM), and biomedicine, as well as mind and body, but also discusses the constructed boundaries obstructing the miscibility of these links in the healthcare context.

1.2.3 The placebo lens

Whether looking at placebos through the lens of clinical practice or culture and society, the subject arises almost exclusively in the medical context. As discussed at the onset, however, placebos are everywhere. From learning to ride a bike, to magic tricks, to brand imaging, everyday placebos resemble their medical counterparts to varying degrees. In order to study and understand how and why people behave the way they do, we need a nuanced, interdisciplinary model—like that of placebo. In the "placebo lens" part of the book, scholars of diverse disciplines apply the framework and vernacular of placebo to their respective fields of study. In each unique chapter, the authors rely on different models and draw from different aspects of the literature to forge new links between their chosen fields and placebo research.

Like medicines, foods are central to human health and possess both physiologically active chemicals (nutritional and drug-like) as well as cultural and symbolic meanings that contribute to our dietary attitudes, behaviors, and experiences. Adapting a placebo model from the medical milieu, Cory Harris and Timothy Johns, in their chapter, develop their concept of the "total food effect," which integrates the nutritional, pharmacological, psychological, social, and cultural dimensions that exist with respect to food and dietary habits. From flavor perception to lactose intolerance to caffeine(-free) highs, they outline how the mind is capable of modifying, if not overriding, biological responses to perceived physical and chemical stimuli. With a global population increasingly burdened by nutrition-related diseases and swamped by food choices and marketing claims, the authors' model offers a valuable interdisciplinary vehicle to investigate how these interacting factors influence health at the individual and collective level.

Whereas the sensory and physiological activity of food constituents provides a fertile setting for the occurrence and study of placebo-related effects, psychological factors such as beliefs, suggestions, and expectations have no such chemistry. In their chapter, psychologists Melanie Takarangi and Elizabeth Loftus describe how memory becomes vulnerable to distortion when people are given suggestive information. Discussing paradigms involving imagination, corroboration, collaboration, and false feedback, they refer to suggestive effects on social behaviors and cognition to uncover the considerable overlap between placebos and false memories. Moreover, by applying their framework to examples of pharmaceuticals, social drugs, food, and popular culture, they highlight the merit of approaching placebo effects from a non-medical perspective. With both false memories and placebos presenting potential physical, psychological, social, economic, and legal consequences, future research on both subjects stand to benefit from a common ground.

Suggestion, although typically understood as framed by external sources, can also arise internally through personal or shared experiences within a particular cultural context. Applying a straightforward model of placebo effects alongside a historical account of contemporary sexual behavior, Edward Shorter forwards the notion of cultural placebos in a new direction. Similar to medical placebos, members of society perceive cultural placebos as active somatic stimuli that elicit physiological responses in the body "even though the stimulus is just the cultural equivalent of a sugar pill". As Shorter articulates, the recent emergence of fetish—a material stimulus to a sexual response—among more historically documented sexual behaviors provides a unique and provocative example of cultural placebos in action.

Tempted by negative connotations transferred from medicine, the idea of placebos in the political arena at first seems obvious. Rhetoric and half-truths to silence an uneasy or suffering public, inept or powerless policies and programs for the mere appearance of action, and national security measures with no impact on safety beyond public perception are but a few examples that come to mind. However, reflecting the tone of previous chapters, Michael Orsini and Paul Saurette disagree with such narrow and superficial interpretations of political placebo effects. In their chapter, the authors build on Moerman's meaning response and Foddy's ethical arguments to develop a more nuanced definition that mirrors our evolving understanding of placebos in medicine. Drawing on recent political events and media coverage, they attempt and succeed at providing novel insights into public responses previously approached by politicians and journalists almost exclusively through rational models. This chapter, like Shorter's and others before it, demonstrates the versatility of placebo as an explanatory model within the social sciences.

1.3 **Looking forward to placebo science**

As Amir Raz describes in his closing remarks in Chapter 15, this book is several years in the making. Over this time, placebo science has continued to expand, and numerous new and exciting findings have taken the field in new directions, with even greater exposure. Like this volume, the recently established and international Society for Interdisciplinary Placebo Studies highlights the need—and our progress toward—an integrated and nuanced approach to understanding placebos, placebo effects, and their potential roles and impacts in the twenty-first century. In reading this volume's vast array of "placebo talk", we invite readers to open their minds to how placebos may speak to their own experiences in health, in healing, and in all other aspects of contemporary life.

References

Benedetti, F. (2014). *Placebo effects.* Oxford: Oxford University Press.

Di Blasi, Z. and Kleijnen, J. (2003). Context effects. Powerful therapies or methodological bias? *Evaluation & the Health Professions*, **26**(2), 166–179.

Fassler, M., Meissner, K., Schneider, A., and Linde, K. (2010). Frequency and circumstances of placebo use in clinical practice—a systematic review of empirical studies. *BMC Medicine*, **8**, 15.

Fournier, J. C., DeRubeis, R. J., Hollon, S. D., et al. (2010). Antidepressant drug effects and depression severity: a patient-level meta-analysis. *Journal of the American Medical Association*, **303**(1), 47–53.

Haake, M., Muller, H. H., Schade-Brittinger, C., et al. (2007). German acupuncture trials (GERAC) for chronic low back pain: randomized, multicenter, blinded, parallel-group trial with 3 groups. *Archives of Internal Medicine*, **167**(17), 1892–1898.

Harris, C. S. and Raz, A. (2012). Deliberate use of placebos in clinical practice: what we really know. *Journal of Medical Ethics*, **38**(7), 406–407.

Kaptchuk, T. J., Friedlander, E., Kelley, J. M., et al. (2010). Placebos without deception: a randomized controlled trial in irritable bowel syndrome. *PLoS One*, **5**(12), e15591.

Khan, A., Leventhal, R. M., Khan, S. R., and Brown, W. A. (2002). Severity of depression and response to antidepressants and placebo: an analysis of the Food and Drug Administration database. *Journal of Clinical Psychopharmacology*, **22**(1), 40.

Kirsch, I., Deacon, B. J., Huedo-Medina, T. B., Scoboria, A., Moore, T. J., and Johnson, B. T. (2008). Initial severity and antidepressant benefits: a meta-analysis of data submitted to the Food and Drug Administration. *PLoS Medicine*, **5**(2), e45.

Linde, K., Niemann, K., and Meissner, K. (2010). Are sham acupuncture interventions more effective than (other) placebos? A re-analysis of data from the Cochrane review on placebo effects. *Forschende Komplementarmedizin*, **17**(5), 259–264.

Louhiala, P. and Puustinen, R. (2008). Rethinking the placebo effect. *Medical Humanities*, **34**(2), 107–109.

Miller, F. G. and Colloca, L. (2009). The legitimacy of placebo treatments in clinical practice: evidence and ethics. *The American Journal of Bioethics*, **9**(12), 39.

Moerman, D. E. (2002). *Meaning, medicine and the "placebo effect": Cambridge studies in medical anthropology.* Cambridge/New York: Cambridge University Press.

Moseley, J. B., O'Malley, K., Petersen, N. J., et al. (2002). A controlled trial of arthroscopic surgery for osteoarthritis of the knee. *New England Journal of Medicine*, **347**(2), 81–88.

Rief, W., Nestoriuc, Y., Weiss, S., Welzel, E., Barsky, A. J., and Hofmann, S. G. (2009). Meta-analysis of the placebo response in antidepressant trials. *Journal of Affective Disorders*, **11**(1–3), 1–8.

Rowling, J. K. (2005). *Harry Potter and the half-blood prince.* London: Bloomsbury.

Sihvonen, R., Paavola, M., Malmivaara, A., et al. (2013). Arthroscopic partial meniscec-tomy versus sham surgery for a degenerative meniscal tear. *New England Journal of Medicine*, **369**(26), 2515–2524.

Silberman, S. (2009). Placebos are getting more effective. Drugmakers are desperate to know why. *WIRED Magazine*, **17**, 1–8.

Temple, R. and Ellenberg, S. S. (2000). Placebo-controlled trials and active-control trials in the evaluation of new treatments. Part 1: ethical and scientific issues. *Annals of Internal Medicine*, **133**(6), 455–463.

Thomas, K. B. (1987). General practice consultations: is there any point in being positive? *British Medical Journal*, **294**(6581), 1200–1202.

Tyrer, P., Oliver-Africano, P. C., Ahmed, Z., et al. (2008). Risperidone, haloperidol, and placebo in the treatment of aggressive challenging behaviour in patients with intellec-tual disability: a randomised controlled trial. *The Lancet*, **371**(9606), 57–63.

Part 2

The practitioner lens

Chapter 2

Antidepressants and the placebo effect

Irving Kirsch

2.1 Introduction

I used to think that antidepressants worked. As a clinical psychologist, I had for years referred some of my clients to psychiatric colleagues who could prescribe antidepressants for them. Sometimes, the antidepressants did not seem to help, but when they did, I assumed that the benefit derived from the chemical properties of the drug. In this chapter, I describe the process by which I came first to doubt and then to disbelieve the hypothesis that antidepressants had a biochemical effect on depression, a process that is more fully documented in my book, *The emperor's new drugs: exploding the antidepressant myth* (Kirsch 2009,2010).

My entry into the world of antidepressant research was serendipitous. I was not particularly interested in evaluating the effects of antidepressants. Instead, I began looking at antidepressant clinical trials because of my long-standing interest in a psychological construct called response expectancy (Kirsch 1985). Response expectancies are anticipations of automatic subjective reactions, like changes in depression, anxiety, and pain. I have argued that response expectancies are self-confirming. The world in which we live is ambiguous, and one of the functions of the brain is to disambiguate it rapidly enough to respond quickly. We do this, in part, by forming expectations. So what we experience at any given time is a joint function of the stimuli to which we are exposed and our beliefs and expectations about those stimuli (Kirsch 1999).

When I first began researching antidepressants, the response expectancy hypothesis was the focus of most of my research. The particular topic areas (hypnosis, psychotherapy, placebo effects, etc.) were chosen merely because they provided a convenient opportunity for examining expectancy effects. It seemed to me that depression ought to be particularly responsive to expectancy effects. This is because hopelessness is a central feature of depression (Abramson et al. 1978) and hopelessness is an expectancy. Specifically, it is the expectancy that a negative state of affairs will not get better, no matter what one does to alleviate it.

Many depressed people will probably tell you that the worst thing in their lives is their depression. They believe that their depression will continue, no matter what they do—a very depressing thought indeed. As John Teasdale (1985) noted, these people are depressed about their depression. If this is the case, then the expectancy of improvement should produce improvement. That is, the belief that one will improve is the opposite of the hopelessness that may be maintaining the depression or, at the very least, is an important component of it. In other words, there ought to be a substantial placebo effect associated with the treatment of depression.

2.2 Listening to Prozac but hearing placebo

In 1998, Guy Sapirstein and I undertook a meta-analysis, the purpose of which was to evaluate the placebo effect in depression (Kirsch and Sapirstein 1998). We searched the literature for studies in which depressed patients had been randomized to receive antidepressant medication, an inert placebo, psychotherapy, or no treatment at all. We included studies of psychotherapy, because those were the only ones in which patients had been randomized to a no-treatment control condition, and we needed that condition to evaluate the placebo effect. The response to a placebo is not the same as the effect of the placebo. The placebo response (as opposed to the placebo effect) may, at least in part, be due to the passage of time, spontaneous remission, the natural history of the disorder, and regression to the mean. Just as the difference between the drug response and the placebo response is deemed to be the drug effect, so the difference between the placebo response and improvement in a no-treatment control group can be interpreted as the placebo effect.

The results of our meta-analysis indicated equal and substantial improvement among patients given medication or psychotherapy. However, patients given placebos also got better, whereas those in no-treatment control groups showed relatively little improvement. We found that approximately 25% of the improvement in the drug group would have occurred without any treatment whatsoever, 50% was a placebo effect, and only 25% was a true drug effect (see Figure 2.1). In other words, the placebo effect (which is the difference between the response to being given a placebo and what would have happened had no treatment been given at all) was twice as large as the drug effect (the response to the drug minus the response to the placebo). This was indeed surprising. Antidepressants had been hailed as miracle drugs that had produced a revolution in the treatment of depression.

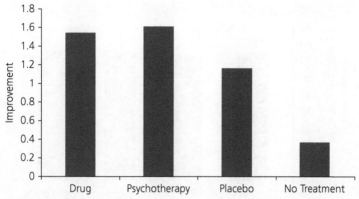

Fig. 2.1 Average improvement on drugs, psychotherapy, placebo, and no treatment. Improvement refers to reduction of symptoms on scales used to measure depression. The numbers are called "effect sizes." They are commonly used when the results of different studies are pooled together. Typically, effect sizes of 0.5 are considered moderate effects, whereas effect sizes of 0.8 are considered large. So, the graph shows that antidepressants, psychotherapy, and placebo all produce a large change in the symptoms of depression, but there is only a relatively small average improvement in people who are not given any treatment at all.

Data from Irving Kirsch and Guy Sapirstein, Listening to Prozac but hearing placebo: A meta-analysis of antidepressant medication, *Prevention and Treatment*, 1 (2), DOI: 10.1037/1522–3736.1.1.12a, 1998.

Our surprise at the outcome of our analysis led us to wonder whether it may have been due to the diversity of antidepressants in the clinical trials we had analyzed. Perhaps some of the medications were very effective and others not, leading us to underestimate the drug effect. To assess this possibility, we returned to our data set and classified the various studies in terms of the type of medication evaluated. We categorized them into four types: tricyclic medications, selective serotonin reuptake inhibitors (SSRIs), miscellaneous other antidepressants, and other medications. The consistency was remarkable. Regardless of the type of medication studied, 75% of the response to the active drugs was duplicated by placebo, leaving a true drug effect of only 25% in each case (Figure 2.2). What makes this particularly surprising is the response to what we have labeled "other medication." These are active drugs that are not regarded as antidepressants (e.g., lithium, barbiturates, and thyroid medication given to depressed patients who were not suffering from depression). They too produced substantial improvement in depression—as great as that produced by tricyclics, SSRIs, and other antidepressants. Joanna Moncrieff has described similar data concerning an even wider range of medications that all surpass placebo in the treatment of depression (Moncrieff 2008), and I have since learned

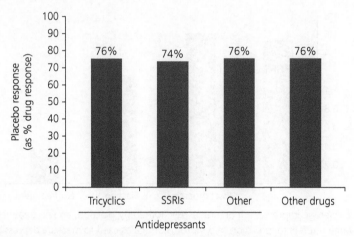

Fig. 2.2 The placebo response as a percentage of the drug response.

Data from Irving Kirsch and Guy Sapirstein, Listening to Prozac but hearing placebo: A meta-analysis of antidepressant medication, *Prevention and Treatment*, 1 (2), DOI: 10.1037/1522–3736.1.1.12a, 1998.

that the same antidepressant effect can be produced by drugs that are supposed to decrease, rather than increase, serotonin levels (Kirsch 2009, 2010). What do you call a substance, the effects of which are independent of its physical properties? I call it a placebo.

The finding of equivalent antidepressant effects of all of these different drugs led us to search for their commonality. One thing they have in common is that they all produce side-effects. Placebos can also produce side-effects, but they do so to a much lesser degree than active medications (Philipp et al. 1999). Why is this important? Imagine that you are recruited to a clinical trial for an anti-depressant medication. As this is a double-blind trial, you are told that you may receive medication or you may receive placebo. You are also told that the active medication has been reported to produce a number of side-effects, such as dry mouth and drowsiness, and that the therapeutic effect may not become evident for some weeks. You are likely to wonder to which group you have been assigned, the active drug group or the placebo control group. You notice that your mouth has become dry and that you feel drowsy. At this point, you are likely to conclude that you have been assigned to the drug condition. Indeed, data indicate that about 80% of patients assigned to the active drug condition in clinical trials of antidepressants break blind and conclude that they are in the active drug condition (Rabkin et al. 1986). Being more certain that you have been assigned to the drug group, you will have a stronger expectancy for improvement which, according to the response expectancy hypothesis, should produce greater improvement. In other words, it is possible that the superiority of active anti-depressant to inert placebo is due to patients breaking blind in the active drug condition. Rather than being a true drug effect, it is an enhanced placebo effect.

The equivalence of active drugs in treating depression shows the importance of including placebos when evaluating new medications. Were these compara-tor trials, rather than placebo-controlled trials, we would have concluded that all of the drugs were highly effective in the treatment of depression. Instead, the data tell us that, except for the large placebo effect they generate, they are all equally ineffective. It is true that conventional randomized controlled trials (RCTs) have various shortcomings, including the problem that patients may break blind because of the side-effects of the active drug, but these weaknesses lead to overestimation of the drug effects, rather than underestimation. Trials that seek to demonstrate drug efficacy by showing equivalence to prior approved drugs are even worse, in that they lead to even greater overestimation of drug effectiveness because, as this chapter shows, previously approved drugs may not be effective at all.

2.3 The emperor's new drugs

Needless to say, our first meta-analysis proved to be quite controversial. Its pub-lication led to heated exchanges. The response from critics was that these data could not be accurate. Perhaps our search had led us to analyze an unrepresen-tative subset of clinical trials. Antidepressants had been evaluated in many trials and their effectiveness had been well established.

In an effort to respond to these critics, we decided to replicate our study with a different set of clinical trials (Kirsch et al. 2002). We used the Freedom of Information Act to request that the Food and Drug Administration (FDA) send us the data that pharmaceutical companies had sent to it in the process of obtaining approval for six new-generation antidepressants that accounted for the bulk of antidepressant prescriptions being written at the time. There are a number of advantages to the FDA data set. First, the FDA requires that the pharmaceutical companies provide information on all of the clinical trials that they have sponsored. Thus, we had data on unpublished trials as well as pub-lished trials. Second, the same primary outcome measure—the Hamilton depression scale (HAM-D)—was used in all of the trials. That made it easy to understand the clinical significance of the drug–placebo differences. Third, these were the data on the basis of which the medications were approved. In that sense, they have a privileged status. If there is anything wrong with them, the decision to approve the medications in the first place can be called into question.

In the data sent to us by the FDA, only 43% of the trials showed a statistically significant benefit of drug over placebo. The results of our analysis indicated that the placebo response was 82% of the response to these antidepressants. Subsequently, my colleagues and I replicated our meta-analysis on a larger number of trials that had been submitted to the FDA (Kirsch et al. 2008). With this expanded data set, we found once again that 82% of the drug response was duplicated by placebo. More important, in both analyses, the mean difference between drug and placebo was less than two points on the HAM-D. The National Institute for Clinical Excellence (NICE), which drafts treatment guidelines for the National Health Service in the United Kingdom, has established a three-point difference between drug and placebo on the HAM-D as a criterion of clinical significance (NICE 2004). Thus, when published and unpublished data are combined, they fail to show a clinically significant advantage for antidepressant medication over inert placebo.

At roughly the same time as our second meta-analysis of the FDA data set was done, Corrado Barbui and his colleagues (Barbui et al. 2008) analyzed the data on paroxetine that had been reported on the GlaxoSmithKline (GSK) website. As part of the settlement of a lawsuit brought against GSK by the State of New York for withholding data showing negative results, the company is required to post summary data from all of its clinical trials of antidepressants, including those that have not been published (Spitzer 2004). Unlike the FDA files, which are limited to pre-approval trial, the GSK website includes post-marketing trials as well. Barbui et al. (2008) found forty placebo-controlled studies of paroxetine for the treatment of major depression, including the sixteen that had been sent to the FDA. Although they analyzed response rates rather than mean symptom change, the results of their analysis of these forty studies were virtually identical to the results of our analysis of the studies that had been sent to the FDA. In their analysis, the placebo was 83% as effective as the real drug. Thus, the failure to find a clinically significant difference between drug and placebo holds for post-marketing as well as pre-marketing trials.

There are two types of design that were used in the clinical trials submitted to the FDA. The most common involved allowing prescribing physicians to adjust the dose as needed during the course of the trial. In addition, approximately one-quarter of trials used a fixed-dose design, in which patients were randomized to receive particular doses of the medication. Thus, we were concerned that the data we had analyzed might have included patients who were assigned to receive an inadequate or subclinical dose of the medication. If this were the case, then we might have underestimated the drug effect.

To check out this possibility, we performed an additional analysis on the fixed-dose clinical trials. Specifically, we compared improvement among patients given the lowest dose used in the trial with improvement among patients given the highest dose. We found that improvement at the lowest dose (9.57 points on the HAM-D) was virtually identical to improvement at the highest dose (9.97 on the HAM-D). Nor was there any apparent advantage for mid-range doses. In fact, out of approximately forty comparisons of different doses of the same antidepressant, only one significant difference was reported. In a study of fluoxetine in moderately to severely depressed patients, the two lower doses were significantly more effective than the high dose, which was not significantly more effective than placebo.

2.4 **The "dirty little secret"**

Whereas the response to our earlier meta-analysis was incredulity, the response to our analysis of the FDA data indicated unanimous acceptance among twelve groups of independent scholars—some of them clinical trialists who had carried out evaluations of antidepressants for pharmaceutical companies—who had been invited to comment on the paper. As one group of commentators put it, "many have long been unimpressed by the magnitude of the differences observed between treatments and controls, what some of our colleagues refer to as the 'dirty little secret' in the pharmaceutical literature" (Hollon et al. 2002).

Perhaps the most disturbing aspect of the keeping of this secret is the complicity of the FDA. Among the data we received using our freedom of information request were copies of internal memos. One of these, written by the Director of the Division of Neuropharmacological Drug Products includes the following revealing information:

> The Clinical Efficacy Trials subsection within the Clinical Pharmacology section not only describes the clinical trials providing evidence of citalopram's antidepressant effects, but make mention of adequate and well controlled clinical studies that failed to do so. I am mindful, based on prior discussions of the issue, that the Office Director is inclined toward the view that the provision of such information is of no practical value to either the patient or prescriber. I disagree. I believe it is useful for the prescriber, patient, and 3rd party payer to know, without having to gain access to official FDA review documents, that citalopram's antidepressant effects were not detected in every controlled clinical trial intended to demonstrate those effects. I am aware that clinical studies often fail to document the efficacy of effective drugs, but I doubt the public, or even the majority of medical community, are aware of this fact. I am persuaded they not only have a right to know, but should know. Moreover, I believe that labelling that selectively describes positive studies and excludes mention of negative ones can be viewed as potentially "false and misleading." (Leber 1998, p. 11)

2.5 **How did these drugs get approved?**

How is it that medications with such weak efficacy data were approved by the FDA? The answer lies in an understanding of the approval criteria used by the FDA. The FDA requires two adequately conducted clinical trials showing a significant difference between drug and placebo. However, there is a loophole: there is no limit to the number of trials that can be conducted in search of these two significant trials. Trials showing negative results simply do not count. Furthermore, the clinical significance of the findings is not considered. All that matters is that the results are statistically significant.

A typical example of the implementation of this criterion is provided by the FDA file on citalopram. Seven controlled efficacy trials were conducted. Two showed small but significant drug–placebo differences. Two were deemed too small to count. Three failing to show any significant benefit for the drug were deemed "adequate" and "well controlled," but were "not counted against citalopram" because there was a "substantial placebo response" (internal memo by T.P. Laughren, FDA Team Leader for Psychiatric Drug Products). Thus, citalopram was approved on the basis of two clinical trials despite negative results in five other trials.

2.6 **The myth of the chemical imbalance**

Depression, we are told over and over again, is a brain disease, a chemical imbalance that can be adjusted by antidepressant medication. I will argue that it is about as close as a theory gets in science to being disproven by the evidence.

When the chemical imbalance theory was introduced more than forty years ago, the main evidence in favor of it was the contention that antidepressants, which were thought to increase the availability of serotonin and/or other neurotransmitters in the brain, seemed to be effective in the treatment of depression. As Alec Coppen wrote in 1967, "one of the most cogent reasons for believing that there is a biochemical basis for depression or mania is the astonishing success of physical methods of treatment of these conditions" (Coppen 1967, p. 1237). The situation has not changed very much since then. People still cite the supposed effectiveness of antidepressants as fundamental support for the chemical imbalance hypothesis. This theory, they say, is supported by "the indisputable therapeutic efficacy of these drugs" (Malhi et al. 2005, p. 97).

Although the therapeutic effectiveness of antidepressants seemed "astonishing" forty years ago and still seems "indisputable" to many today, it is, in fact, an illusion. When the unpublished as well as published data are analyzed, the difference between the effects of antidepressants and placebos is clinically insignificant, despite clinical trial methods that ought to enhance it. However, strangely enough, it is not the ineffectiveness of antidepressants that seals the fate of the chemical imbalance theory but rather, it is their effectiveness. The problem is that too many different types of antidepressants work too well for the theory to make physiological sense.

Different types of antidepressants are supposed to work by different means. SSRIs are supposed to increase serotonin levels. NDRIs (norepinephrine dopamine reuptake inhibitors) are supposed to increase norepinephrine and dopamine, rather than serotonin. These two types of antidepressants are supposed to be "selective," affecting the designated neurotransmitters without affecting the others. The strange thing is that these two types of antidepressants are equally effective in treating depression. Using data reported in a recent meta-analysis that was published in the prestigious medical journal *The Lancet*, I have calculated that 60% of patients respond to SSRIs and 59% of patients respond to NDRIs (Cipriani et al. 2009).

"So what is wrong with that?" you might ask. Maybe some people do not have enough serotonin and others do not have enough norepinephrine or dopamine. The problem is that besides the remarkable coincidence of the response rates being virtually identical, we have accounted for too many people. Adding together 60% and 59%, we get 119%, which is 19% too much. That may not be a big problem. It could be that some depressed people do not have a chemical imbalance and would respond to anything—even a placebo—whereas others get better only when you give them the right medication. However, if this were true, then switching people to a different type of medication ought to make a difference. In fact, some people who have not responded to a particular antidepressant do indeed get better when you switch them to another antidepressant. The problem for the chemical imbalance theory is that it does not matter what the other antidepressant is. In the STAR*D (Sequenced Treatment Alternatives to Relieve Depression) trial, which was designed to be especially representative of what happens in real-world clinical practice, switching unresponsive depressed people from one SSRI to another was exactly as effective as switching them to an NDRI. When depressed people who do not respond to an SSRI are given an NDRI, 26% of them get better, but 27% of them also get better if the drug they are switched to is just another SSRI (Rush et al. 2006a). Once again, we have the remarkable coincidence of identical effects from different drugs.

The STAR*D trial is not alone in finding that all antidepressants are created equal. In meta-analyses of head-to-head comparisons of different antidepressants, statistically significant differences are occasionally found, but these tend to be very small—smaller even than the clinically insignificant drug–placebo difference that we have found in our meta-analyses of the FDA data set. If the difference between antidepressant and placebo is small, the differences between one antidepressant and another are virtually non-existent. As the authors of one of these analyses concluded, "overall, second-generation antidepressants probably do not differ substantially for treatment of major depressive disorder" (Hansen et al. 2005). Furthermore, when small differences are found, they may be at least partly due to the biases in the studies. A team of researchers at the Beth Israel Medical Center in New York looked at the outcome of clinical trials as a function of who had sponsored the trial. They found that studies funded by a drug company generally reported positive results for that company's drug and negative results for drugs manufactured by competitors (Kelly et al. 2006).

The most common interpretation of the failure to find clinically meaningful differences between the effects of different antidepressants is that "choosing the agent that is most appropriate for a given patient is difficult" (Hansen et al. 2005). This presupposes that there is a right drug for a particular patient, but the data on which this conclusion is based suggest exactly the opposite. Let us suppose that some patients have a serotonin deficiency, others have a norepinephrine deficiency, and still others have a shortage of both neurotransmitters in their brains. It seems a rather remarkable coincidence that the number of people suffering from all three types of imbalance is exactly the same. However, even this level of improbability underestimates how subversive the equivalence data are for the chemical imbalance hypothesis. If some people suffer from a shortage of serotonin, others from a shortage of norepinephrine, and still others from both, then SNRIs (serotonin norepinephrine reuptake inhibitors)—which are designed to increase the availability of both neurotransmitters—should provide a clinical benefit to substantially more people than either of the more selective treatments. However, they do not. The effects of SNRIs are not much better than the effects of SSRIs or than drugs like bupropion that do not affect serotonin at all (Rush et al. 2006b).

It is difficult to even imagine a convincing biochemical explanation of the virtual equivalence of different types of antidepressants. The tailoring hypothesis (the idea that the right antidepressant can be found for each patient's particular chemical imbalance) certainly does not work. There are just too many drugs that produce response rates of 50% or better in the treatment of depression, and these are not limited to antidepressants. Other drugs that work better than placebo in treating depression include sedatives, stimulants, opiates, antipsychotic drugs, and the herbal remedy, St John's wort (Kirsch 2003; Kirsch and Sapirstein 1998; Moncrieff 2008). I do not think anyone would argue that there is a common chemical mechanism by which all of these very different drugs work. There may indeed be different subtypes of depression, and it is plausible to suppose that different treatments might be effective for these different subtypes of the disorder. However, the proportion of people having each subtype of depression cannot add up to more than 100%. Yet that is exactly what the data tell us, if we assume that the tailoring hypothesis is right.

Although the tailoring hypothesis does not fit the data, there is another hypothesis that works just fine. It is the idea that antidepressants are active placebos. That is, they are active drugs, complete with chemically induced side-effects, but their therapeutic effects are based on the placebo effect rather than their chemical composition. Their small advantage in clinical trials derives from the production of side-effects, which leads patients to realize that they have been given the active drug, thereby increasing their expectancy for improvement.

2.7 Selective serotonin reuptake enhancers: the last nail in the coffin

Different types of antidepressants are supposed to affect different neurotransmitters. Some are supposed to affect only serotonin, others are supposed to affect both serotonin and norepinephrine, and still others are supposed to affect norepinephrine and dopamine. However, there is a relatively new antidepressant that has a completely different mode of action. It is a most unlikely medication, and the evidence for its effectiveness puts the last nail in the coffin of the chemical imbalance theory of depression.

The name of this new antidepressant is tianeptine. It was developed in France, where it is licensed as an antidepressant and marketed under the name Stablon. It is also prescribed as an antidepressant in a number of other countries, sometimes under the names Coaxil or Tatinol. Tianeptine is a selective serotonin reuptake *enhancer* (SSRE). Instead of *increasing* the amount of serotonin in the brain—as SSRIs and SNRIs are supposed to do—tianeptine *decreases* it (Preskorn 2004; Sarek 2006). If the monoamine imbalance theory is right, tianeptine ought to induce depression, rather than ameliorate it. However, the clinical trial data show exactly the opposite. Tianeptine is significantly more effective than placebo and as effective as SSRIs and tricyclic antidepressants (Kasper and McEwen 2008; Uzbay 2008; Wagstaff et al. 2001). In head-to-head comparisons of tianeptine with SSRIs and with the earlier tricyclic antidepressants, all three produced virtually identical response rates (Figure 2.3). In these studies, 63% of patients responded to tianeptine, compared to 62% of patients on SSRIs and 65% of patients on tricyclics (Wagstaff et al. 2001).

I suppose that some ingenious minds will be able to find a way of accommodating the chemical balance hypothesis to these data, but I suspect that the accommodation will require convoluted circumventions like those used by the

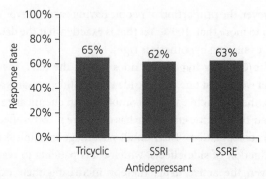

Fig. 2.3 Response rates for tricyclic antidepressants, SSRIs, and SSREs in head-to-head comparator trials.

Flat Earth Society in their efforts to maintain their defunct theory in the face of photographic evidence from space. If drugs that increase serotonin, decrease it, or do not affect it at all, can equally affect depression, then the benefits of these drugs cannot be due to their specific chemical activity. Additionally, if the therapeutic benefits of antidepressants are not due to their chemical composition, then the widely proffered chemical imbalance theory of depression is without foundation. It is an accident of history produced serendipitously by the placebo effect.

2.8 Clinical conclusions

To summarize, there is a strong therapeutic response to antidepressant medication. However, the response to placebo is almost as strong. This presents a therapeutic dilemma. The drug effect of antidepressants is not clinically significant, but the placebo effect is. What should be done clinically in light of these findings?

One possibility would be to prescribe placebos, but this entails deception. Although some have argued that it is ethically justifiable to knowingly prescribe placebos (see Chapter 4), and it has been shown to be a rather common habit (Raz et al. 2011), I disagree with this practice. Research indicates that the therapeutic relationship is an important component in the effectiveness of medical treatment (Di Blasi et al. 2001; Kaptchuk et al. 2008). The therapeutic relationship is founded on trust; trust must first be earned in order to be maintained. Violating trust entails the risk of losing trust, and a loss of trust between patient and clinician deprives the clinician of one of the most potent weapons in his or her therapeutic arsenal. If placebos are to be used ethically in clinical practice, a means must be found to do so without deception, either explicit or implicit.

Surprisingly, there are some data to suggest that placebos can in fact be given openly without losing their effectiveness (Kaptchuk et al., 2010).

Another possibility that has been proposed is to use antidepressants as active placebos (Hollon et al. 2002; Moerman 2002), but the risks of side-effects, suicide, withdrawal symptoms, and drug interactions render this alternative problematic.

A third possibility is the use of alternative treatments. Physical exercise, for example, has been shown to produce clinical benefit in moderately depressed people (reviewed in Kirsch 2009, 2010). This might also be a placebo effect, but the difference in the side-effect profile can be considered. Side-effects of antidepressants include sexual dysfunction, insomnia, diarrhea, nausea, anorexia, bleeding, forgetfulness, seizures, and increased suicide risk. Side-effects of physical exercise include enhanced libido, better sleep, decreased body fat, improved muscle tone, longer life, increased strength and endurance, and improved cholesterol levels.

The best-researched alternative to antidepressant drugs is psychotherapy and, in particular, a form of psychotherapy called cognitive behavior therapy (CBT). On the basis of the existing data, psychotherapy should be considered as a first-choice treatment for depression. The data indicate that it is as effective as medication in the short run and that CBT, in particular, is considerably more effective when relapse rates are assessed, even for severely and chronically depressed patients (see Kirsch 2009, 2010). As an intervention that is psychological rather than physical, psychotherapy is, by definition, a placebo in the strictest sense of the term. Psychotherapies of all varieties deal with the meaning that events have for people. In this sense, they are all openly eliciting what Dan Moerman refers to as the meaning response (see Chapter 7).

Finally, the social and economic causes of depression need to be addressed. Depression is correlated with unemployment, poverty, poor education, and unaffordable housing, and the people who benefit most from antidepressant or psychotherapeutic interventions tend to be white, well paid, and well educated (Kirsch 2009, 2010). Treating depression is not enough. We also need to prevent it by changing the social conditions that increase the risk of becoming depressed.

Since the publication of our meta-analyses of the FDA data files, a number of changes have occurred. The problem of hidden data is now widely recognized, and some steps have been taken to remedy it (e.g., the requirement to register clinical trials). Citing our analyses, as well as others, NICE issued a new set of guidelines for the treatment of depression, in which psychotherapy was emphasized as an alternative or addition to drug treatment (NICE 2004). Subsequently, the UK government initiated a program to train 10,000 new therapists to administer these treatments. Finally, three months after the publication of our

2008 analysis (Kirsch et al. 2008), a poll of British physicians indicated that 44% of them would now consider alternatives to medication for the treatment of depression (*OnMedica* 2008).

It takes time for scientific findings to lead to practical changes, especially where substantial financial interests are at stake, but it is encouraging to note that change has finally begun. I look forward to the day when the prescription of current antidepressants is regarded as a curiosity of medical history, much as blood-letting is considered after centuries of clinical practice were thought to have proven its efficacy.

References

Abramson, L. Y., Seligman, M. E. P., and Teasdale, J. D. (1978). Learned helplessness in humans: critique and reformulation. *Journal of Abnormal Psychology*, **87**(1), 49–74.

Barbui, C., Furukawa, T. A., and Cipriani, A. (2008). Effectiveness of paroxetine in the treatment of acute major depression in adults: a systematic re-examination of published and unpublished data from randomized trials. *Canadian Medical Association Journal*, **178**(3), 296–305. DOI: 10.1503/Cmaj.070693

Cipriani, A., Furukawa, T. A., Salanti, G., et al. (2009). Comparative efficacy and acceptability of 12 new generation antidepressants: a multiple treatments meta-analysis. *The Lancet*, **273**(9665), 746–758. DOI: 10.1016/S0140-6736(09)60046–60045

Coppen, A. (1967). The biochemistry of affective disorders. *British Journal of Psychiatry*, **113**, 1237–1264.

Di Blasi, Z., Harkness, E., Ernst, E., Georgioud, A., and Kleijnen, J. (2001). Influence of context effects on health outcomes: a systematic review. *The Lancet*, **357**(9258), 757–762.

Hansen, R. A., Gartlehner, G., Lohr, K. N., Gaynes, B. N., and Carey, T. S. (2005). Efficacy and safety of second-generation antidepressants in the treatment of major depressive disorder. *Annals of Internal Medicine*, **143**(6), 415–426.

Hollon, S. D., DeRubeis, R. J., Shelton, R. C., and Weiss, B. (2002). The emperor's new drugs: effect size and moderation effects. *Prevention and Treatment*, **5**, article 27.

Kaptchuk, T. J., Friedlander, E., Kelley, J. M., Sanchez, M. N., Kokkotou, E., Singer, J. P., Kowalczykowski, M., Miller, F. G., Kirsch, I., Lembo, A. J. (2010). Placebos without Deception: A Randomized Controlled Trial in Irritable Bowel Syndrome. *PLoS One*, **5**(12), e15591.

Kaptchuk, T. J., Kelley, J. M., Conboy, L. A., et al. (2008). Components of the placebo effect: a randomized controlled trial in irritable bowel syndrome. *British Medical Journal*, **336**, 998–1003.

Kasper, S. and McEwen, B. S. (2008). Neurobiological and clinical effects of the antidepressant tianeptine. *CNS Drugs*, **22**(1), 15–26.

Kelly Jr., R. E., Cohen, L. J., Semple, R. J., et al. (2006). Relationship between drug company funding and outcomes of clinical psychiatric research. *Psychological Medicine*, **36**(11), 1647–1656. DOI: 10.1017/S0033291706008567

Kirsch, I. (1985). Response expectancy as a determinant of experience and behavior. *American Psychologist*, **40**(11), 1189–1202.

Kirsch, I. (1999). *How expectancies shape experience* (1st edn.). Washington, DC: American Psychological Association.

Kirsch, I. (2003). St John's wort, conventional medication, and placebo: an egregious double standard. *Complementary Therapies in Medicine*, **11**(3), 193–195. DOI: 10.1016/S0965-2299(03)00109-2

Kirsch, I. (2009). *The emperor's new drugs: exploding the antidepressant myth*. London: The Bodley Head.

Kirsch, I. (2010). *The emperor's new drugs: exploding the antidepressant myth*. New York: Basic Books.

Kirsch, I., Deacon, B. J., Huedo-Medina, T. B., Scoboria, A., Moore, T. J., and Johnson, B. T. (2008). Initial severity and antidepressant benefits: a meta-analysis of data submitted to the Food and Drug Administration. *PLoS Medicine*, **5**(2).

Kirsch, I., Moore, T. J., Scoboria, A., and Nicholls, S. S. (2002). The emperor's new drugs: an analysis of antidepressant medication data submitted to the U.S. Food and Drug Administration. *Prevention and Treatment*, **5**(23).

Kirsch, I. and Sapirstein, G. (1998). Listening to Prozac but hearing placebo: a meta-analysis of antidepressant medication. *Prevention and Treatment*, **1**, article 0002a. DOI: 10.1037/1522-3736.1.1.12a

Leber, P. (May 4, 1998). Approvable action on Forrest Laboratories, Inc. NDA 20–822 Celexa (citalopram HBr) for the management of depression. Memorandum to the Department of Health and Human Services, Public Health Service, Food and Drug Administration, Center for Drug Evaluation and Research. Washington, DC.

Malhi, G. S., Parker, G. B., and Greenwood, J. (2005). Structural and functional models of depression: from sub-types to substrates. *Acta Psychiatrica Scandinavica*, **111**(2), 94–105. DOI: 10.1111/J.1600-0447.2004.00475.X

Moerman, D. E. (2002). "The loaves and the fishes": a comment on "The emperor's new drugs: an analysis of antidepressant medication data submitted to the U.S. Food and Drug Administration." *Prevention and Treatment*, **5**, article 29.

Moncrieff, J. (2008). *The myth of the chemical cure*. Basingstoke: Palgrave Macmillan.

NICE (2004). Depression: management of depression in primary and secondary care. Clinical practice guideline no. 23.

OnMedica (2008-05-23). Doctors change prescribing habits on back of SSRI study. *OnMedica News*, May 23, 2008. Retrieved from http://www.onmedica.com/newsArticle.aspx?id=ae98220c-10e5-4350-8a9b-c85d534c79ea.

Philipp, M., Kohnen, R., and Hiller, K. O. (1999). Hypericum extract versus imipramine or placebo in patients with moderate depression: randomised multicentre study of treatment for eight weeks. *British Medical Journal*, **319**(7224), 1534–1539.

Preskorn, S. H. (2004). Tianeptine: a facilitator of the reuptake of serotonin and norepinephrine as an antidepressant? *Journal of Psychiatric Practice*, **10**(5), 323–330.

Rabkin, J. G., Markowitz, J. S., Stewart, J. W., et al. (1986). How blind is blind? Assessment of patient and doctor medication guesses in a placebo-controlled trial of imipramine and phenelzine. *Psychiatry Research*, **19**, 75–86.

Raz, A., Campbell, N., Guindi, D., Holcroft, C., Déry, C., and Cukier, O. (2011). Placebos in clinical practice: a pan-Canadian review of attitudes and patterns of use between academic psychiatrists and non-psychiatrists. *Canadian Journal of Psychiatry*, **56**(4), 198–208.

Rush, A. J., Trivedi, M. H., Wisniewski, S. R., et al. (2006a). Acute and longer-term outcomes in depressed outpatients requiring one or several treatment steps: a STAR*D report. *American Journal of Psychiatry*, **163**, 1905–1917.

Rush, A. J., Trivedi, M. H., Wisniewski, S. R., et al. (2006b). Bupropion-SR, sertraline, or venlafaxine-XR after failure of SSRIs for depression. *New England Journal of Medicine*, **354**(12), 1231–1242.

Sarek, M. (2006). Evident exception in clinical practice not sufficient to break traditional hypothesis. *PLoS Medicine*, **3**(2), e120. DOI: 10.1371/journal.pmed.0030120

Spitzer, E. (2004). Major pharmaceutical firm concealed drug information: GlaxoSmith-Kline misled doctors about the safety of drug used to treat depression in children. Press release: Office of the New York State Attorney General, June 2, 2004. Retrieved from http://www.badfaithinsurance.org/reference/PH/0002a.htm.

Teasdale, J. D. (1985). Psychological treatments for depression: how do they work? *Behaviour Research and Therapy*, **23**, 157–165.

Uzbay, T. I. (2008). Tianeptine: potential influences on neuroplasticity and novel pharmacological effects [review]. *Progress in Neuropsychopharmacology and Biological Psychiatry*, **32**(4), 915–924. DOI: 10.1016/j.pnpbp.2007.08.007

Wagstaff, A. J., Ormrod, D., and Spencer, C. M. (2001). Tianeptine: a review of its use in depressive disorders. *CNS Drugs*, **15**(3), 231–259.

Chapter 3

Active expectations: insights on the prescription of sub-therapeutic doses of antidepressants for depression

Veronica de Jong and Amir Raz

3.1 **Introduction**

In many places around the world, so-called non-alcoholic or de-alcoholized beer can contain up to 0.5% alcohol by law. These types of beverages are said to contain no, or only small traces of, ethanol-based alcohols. However, the distinction between no alcohol and small traces of it may not be as trivial as consumers assume.

In the medical domain, the difference between a pure placebo and a drug is the dose of active ingredient—from zero to a therapeutically active amount. At the margins of pharmacological efficacy, we venture into the domain of active placebos. Active placebos are interventions that may be active in principle but without sufficient or specific activity for the condition being treated (also known as "impure placebos" or "pseudoplacebos") (Ernst 2001; Raz et al. 2011; Shapiro and Shapiro 1999). In the classic sense, a placebo is inert (e.g., sugar pill, saline injection), but a more nuanced definition of placebo also includes active ones (e.g., inefficacious medication or medication used at an inefficacious dosage) (Shapiro and Shapiro 1999).[1] With either inert or active placebos, benefits are not inherent to the properties of the named substance but are instead a product of the complex set of factors that surround (and include) their administration (i.e., placebo effects).

Throughout this volume we see how expectation can exert incredible influences on our experiences. In medicine, these influences are most often built on the premise of taking or receiving a helpful medical intervention (Altman 1991); the expectation accompanying active placebos, however, has many complexities that relatively few have explored.

The act of taking medication, regardless of the dose, instills "top–down" effects through the reward expectation pathway that can lead to therapeutic benefit in diseases susceptible to such effects (Diederich and Goetz 2008). Some medications, thanks to biomedical advancement, also produce powerful "bottom–up," biochemically mediated effects. In certain diseases, moreover, the brain regions activated by top–down and bottom–up effects overlap (Faria et al. 2008). In general, top–down processes seem to underlie placebo effects by generating and maintaining cognitive expectancies (Faria et al. 2008).

Consider then the relative influence of top–down and bottom–up effects when sipping a beverage of minimal percentage alcohol. Is there a suggestive role to the 0.5% label adorning a "non-alcoholic" beverage? Is it our intrinsic physiology alone that decides how we react to 0.5% as opposed to 5% alcohol content (the alcohol content of an average beer)? Our cells may sense the difference in concentration but do our cognitive processes? What if an individual has never had prior experience drinking alcohol, or has never paid attention to relative alcohol percentages? From the bottle to the taste, "non-alcoholic" beer is meant to recreate the true drinking experience with everything minus the "active" ingredient. However, does the presence of alcohol in negligible quantities make it an inactive contributor?

Studies have shown that subjects who think they are drinking alcohol show signs of intoxication even when there is nothing more than tonic water and lime in their seemingly "alcoholic" beverages (Marlatt and Rohsenow 1981). Through outcome expectancy effects, subjects display typical drinking behaviors such as motor impairment and sexual dysfunction based merely on the belief that they are consuming alcohol (Marlatt and Rohsenow 1980). These types of psychobiological outcomes demonstrate that there is much more to drinking alcohol than the physiological interaction of the contents of the drink with our cells (see Chapters 11 and 12).

In this chapter, we seek to shed light on the hollows between active drugs and pure placebos in the context of a medical condition not only central to this book but also of rising global concern: depression.

Formally defined, "sub-therapeutic" means "below the dosage levels used to treat diseases" (American Heritage Dictionary of the English Language 2000) or "indicating a dosage . . . less than the amount required for a therapeutic effect" (Dictionary.com 2011). A standard starting dose represents the lowest tested amount that elicits a statistically significant benefit over placebo (Sheiner et al. 1989), and anything below this benchmark is conventionally considered sub-therapeutic. The small quantity of biochemically active material in such doses is likely to cause no clinical outcome—homeopathic dilutions being an extreme case. The complex patient variability in responses to antidepressant medication, however, seems to complicate these definitions. In other words, a dose exerting no therapeutic effect for the majority of patients may be therapeutically active in some individuals. For the purposes of this discussion, however, we adapt the term "sub-therapeutic" from the formal definitions and use it more specifically in reference to any dose below the minimal effective dose, as stated in the published literature (e.g., drug product monograph, pharmacology reference books, evidence-based practice guidelines, systematic reviews or meta-analyses).

Psychiatrists who opt to treat depression with antidepressant medication typically "start low and go slow"—initially prescribing modest doses and then gradually increasing them (de Jong and Raz 2011). General practitioners, moreover, tend to prescribe low, even sub-therapeutic maintenance doses of antidepressants (Beaumont et al. 1996; Gilbody et al. 2006; Katon et al. 1992). Indeed, some patients report clinical improvements even when taking extremely low-dose medication. For such situations, limited evidence exists to support whether or not dose titration should continue to a dose of proven efficacy. Interestingly, however, some clinical guidelines (Anderson et al. 2008) encourage upward titration despite both the lack of evidence and the fact that side-effects are clearly dose-dependent (Bollini et al. 1999).

In a recent effort to assess the controversial topic of placebos and placebo-like treatments in medical practice, Raz et al. (2011) surveyed over 600 Canadian physicians about their use of certain treatments in situations without demonstrated or expected benefits. Results revealed that 38% of psychiatrists administer sub-therapeutic doses of medication, a frequency over six times that of non-psychiatrists. Interestingly, only 6% of the surveyed psychiatrists both administer sub-therapeutic doses and admit to having used a placebo in routine clinical practice. Moreover, only 2% of the 257 psychiatrist respondents deemed placebos of no clinical benefit. These intriguing findings raise several questions that are especially relevant to antidepressant prescriptions.

The biologically active ingredients in quantities too low to exert therapeutic benefits—although they may still exert side-effects—render sub-therapeutic doses a type of active placebo. In the case of depression, much evidence depicts standard antidepressant medication as a characteristic example of an active placebo, which, predictably, has created a complicated medical and ethical situation (Abi-Jaoude 2011; Kirsch 2009). Several meta-analytic findings (Fournier et al. 2010; Khan et al. 2002, 2008; Rief et al. 2009) support the results of Kirsch and colleagues (see Chapter 2) suggesting a negligible clinical benefit of antidepressants over placebos for the treatment of mild to moderate depression. Conversely, an independent line of research (Cohen 2001b, 2004; McCormack et al. 2011) has shown a clinically meaningful difference between antidepressants and placebo, but suggests that antidepressants can often achieve this difference at doses much lower than those currently recommended.

In light of the contentious state of research concerning antidepressant medication, we recently investigated how Canadian academic clinicians, all experienced in direct patient care, treat depression (de Jong and Raz 2011). Through interviews with academic psychiatrists, we utilized sub-therapeutic doses and non-drug effects as vehicles for probing underlying conceptualizations of pharmacological treatments for depression. Insights gleaned from the interviews, together with an appraisal of the relevant literature, uncover tacit attitudes and sketch conceptual challenges associated with the use of antidepressants.

3.2 **The current state of affairs**

In the last decade, the efficacy of antidepressant medication—considered a backbone drug of modern psychiatry (Ioannidis 2008)—has come under intense scrutiny (Pigott et al. 2010). The rationale behind the "anti" prefix in *anti*depressant is grounded in the chemical imbalance theory (Moncrieff 2007), a controversial view that purports depression as a consequence of a neurotransmitter shortage. The scarcity of scientific evidence supporting the chemical imbalance theory as a comprehensive theory for depression (Ioannidis 2008; Kirsch 2009; Ruhé et al. 2007) raises uncertainty with respect to the biological nature of depression (Beck and Alford 2009; Lacasse and Leo 2005). Nonetheless, most clinicians appear comfortable prescribing antidepressants to patients and clinical guidelines (American Psychiatric Association 2010; Lam et al. 2009) fully support this practice.

Mounting evidence from psychological science, neuroimaging, and clinical trials sheds light on the role of placebos in treating depression (Ankarberg and Falkenström 2008; Kirsch 2009; Mayberg et al. 2002). One of the most contentious set of research results has emerged from a trail-blazing trajectory of meta-analytic studies that examined placebo-controlled clinical trials of antidepressant medications. Findings from multiple independent meta-analyses (Fournier et al. 2010; Khan et al. 2002, 2008; Kirsch and Sapirstein 1998; Kirsch et al. 2008, 2002; Rief et al. 2009) suggest that antidepressants and placebos hardly differ in clinical benefit, especially for the treatment of mild to moderate depression. Notably, both interventions seem to improve depression ratings when compared to no treatment (Kirsch and Sapirstein 1998).

Depression is a heterogeneous condition, characterized in part by a spectrum of severity (Chen et al. 2000; Weissman et al. 1986). Kirsch and colleagues' meta-analysis (2002) did not consider the potential relationship between initial depression severity and drug versus placebo benefits (Elkin et al. 1989; Wilcox et al. 1992). Subsequent independent meta-analyses sought out this relationship (Fournier et al. 2010; Khan et al. 2002; Kirsch et al. 2008) and found such a link. Findings demonstrate, however, that the increasing benefit of antidepressants over placebos only reaches clinical significance in severely depressed individuals (Fournier et al. 2010; Kirsch et al. 2008).

One interpretation for why antidepressants seem to work better than placebos in patients with severe depression argues for decreased responsiveness to placebo, rather than increased responsiveness to medication (Kirsch et al. 2008). A related argument suggests that any antidepressant–placebo difference may be at least partly accounted for by patients breaking blind. This is a frequent occurrence due to the absence of common side-effects from inert placebo pills (Gaudiano and Herbert 2004; Kirsch 2009; Kirsch and Rosadino 1993; Moncrieff et al. 2010; White et al. 1992). However, future studies would need to corroborate this interpretation in patients with severe depression.

As described in the previous chapter by Kirsch (see Chapter 2), an analysis of the antidepressant meta-analytic literature fails to find a correlation between dosage and level of improvement in depression ratings (Kirsch et al. 2002). This finding contradicts the principle of a dose–response relationship. In fact, for the majority of the commonly prescribed selective serotonin reuptake inhibitors (SSRIs) (Hemels et al. 2002), no dose–response relationship has been clearly established (Berney 2005; Bijl et al. 2008; Khan et al. 2003; Wood and Gram 1994). Further, for antidepressants such as fluoxetine, a lower limit of effective dose evades documentation. These findings, or lack thereof, fall short in supporting a pharmacological explanation for antidepressant action in the "depressed brain."

Another controversial account proposes that antidepressants are clinically effective at sub-standard doses (Cohen 2001b; Furukawa et al. 2002; McCormack et al. 2011; Zilberman et al. 2010). Reconsideration of early fluoxetine (Prozac) studies (Cain 1992; Louie et al. 1993; Wernicke et al. 1988) and reviews (Salzman 1990; Schatzberg 1991; Schatzberg et al. 1987; Stewart et al. 1992; Wood and Gram 1994) supports the idea of "starting low," as low as one quarter (McCormack et al. 2011) or even one eighth (Cohen 2001b) of the recommended initial dose found in clinical practice guidelines such as those published by the American Psychiatric Association. Cohen reported (2001b, 2004) that when establishing the dosing recommendations, members of industry and regulatory agencies suppressed or ignored these early low-dose fluoxetine studies and reviews. Along with the intent of minimizing costs and harms, the low-dose proponents base their recommendations on evidence of equivalent efficacy among different antidepressant doses. For example, a review of fluoxetine trials

(Wood and Gram 1994) demonstrated equivalent efficacy among 40-mg, 20-mg (the current convention for minimal effective dose), and 5-mg doses. A recent analysis (McCormack et al. 2011) further asserts that prescribing very low dosages may prove maximally useful, by enlisting both the benefits of a placebo effect and the provision of a veridical drug. In the clinic, however, it would be very difficult to discern whether psychology or pharmacology is responsible for the majority of antidepressant benefits.

The evidence that placebos replicate the bulk of antidepressant drug effects withstanding, fractional dose treatments are likely to also employ placebo mechanisms to exert their effects. Teasing apart the pharmacological influence of sub-therapeutic dose from non-drug effects reifies the precarious relationship between low dose and placebo. Outside a certain dose range, drug concentration is too low to exert an effect above and beyond placebo. If no such limit exists for antidepressants, we can further contextualize their lack of chemical specificity on depressed mood. The ongoing "antidepressants versus placebos" conundrum begs the question: How do physicians who treat depression mobilize these contradictory lines of research when rationalizing antidepressant prescription?

Establishing a clear consensus for what constitutes a sub-therapeutic dose may elucidate why physicians prescribe them. One possibility is that physicians questioning the need or the benefit of certain drugs for certain patients may use these treatments as "convenient placebos." It is not uncommon for physicians to engage in non-scientific prescribing (Fassler et al. 2010; Raz et al. 2011), most often due to patient demand or benefit from placebo effects (Schwartz et al. 1989). For practical reasons, a "pure" placebo is not as easy for a physician to acquire as one may assume, says an anonymous former Dean of Medicine in Montreal, Canada (personal communication, October 13, 2010). Not all pharmacy outlets will agree, let alone have the capacity to fabricate placebos. Beyond such practicalities, deliberate placebo prescribing is a contentious ethical issue, often associated with bad clinical form (American Medical Association 2008, p. 254). The use of active placebos is much more difficult to detect (Kolber 2007); some physicians do not even associate such treatments with the word "placebo" (Fassler et al. 2010). The ethical repercussions of prescribing them, however, raise their own series of questions and little resources exist to address them.

A very low dose of medication occupies an unchartered space between a pure placebo and a full dose of pharmacologically active therapy. The use of sub-therapeutic doses, unlike pure placebos, would not require deception in terms of the identity of the intervention; the side-effect warnings, the chemical formula, the appearance, and name are all truthful elements that contribute to the aura and suggestion of taking a drug. Could prescribing sub-therapeutic doses be a way of benefitting from the attributes of active placebos while avoiding the dubious domain of handing out pure placebos? If this was the tendency, how do physicians explain their rationale and expectation of drug action to their patients? Would this process now imply a degree of deception? And could an expectation-mediated therapeutic benefit ever outweigh the ethical dilemmas associated with using active medications for their placebo-like qualities?

Other explanations certainly exist for why physicians prescribe what we consider active placebos. The use of sub-therapeutic doses could signal attempts at capturing insights from the low-dose literature with the aim of achieving therapeutic efficacy at below conventional doses. This motivation is not void of ethical concern because no matter the rationale, antidepressants at any dose may not perform better—albeit with worse side-effects—than placebos. An analysis of the results from psychiatrist interviews sheds light on these ethically charged questions while unearthing clinical realities of the treatment of depression.

3.3 Psychiatrist interviews

We conducted interviews with fifteen university affiliated psychiatrists. Addressing current conceptualizations of sub-therapeutic doses of antidepressants, rationales for prescribing them, as well as communication, and expectation tactics surrounding dose, we provide a review of the pertinent interview results. A complete description of the study methods and a discussion of the results are available online (de Jong and Raz 2011).

Determining how physicians conceptualize sub-therapeutic doses is crucial to understanding the role of such treatments in clinical practice. When we asked participant psychiatrists to define the term "sub-therapeutic dose," the question was often met with an extended pause; participants did not seem to have a formal medical definition to readily draw upon. To some, the term was inherently contradictory and makes no practical sense. When pressed further, the most common definition was the one we have adopted: *any dose below the established minimum effective dose from the published literature.*

Most participants indicated caveats to the definitions or provided additional comments in light of the antidepressant context. A major issue was inter-individual variability in response to antidepressants, attributed largely to differences in metabolism. In light of this issue, participants provided a second definition: *any dose where no therapeutic benefit can be observed in the individual patient.* Participants often highlighted the difficulties in predicting patient sensitivity to a new prescription, although some said they could approximate the sensitivity of a patient to a new drug based on drug history, since patterns of similar responses often exist between drug classes. Regardless of being able to predict sensitivity, almost all participants reported occurrences of unexpected improvement at doses of antidepressants that are below established levels of therapeutic efficacy.

When questions concerning the limits of a sub-therapeutic dose arose, it became apparent that its lower limit is, as yet, undefined. In particular, participants were unable to provide clear responses to how one could distinguish between a sub-therapeutic dose, a homeopathic remedy, and a placebo. Difficulties also arose with respect to defining what, if any, is the range of sub-therapeutic "efficacy." A small handful of participants volunteered explanations for our limited knowledge, citing that only a subset of doses are clinically tested and appear in the published literature, and an even smaller subset are commercially available.

Mixed attitudes toward what constitutes a placebo persist among physicians and the public at large. When we asked participant psychiatrists whether administering a sub-therapeutic dose of antidepressant can equate to giving a placebo, the consistent response was "no." This sentiment was well summarized by a participant who said, "If [a sub-therapeutic dose] were the same as a placebo, then you could give just about anything."

As it did not seem that participants were intentionally prescribing sub-therapeutic doses for their placebo-like qualities, we investigated other potential rationales they may hold. Most participants cited the "start low, go slow" titration technique as a frequent motivation for prescribing sub-therapeutic antidepressant doses. Two-thirds of participants emphasized tolerance building to minimize the antidepressant side-effects as a rationale for slowly increasing the dose from a low level. Twenty percent of participants stated that starting at lower doses could also provide a level of comfort or allay anxiety. Striving for the lowest effective dose, regardless if it were below standard levels, was the rationale for starting low for only two participants. With the exception of these participants, the majority concurred that no clinical benefit was expected outside of the established therapeutic dose range of a drug. Interestingly, most participants reported situations of unexpected responses to sub-therapeutic doses, and so we sought potential explanations.

Sixty percent of the participants arrogated sub-therapeutic dose responses in physiological terms: the patient must "lie on the lower end of the response curve," or be "sensitive to the medication," or be "a poor metabolizer." Slightly less than half of the participants acknowledged that the response could be due to placebo effects, but argued that such effects may also be coupled with other factors at play. Participants did not comfortably attribute sustained sub-therapeutic dose improvements solely to placebo effects; placebo effects were often conceived of as transitory and short-term in comparison to pharmacological effects. Even with improvement on a sub-therapeutic dose, one-third of participants mentioned that they would increase the dose to the minimum established therapeutic level. Other participants belittled the need to pinpoint the cause of a satisfactory therapeutic response, especially through unfavorable genetic testing.

Participants suggested that the majority of patients do not understand that different drug potencies relate to different doses. For example, an average 20-mg dose of fluoxetine seems much less potent than 125 mg of buproprion (a below average dose of this antidepressant). Transparency is necessary, participants contended, but they must take a nuanced approach. For instance, as one participant explained, if a patient thinks that he is taking a very high dose, he may feel that his illness is more severe and is thus less likely to recover. Alternately, if a patient understands his dose as very small and thereby holds low expectations of the drug's therapeutic ability, this knowledge can elicit a nocebo (negative placebo) effect. As a result, some participants (10%) prefer to leave dosage information out of the conversation as much as possible. To avoid the negative influence that dose may have on patients, one participant often emphasizes, "The fact you need a high or low dose has nothing to do with being more or less ill; it is about what your body needs. Some patients need high doses of medication, and that is okay, they may just have a fast metabolism."

In situations where patients are anxious about taking medications, certain participants said that they will carefully craft their wording and use phrases such as, "I am putting you on a microscopic dose," "some people take ten times this dose and are just fine," or "we are still not at the maximum dose level." On occasion, participants will prescribe a lower dose solely because a patient is hesitant to begin drug treatment. Participants also depicted patient anxiety about drug weaning. In most instances, psychiatrists will proceed slowly. One participant divulged treatment adaptations for patients with dependency toward drugs, explaining that it was not unusual to maintain them on a dose "that does not make sense [in terms of a] pharmacological effect but provides comfort for them." In such cases, the routine of coming to the clinic and receiving the low-dose prescription can continue for years.

All participants highlighted the therapeutic importance of factors involved in the clinical encounter that are not specific to the treatment modality. Participants consistently stressed the importance of patient choice and willingness to use pharmacological treatments. On the one hand, participants emphasized that treatment effects are likely to diminish if a patient does not believe in the treatment modality. One of these participants often explains this sentiment to patients: "If you think it is going to work, it is probably going to have a different effect than if you take it reluctantly. It is important to talk about whether you think I am shoving this down your throat, or if you actually believe in it." He elaborated: "Even the strongest doses of medications will have little chance of producing satisfactory outcomes if the patient is not convinced that they will work." Another participant reported taking pride in being able to convince patients and "get them on board" with the treatment.

On the other hand, many participants cautioned against over-inflating the efficacy of drug treatments to patients in order to ensure realistic goals. When prescribing initial doses, certain participants (40%) adopt a cautionary approach and express to patients that they do not expect any therapeutic benefits. One participant reported that he advises patients that "if they start to feel the side- effects, they may be fortunate enough to receive the therapeutic effects; at least the drug is doing something!" These participants explained that they are careful not to instill false hope about the medications, largely to prevent patient discouragement if the prescription does not work. Two participants went on to say that they rarely promote the placebo effect or attempt to harness it in their practice.

According to participants, a sub-group of patients seek out drug treatment or rely heavily on notions of using medications to "fix" chemical imbalances. Pamphlets adorning waiting rooms clearly communicate this explanation to patients. One such pamphlet ("made possible by an unconditional grant from Wyeth Canada") states:

> Depression is often described as a "chemical imbalance" in the brain. What this means is that certain neurotransmitters (your brain chemicals) are not at the levels they should be to maintain a positive mood . . . The most common treatment for depression involves medication designed to increase the levels of these neurotransmitters and thus, improve your mood. (Mood Disorders Society of Canada 2009)

Throughout the interviews, very few participants broached the subject of antidepressant neurochemical mechanisms. One such iteration was an explanation of how SSRIs can produce an instant "serotonin kick" in the brain but not always treat the target. A few participants also commented that elaborating on the scientific underpinnings of their decisions helps the patient understand what to expect from the medication.

3.4 Discussion

The mixed conceptualizations and lack of clarity surrounding sub-therapeutic antidepressants are largely a reflection of contradictory lines of research, whether or not psychiatrists are explicitly aware of them. Environmental, pathophysiological, and genetic factors contribute to the inter-individual variability in drug response; nonetheless, the drug literature demarcates threshold doses by averaging individual responses. Variation in the efficacy of drug metabolizing enzymes is a key differentiating factor (Meyer and Zanger 1997). For example, 5–10% of the Caucasian population have genetic polymorphisms in the cytochrome P450 enzyme, CYP2D6, that render them poor metabolizers of several commonly prescribed antidepressants (Sachse et al. 1997). However, uncertainty lingers as to how and whether these phenomena wield clinical effects (Bijl et al. 2008). When it comes to depression *outcomes*, the data have yet to substantiate a clear influence of the most frequent CYP2D6 polymorphisms on clinical responses to antidepressants, especially SSRIs. As such, genetic screening to optimize treatment outcomes remains elusive (Bijl et al. 2008) and serum drug level testing is rare.

The opinion among participants that placebos are not equivalent to subtherapeutic doses parallels recent findings suggesting that the majority (84%) of psychiatrists who have administered sub-therapeutic doses in situations of no expected clinical efficacy claim to have never used a placebo in clinical care (Raz et al. 2011). Despite this, few psychiatrists actually define placebos simply as inert or innocuous substances. From our discussions, it seems that psychiatrists differentiate between pure placebos and sub-therapeutic doses in terms of their intentions: although a placebo effect may be responsible for the improvement of patients on a minimal dose, this is rarely the intended mechanism of action. As documented here and elsewhere (Abi-Jaoude 2011; Shapiro and Shapiro 1999), however, the clinician has little drive or means (i.e., controlled setting) to decipher the underlying mechanism of action of an intervention, so long as it is working.

The strongly held notion that placebo effects in depression are only shortlived—although findings refute this assumption (Khan et al. 2008)—seems to create reluctance in attributing antidepressant responses (let alone those to subtherapeutic doses) to such effects alone. Instead, participants utilize placebo effects in more subtle ways in order to enhance the effectiveness of drug treatment. Engaging in patient belief systems to recruit conviction in the treatment seems critical to maximizing therapeutic outcomes; at least one empirical study would support this notion in terms of improving adherence to antidepressants (Aikens et al. 2005).

Neurochemical-based beliefs in depression etiology and treatment, borne out of the popular chemical imbalance theory of depression, are likely ingrained in many patients (Leo and Lacasse 2008). From the interviews we conducted, it was not entirely clear whether Canadian academic psychiatrists have completely rejected this theory. It is possible that despite uncertainty in the field, clinicians perpetuate this theory, at least indirectly, by using it as a simple explanation for the proposed drug treatment. Whether communicated subtly or overtly, accurately or imprecisely, the meaning imbued in the ability of drugs to fix mental illness seems to be a powerful therapeutic ally.

3.5 **Concluding thoughts**

Communication is integral to the art of medicine and vital to good physician-ship. We typically consider dose, with its exact milligram quantities of potent ingredients, as a key component of the science of medicine. Through the exploration of dose-related questions, it is evident that dose modification and communication represent an interface between the art and science of psychiatric practice.

Clinicians seem to foster placebo effects through nuanced psychological manipulation of dose communication and by employing expectancy-shaping techniques. In certain situations, moreover, dose alterations sustain psychological manipulations. The prescription of micro-doses, for example, helps to allay patient anxiety involved in starting or stopping a medication. The pharmacological treatment of depression provides an opportunity to tailor dose, or the communication of dose, in order to tilt the clinical situation in favor of positive patient expectancies. In doing so, however, the clinician may have to entertain a degree of deception.

Most psychiatrists do not start antidepressant prescriptions at a low dose based on expectations of efficacy. Rather, most do not expect measureable improvement in the patient's condition until the established therapeutic dose has been reached. Moreover, many psychiatrists openly convey these expectations to their patients. According to the Cohen low-dose literature (2001a, b, 2004), at such dose levels, the patient may already be taking eight times what he or she needs. In light of the influential role of physicians' positive expectations (Thomas 1987), another concern is that clinicians may not mobilize their full capacities as healers when prescribing initial low doses. Maintaining an optimistic front about the therapeutic potential of a sub-therapeutic dose would entail an element of deception if the clinician were certain such a dose would have no effect. It is clear, however, how expectations of improvement do not always align with patient outcomes.

The expectation effects brought on by antidepressant side-effects add another layer of complexity that warrants consideration. Rationales for prescribing sub-therapeutic doses seem grounded more in minimizing side-effects than in harnessing either placebo or targeted drug effects. As mentioned earlier (see "The current state of affairs"), unlike the evidence for the serotonergic "anti"-depressant effects, their side-effects do adhere to a dose–response relationship. In addition to the noxious physiological symptoms brought on by these side-effects, a series of clinical trial research (Gaudiano and Herbert 2004; Moncrieff et al. 2010; White et al. 1992) has pointed to their positive psychological influence on treatment outcomes. In other words, experiencing the side-effects associated with the antidepressant provides self-confirmation that the drug is exerting a physiological and assumed "beneficial" effect, a concept that an interview psychiatrist also alluded to. Taken together, we see the possibility of a side-effect dose–response relationship mediating the expectation effects of antidepressants; an interesting interface of top–down and bottom–up effects with consequences for the manipulation of dose escalation in the antidepressant context.

Clinicians do not control for the non-drug effects of their prescriptions by comparing them to placebos. Yet in the interest of medical science, it is crucial that the therapeutic benefits clinicians and patients may observe following an increase in dosage are not blindly attributed to the drug's biochemical properties. Unfortunately, this is often the case; the correlation between dosage and illness severity is often cited as evidence for the efficacy of antidepressants. Recent research, however, has provided evidence that in depression (Benkert et al. 1997) and other conditions (De Craen et al. 1999; Sandler et al. 2010) placebos and placebo effects elicit their own dose–response relationships. In other words, two placebos are better than one for many conditions and the perception of an antidepressant dose increase can produce comparable benefits to an actual increase in dose (Benkert et al. 1997; Kirsch and Sapirstein 1998).

Exploring the nuances of sub-therapeutic dosing reveals subtleties in clinician behaviors that give merit to the role of placebo effects in the treatment of depression. Psychiatrists are often in the position of interpreting controversial research while exuding the clinical confidence of a reliable caregiver. Converging on the clinically optimal dose requires mastery of the highly contentious scientific literature concerning dose–response relationships for antidepressants, while mediating the influence of individual patient variability. In addition, clinicians must consider the commonly accepted, yet cautiously entrusted, role of placebo effects in the recovery from depression. The factors that shape both patient and clinician choices and expectations are innumerable. Even the chemical imbalance theory of depression, though it has been widely disputed and scarcely validated in empirical research, may play a role in this process. As highlighted in this chapter and validated elsewhere in the scientific literature, the contributions of patient choice (McPherson 1994), knowledge (Entwistle et al. 1998), expectancy (Kirsch 1999), and belief (Aikens et al. 2005) to treatment outcomes may benefit from *notions* of specific neurochemical antidepressant action while collectively outperforming *actual* pharmacological action.

Sound clinical practice entails holding prescription rationales that align with drug action and outcome. That the use of sub-therapeutic doses is not infrequently met with a therapeutic response calls for systematic evaluation of the mechanisms by which these low doses exert their effects. Furthermore, that sub-standard dosing for promoting side-effect tolerance is common in clinical practice warrants further investigation of the clinical merit of this practice, especially in the context of newer and safer antidepressants. Within the current evidence base, clinical practice would stand to benefit from a greater appreciation among physicians and policy makers that at low, if not any, dose, antidepressants may be closer to active placebos than efficacious drugs. Placebo science would gain from empirical investigation into the influence of the mere presence of a substance construed or understood as efficacious, a novel arena that we have but scratched the surface of here.

Acknowledgement

This chapter was originally published as: de Jong, V. and Raz, A. (2011). Sub-therapeutic doses in the treatment of depression: the implications of Starting low and going Slow. *The Journal of Mind–Body Regulation*, 1 (2), pp. 73–84, © The Authors, 2011.

Note

1 Unlike Shapiro and Shapiro's definition that uses the term "ineffective," we use the term "inefficacious" based on the following definitions. In clinical terms, efficacy refers to the ability of a treatment such as a medication to produce a desired effect through a particular mechanism of action. Effectiveness refers to the actual utility of a substance. Research has often provided examples of efficacy without effectiveness (Glasgow et al. 2003); pharmaceutical agents, for example, sometimes produce side-effects that are more noxious than the condition they are meant to treat, thereby rendering them ineffective. In contrast, evidence also suggests that, in some cases, a substance such as a placebo may prove effective without being efficacious.

References

Abi-Jaoude, E. (2011). Are SSRI antidepressants little more than active placebo? A critical exploration. *The Journal of Mind–Body Regulation*, **1**(2), 100–105.

Aikens, J. E., Nease, D. E., Jr., Nau, D. P., Klinkman, M. S., and Schwenk, T. L. (2005). Adherence to maintenance-phase antidepressant medication as a function of patient beliefs about medication. *Annals of Family Medicine*, **3**(1), 23–30. DOI: 10.1370/afm.238

Altman, D.G. (1991). *Practical statistics for medical research*. London: Chapman & Hall.

American Medical Association (2008). Opinion 8.083—placebo use in clinical practice. In: *Code of medical ethics: current opinions with annotations*. Chicago, IL: AMA, pp. 254.

American Psychiatric Association (2010). Practice guideline for the treatment of patients with major depressive disorder (3rd edn.). *American Journal of Psychiatry*, **167** (Supp.10), 1–124.

Anderson, I. M., Ferrier, I. N., Baldwin, R. C., et al. (2008). Evidence-based guidelines for treating depressive disorders with antidepressants: a revision of the 2000 British

Association for Psychopharmacology guidelines. *Journal of Psychopharmacology*, **22**(4), 343–396. DOI: 10.1177/0269881107088441

Ankarberg, P. and Falkenström, F. (2008). Treatment of depression with antidepressants is primarily a psychological treatment. *Psychotherapy: Theory, Research, Practice, Training*, **45**(3), 329.

Beaumont, G., Baldwin, D., and Lader, M. (1996). A criticism of the practice of prescribing subtherapeutic doses of antidepressants for the treatment of depression. *Human Psychopharmacology: Clinical and Experimental*, **11**(4), 283–291. DOI: 10.1002/(sici)1099-1077(199607)11:4<283::aid-hup770>3.0.co;2-2

Beck, A. T. and Alford, B. A. (2009). *Depression: causes and treatment* (2nd edn.). Philadelphia: University of Pennsylvania Press.

Benkert, O., Szegedi, A., Wetzel, H., Staab, H. J., Meister, W., and Philipp, M. (1997). Dose escalation vs. continued doses of paroxetine and maprotiline: a prospective study in depressed out-patients with inadequate treatment response. *Acta Psychiatrica Scandinavica*, **95**(4), 288–296. DOI: 10.1111/j.1600-0447.1997.tb09634.x

Berney, P. (2005). Dose–response relationship of recent antidepressants in the short-term treatment of depression. *Basic Research*, **7**, 249–262.

Bijl, M. J., Visser, L. E., Hofman, A., et al. (2008). Influence of the CYP2D6* 4 polymorphism on dose, switching and discontinuation of antidepressants. *British Journal of Clinical Pharmacology*, **65**(4), 558–564.

Bollini, P., Pampallona, S., Tibaldi, G., Kupelnick, B., and Munizza, C. (1999). Effectiveness of antidepressants: meta-analysis of dose–effect relationships in randomised clinical trials. *British Journal of Psychiatry*, **174**(4), 297–303. DOI: 10.1192/bjp.174.4.297

Cain, J. W. (1992). Poor response to fluoxetine: underlying depression, serotonergic overstimulation, or a "therapeutic window"? *Journal of Clinical Psychiatry*, **53**(8), 272–277.

Chen, L., Eaton, W. W., Gallo, J. J., and Nestadt, G. (2000). Understanding the heterogeneity of depression through the triad of symptoms, course and risk factors: a longitudinal, population-based study. *Journal of Affective Disorders*, **59**(1), 1–11. DOI: 10.1016/s0165-0327(99)00132-9

Cohen, J. S. (2001a). Dose discrepancies between the Physicians' Desk Reference and the medical literature, and their possible role in the high incidence of dose-related adverse drug events. *Archives of Internal Medicine*, **161**(7), 957.

Cohen, J. S. (2001b). How drug-company policies cause problems for 50 to 75% of patients taking Prozac. In: *Overdose: the case against the drug companies*. New York: Tarcher-Putnam, pp. 36–49.

Cohen, J. S. (2004). Antidepressants: an avoidable and solvable controversy. *Annals of Pharmacotherapy*, **38**(10), 1743–1746. DOI: 10.1345/aph.1E240

De Craen, A. J. M., Moerman, D. E., Heisterkamp, S. H., Tytgat, G. N. J., Tijssen, J. G. P., and Kleijnen, J. (1999). Placebo effect in the treatment of duodenal ulcer. *British Journal of Clinical Pharmacology*, **48**(6), 853–860. DOI: 10.1046/j.1365-2125.1999.00094.x

de Jong, V. and Raz, A. (2011). Sub-therapeutic doses in the treatment of depression: the implications of starting low and going slow. *Journal of Mind–Body Regulation*, **1**(2), 73–84. Available at: http://mbr.synergiesprairies.ca/mbr/index.php/mbr/article/view/495 [accessed: January 30, 2012].

Diederich, N. J. and Goetz, C. G. (2008). The placebo treatments in neurosciences. *Neurology*, **71**(9), 677–684. DOI: 10.1212/01.wnl.0000324635.49971.3d

Elkin, I., Shea, M. T., Watkins, J. T., et al. (1989). National Institute of Mental Health treatment of depression collaborative research program: general effectiveness of treatments. *Archives of General Psychiatry*, **46**(11), 971.

Entwistle, V. A., Sheldon, T. A., Sowden, A., and Watt, I. S. (1998). Evidence-informed patient choice: practical issues of involving patients in decisions about health care technologies. *International Journal of Technology Assessment in Health Care*, **14**(2), 212–225.

Ernst, E. (2001). Towards a scientific understanding of placebo effects. In: *Understanding the placebo effect in complementary medicine: theory, practice and research* (ed. D. Peters). New York: Churchill Livingstone, pp. 20–21.

Faria, V., Fredrikson, M., and Furmark, T. (2008). Imaging the placebo response: a neurofunctional review. *European Neuropsychopharmacology*, **18**(7), 473–485. DOI: 10.1016/j.euroneuro.2008.03.002

Fassler, M., Meissner, K., Schneider, A., and Linde, K. (2010). Frequency and circumstances of placebo use in clinical practice: a systematic review of empirical studies. *BioMed Central Medicine*, **8**(1), 15–25. DOI: 10.1186/1741-7015-8-15

Fournier, J. C., DeRubeis, R. J., Hollon, S. D., et al. (2010). Antidepressant drug effects and depression severity: a patient-level meta-analysis. *Journal of the American Medical Association*, **303**(1), 47–53. DOI: 10.1001/jama.2009.1943

Furukawa, T. A., McGuire, H., and Barbui, C. (2002). Meta-analysis of effects and side effects of low dosage tricyclic antidepressants in depression: systematic review. *British Medical Journal*, **325**(7371), 991–1000. DOI: 10.1136/bmj.325.7371.991

Gaudiano, B. A. and Herbert, J. D. (2004). Methodological issues in clinical trials of antidepressant medications: perspectives from psychotherapy outcome research. *Psychotherapy and Psychosomatics*, **74**(1), 17–25.

Gilbody, S. M., Sheldon, T., and Wessely, S. (2006). Should we screen for depression? *British Medical Journal*, **332**(7548), 1027–1030. DOI: 10.1136/bmj.332.7548.1027

Glasgow, R. E., Lichtenstein, E., and Marcus, A.C. (2003). Why don't we see more translation of health promotion research to practice? Rethinking the efficacy-to-effectiveness transition. *American Journal of Public Health*, **93**(8), 1261.

Hemels, M. E., Koren, G., and Einarson, T. R. (2002). Increased use of antidepressants in Canada: 1981–2000. *Annals of Pharmacotherapy*, **36**(9), 1375–1379. DOI: 10.1345/aph.1A331

Ioannidis, J. (2008). Effectiveness of antidepressants: an evidence myth constructed from a thousand randomized trials? *Philosophy, Ethics, and Humanities in Medicine*, **3**(1), 14.

Katon, W., Von Korff, M., Lin, E., Bush, T., and Ormel, J. (1992). Adequacy and duration of antidepressant treatment in primary care. *Medical Care*, **30**(1), 67–76.

Khan, A., Khan, S. R., Walens, G., Kolts, R., and Giller, E. (2003). Frequency of positive studies among fixed and flexible dose antidepressant clinical trials: an analysis of the Food and Drug Administration summary basis of approval reports. *Neuropsychopharmacology*, **28**(3), 552–557.

Khan, A., Leventhal, R. M., Khan, S. R., and Brown, W. A. (2002). Severity of depression and response to antidepressants and placebo: an analysis of the Food and Drug Administration database. *Journal of Clinical Psychopharmacology*, **22**(1), 40–45.

Khan, A., Redding, N., and Brown, W. A. (2008). The persistence of the placebo response in antidepressant clinical trials. *Journal of Psychiatric Research*, **42**(10), 791–796. DOI: 10.1016/j.jpsychires.2007.10.004

Kirsch, I. (ed.) (1999). *How expectancies shape experience.* Washington, DC: American Psychological Association.

Kirsch, I. (2009). *The emperor's new drugs: exploding the antidepressant myth.* London: Bodley Head.

Kirsch, I. and Rosadino, M. J. (1993). Do double-blind studies with informed consent yield externally valid results? *Psychopharmacology,* **110**(4), 437–442.

Kirsch, I. and Sapirstein, G. (1998). Listening to Prozac but hearing placebo: a meta-analysis of antidepressant medication. *Prevention & Treatment,* **1**(8).

Kirsch, I., Deacon, B. J., Huedo-Medina, T. B., Scoboria, A., Moore, T. J., and Johnson, B. T. (2008). Initial severity and antidepressant benefits: a meta-analysis of data submitted to the Food and Drug Administration. *PLoS Medicine,* **5**(2), 260–268.

Kirsch, I., Moore, T. J., Scoboria, A., and Nicholls, S. S. (2002). The emperor's new drugs: an analysis of antidepressant medication data submitted to the US Food and Drug Administration. *Prevention & Treatment,* **5**(1), 23a.

Kolber, A. J. (2007). A limited defense of clinical placebo deception. *Yale Law & Policy Review,* **26**(1), 75–134.

Lacasse, J. R. and Leo, J. (2005). Serotonin and depression: a disconnect between the advertisements and the scientific literature. *PLoS Medicine,* **2**(12), e392. DOI: 10.1371/journal.pmed.0020392

Lam, R. W., Kennedy, S. H., Grigoriadis, S., et al. (2009). Canadian Network for Mood and Anxiety Treatments (CANMAT): clinical guidelines for the management of major depressive disorder in adults. III: Pharmacotherapy. *Journal of Affective Disorders,* **117**, S26–S43.

Leo, J. and Lacasse, J. R. (2008). The media and the chemical imbalance theory of depression. *Society,* **45**(1), 35–45. DOI: 10.1007/s12115–12007–9047–9043

Louie, A. K., Lewis, T. B., and Lannon, R. A. (1993). Use of low-dose fluoxetine in major depression and panic disorder. *Journal of Clinical Psychiatry,* **54**(11), 435.

Marlatt, G. A. and Rohsenow, D. J. (1980). Cognitive processes in alcohol use: expectancy and the balanced placebo design. *Advances in Substance Abuse,* **1**, 159–199.

Marlatt, G. A. and Rohsenow, D. J. (1981). The think–drink effect. *Psychology Today,* December Issue, 60–69.

Mayberg, H. S., Silva, J. A., Brannan, S. K., et al. (2002). The functional neuroanatomy of the placebo effect. *American Journal of Psychiatry,* **159**(5), 728–737.

McCormack, J. P., Allan, G. M., and Virani, A. S. (2011). Is bigger better? An argument for very low starting doses. *Canadian Medical Association Journal,* **183**, 65–69.

McPherson, K. (1994). The best and the enemy of the good: randomised controlled trials, uncertainty, and assessing the role of patient choice in medical decision making. *Journal of Epidemiology and Community Health,* **48**(1), 6–15.

Meyer, U. A. and Zanger, U. M. (1997). Molecular mechanisms of genetic polymorphisms of drug metabolism. *Annual Review of Pharmacology and Toxicology,* **37**(1), 269–296.

Moncrieff, J. (2007). *The myth of the chemical cure: a critique of psychiatric drug treatment.* New York: Palgrave Macmillan.

Moncrieff, J., Wessely, S., and Hardy, R. (2010). Active placebos versus antidepressants for depression. *The Cochrane Library,* (1), 1–30.

Mood Disorders Society of Canada (2009). What is Depression? In: *Mood Disorders Society of Canada, Wyeth Canada* (1st edn.). Guelph, Ontario.

Pigott, H. E., Leventhal, A. M., Alter, G. S., and Boren, J. J. (2010). Efficacy and effectiveness of antidepressants: current status of research. *Psychotherapy and Psychosomatics*, 79(5), 267–279.

Raz, A., Campbell, N., Guindi, D., Holcroft, C., Dèry, C., and Cukier, O. (2011). Placebos in clinical practice: comparing attitudes, beliefs, and patterns of use between academic psychiatrists and nonpsychiatrists. *Canadian Journal of Psychiatry*, 56(4), 198.

Rief, W., Nestoriuc, Y., Weiss, S., Welzel, E., Barsky, A. J., and Hofmann, S. G. (2009). Meta-analysis of the placebo response in antidepressant trials. *Journal of Affective Disorders*, 118(1–3), 1–8.

Ruhé, H. G., Mason, N. S., and Schene, A. H. (2007). Mood is indirectly related to serotonin, norepinephrine and dopamine levels in humans: a meta-analysis of monoamine depletion studies. *Molecular Psychiatry*, 12(4), 331–359.

Sachse, C., Brockmöller, J., Bauer, S., and Roots, I. (1997). Cytochrome P450 2D6 variants in a Caucasian population: allele frequencies and phenotypic consequences. *American Journal of Human Genetics*, 60(2), 284.

Salzman, C. (1990). Practical considerations in the pharmacologic treatment of depression and anxiety in the elderly. *Journal of Clinical Psychiatry*, 51(Supp.), 40–43.

Sandler, A. D., Glesne, C. E., and Bodfish, J. W. (2010). Conditioned placebo dose reduction: a new treatment in attention-deficit hyperactivity disorder? *Journal of Developmental & Behavioral Pediatrics*, 31(5), 369–375.

Schatzberg, A. F. (1991). Dosing strategies for antidepressant agents. *Journal of Clinical Psychiatry*, 52(Supp.), 14–20.

Schatzberg, A. F., Dessain, E., O'Neil, P., Katz, D. L., and Cole, J. O. (1987). Recent studies on selective serotonergic antidepressants: trazodone, fluoxetine, and fluvoxamine. *Journal of Clinical Psychopharmacology*, 7(6), 50S.

Schwartz, R. K., Soumerai, S. B., and Avorn, J. (1989). Physician motivations for nonscientific drug prescribing. *Social Science & Medicine*, 28(6), 577–582.

Shapiro, A. K. and Shapiro, E. (1999). The placebo: is it much ado about nothing? In: *The placebo effect: an interdisciplinary exploration* (ed. A. Harrington). Boston: Harvard University Press, pp. 12–36.

Sheiner, L. B., Beal, S. L., and Sambol, N. C. (1989). Study designs for dose-ranging. *Clinical Pharmacology & Therapeutics*, 46(1), 63–77.

Stewart, J. W., Quitkin, F. M., and Klein, D. F. (1992). The pharmacotherapy of minor depression. *American Journal of Psychotherapy*, 46(1), 23–36.

[Sub-therapeutic: definition] (2000). *The American heritage dictionary of the English language* (4th edn.). Boston, MA: Houghton Mifflin.

[Subtherapeutic: definition] (2011). *Dictionary.Com*, available at http://dictionary.reference.com/browse/subtherapeutic [accessed: January 19, 2011].

Thomas, K. B. (1987). General practice consultations: is there any point in being positive? *British Medical Journal*, 294(6581), 1200–1202.

Weissman, M. M., Merikangas, K. R., Wickramaratne, P., et al. (1986). Understanding the clinical heterogeneity of major depression using family data. *Archives of General Psychiatry*, 43(5), 430–434. DOI: 10.1001/archpsyc.1986.01800050028003

Wernicke, J. F., Dunlop, S. R., Dornseif, B. E., Bosomworth, J. C., and Humbert, M. (1988). Low-dose fluoxetine therapy for depression. *Psychopharmacology Bulletin*, **24**(1), 183–188.

White, K., Kando, J., Park, T., Waternaux, C., and Brown, W. A. (1992). Side effects and the "blindability" of clinical drug trials. *American Journal of Psychiatry*, **149**(12), 1730–1731.

Wilcox, C. S., Cohn, J. B., Linden, R. D., et al (1992). Predictors of placebo response: a retrospective analysis. *Psychopharmacology Bulletin*, **28**(2), 157–162.

Wood, A. J. J. and Gram, L. F. (1994). Fluoxetine. *New England Journal of Medicine*, **331**(20), 1354–1361. DOI: 10.1056/NEJM199411173312008

Zilberman, M. L., Gorenstein, C., and Gentil, V. (2010). The utility of low-dose antidepressants. In: *Clinical trials in psychopharmacology: a better brain* (2nd edn.) (eds. M. Hertzman and L. Adler). West Sussex, UK: John Wiley & Sons, pp. 179–188.

Chapter 4

Justifying deceptive placebos

Bennett Foddy

4.1 **Introduction**

Imagine a patient, Eric, who suffers from *neuropathic itch*, a neurological disorder that causes an itching sensation in his arms. Because this disorder is poorly understood, and because it has no identifiable physical cause, there is no treatment currently available. Molly, Eric's doctor, has read a recent paper by van Laarhoven and colleagues which suggests that an inert substance, or "placebo," could alleviate the sensation of itching (van Laarhoven et al. 2011). So she hands Eric a small unlabeled tube of topical cream, which she knows is made with an ingredient—witch hazel—that cannot have any pharmacological effect on Eric's neuropathic symptoms. She asks Eric to apply the cream to his arms, saying, "The cause of your itching is not fully understood, so I do not have a medicine that will cure it. However, this cream should reduce the sensation of itching and make you more comfortable."

Molly believes that what she is saying is correct: by means of a psychological association, which we call the *placebo effect*, the cream will reduce Eric's discomfort. However, this effect demands that Eric strongly associates the cream with topical medicines he has used successfully in the past. If Eric believes that the cream works through a psychological effect alone, the effect will be much weaker. So Molly simply omits to tell Eric *how* she thinks the cream will work, and he happily accepts the medicine without asking for more information, having no interest in, or understanding of, medical science.

One of the oldest debates in medical ethics concerns the deceptive prescription of pharmacologically inert medicines, or "placebos," to patients in the clinic. Doctors have long understood that the suffering of patients could be ameliorated by sham treatments, but the deceptive nature of these treatments, at least on the face of it, contravenes the strong prohibition against the deception of patients contained in the norms, guidelines, and laws that constitute modern medical ethics. If a doctor like Molly were to prescribe Eric a placebo without revealing its true nature, she would be acting against her obligations as a physician.

In this paper, I will seek to resolve the ethical debate over clinical placebo use by showing that it involves a special case of deception, which is not subject to the same ethical objections as other forms of clinical deception. There remain a number of specific objections to placebo use that do not relate to the general impermissibility of deception; I will show that these objections ought to *limit* our use of placebos in certain ways, but not *prohibit* it entirely. I will explain that clinical deception should only be considered paternalistic or coercive when it strays outside these ethical limits, and I will show that one very common case—the case of depression—represents an everyday clinical scenario in which the use of deceptive placebos is both appropriate and ethical.

These arguments require that we first agree, at least for the sake of argument, that placebos are usually efficacious, and that deception is required to maximize their efficacy. I will begin by addressing these issues.

4.2 **The efficacy of placebo therapies**

In addition to the ethical controversy, there is an enduring scientific controversy over whether placebos can be effective as a clinical treatment, and whether or not they can be made to work when the patient knows he is getting a placebo. For the sake of brevity, I am going to begin by assuming that placebos are effective at least for relief of felt symptoms, that they are rarely or never harmful in the clinic,[1] and that their effectiveness depends, at least in part, on the patient being unaware that he is receiving a placebo.

Whether or not these presumptions are correct is largely an empirical question. In a previous paper, I reviewed some of the available data (Foddy 2009). Evidence from sources such as Irving Kirsch's study in this volume (see Chapter 2) or Bingel's recent fMRI (functional magnetic resonance imaging) study, give us reason to believe that clinical placebos can be both effective and beneficial (Bingel et al. 2011; Kirsch 2012). Yet there is very little in the way of direct evidence concerning either the usefulness of placebo in the clinic or the effect of deception on the magnitude of the placebo effect. Why is this?

One reason is that when placebos are given in a research context, it is almost always because researchers need to *control for* the placebo effect—they are not trying to elicit or maximize it. They tell their subjects that they will receive either an active medication or an entirely inert one, and as Kirsch suggests, patients can frequently tell whether or not they have received a placebo because only the active medication produces side-effects (Kirsch 2012). For these reasons, the magnitude of the placebo effect measured in clinical trials is certainly underestimated, though to what degree, it is impossible to guess.

There are very few empirical studies of the clinical use of "deceptive" placebo, wherein a doctor prescribes a placebo without telling the patient that he may receive an inert substance. The reason for this is twofold. First, the deception of research subjects is prohibited in medical research by the doctrine of informed consent (Wear 1998). Research subjects can be deceived, but they must give prior consent to any deception that is made in the course of the research. Second, the use of deceptive placebos is explicitly prohibited in the clinic, rendering the results of such studies moot (American Medical Association's Council on Ethical and Judicial Affairs 2006–2007). Since deceptive placebo use cannot be studied, the difference between deceptive and non-deceptive placebo use cannot be measured within the ethical guidelines governing modern medical research.

Aside from the difficult empirical questions of whether placebos are effective and whether deception is required, however, there is a separate philosophical question concerning whether and when a doctor may prescribe a deceptive, albeit beneficial and efficacious, placebo in the clinic. It is this question with which I am concerned in this paper.

4.2.1 Are placebos necessarily deceptive?

In using a placebo to treat a patient, the doctor's primary aim is to make the patient believe something that she (as a physician) believes to be true: that the patient will feel better if he takes the placebo. It is worth examining what is usually assumed—that the prescription of placebo deceives a patient into holding this belief.

Consider the placebo vignette I presented at the beginning. To use the formulation of Igor Primoratz, when we lie we make "a statement believed to be false, with the intention of getting another to accept it as true" (1984). The only overt statement Molly makes in this case is one she believes to be true. She sincerely predicts that using the placebo cream twice a day will reduce the discomfort in Eric's arms. She has not told a lie but has, in telling the truth, led Eric to hold two true beliefs and one false belief. He comes to believe correctly that he will feel better, and that using the cream will make him feel better, but he also now holds the false belief that the cream works through a similar mechanism to topical medicines he has used. Since she deliberately leads him into this false belief, Molly has *deceived* Eric.

Patients seek out doctors expecting to have their diseases cured, and when that cannot be done, they expect to have their unwanted symptoms alleviated. Sometimes, the only way that the symptoms can be treated is through the use of the placebo effect (Foddy 2009) and in order to harness the placebo effect, the patient needs to believe, at some deep level, that the treatment will make him feel better.

At one level, it is thoroughly rational to believe that taking a placebo will make us feel better. Patients ought to believe that they will feel better, since their goal—the alleviation of their symptoms—will be met, to some extent, just so long as they believe it will be met.

Unfortunately, as Gibbard points out, "Beliefs seem like prime examples of what we can appraise as rational or irrational, but beliefs, like emotions, cannot be had or cast off at will. We may be able to 'make believe' at will, but that is not the same as really believing at will" (Gibbard 1990). I might believe, on reflection, that I will feel better just so long as I believe I will feel better. However, I cannot just make believe that I will feel better, and I cannot simply will myself into believing what I realize to be true.

In any case, the placebo effect does not seem to harness a high-level, reflective expectation that one will feel better. Instead, it harnesses conditioned associations between medicines and medical benefits (Benedetti 2006; Colloca and Benedetti 2006). Because of this, it would not be enough to believe that I will get better through the placebo effect, even if I could deliberately form such a belief. I need to believe, sincerely, that what I am getting is similar to the treatments that have made me feel better in the past.

Clearly, it is impossible to form a false belief such as this by oneself. An accomplice is needed. The accomplice must recognize and respect my goal—that is, to feel better—but I can never explicitly ask the accomplice to deceive me, or else I will not form the right kind of false belief. The relationship between doctor and patient is the exact kind of structure that can make possible this type of epistemic sleight of hand; since the doctor (or some other doctor) has given me efficacious therapies in the past, I will associate whatever treatment she gives me with past pharmacological benefits. When a doctor leads a patient into holding a beneficial false belief in this way, that is (by definition) deception.

It is possible that we can harness the *unconscious* association between pills and benefits that many people have formed. Perhaps if I give myself a placebo, or if a doctor gives me a placebo openly, letting me know that she expects to elicit a placebo effect, it will not matter that I do not consciously expect a pharmacological effect. Perhaps my unconscious expectation of an effect will be enough to produce a benefit. This suggestion is made by the American Medical Association in its policy which prohibits deceptive placebo use, and it was explored in one study by Park and Covi in 1965, which is now thought to be flawed (American Medical Association's Council on Ethical and Judicial Affairs 2006–2007; Klein 1994; Park and Covi 1965).

A recent paper by Kaptchuk et al. provides new evidence for the effectiveness of such "open" or "non-blind" placebos compared to the absence of treatment (2010). Patients suffering from irritable bowel syndrome (IBS) were assigned either to a group receiving no treatment or to a group that was prescribed "open-label" placebo, with a label reading "placebo pills." The prescribing doctor or nurse explained the placebo effect to the placebo group, telling them that the effect was "powerful" and that the pills contained no medicine. The placebo group improved significantly more than the no-treatment group on a range of IBS measures.

The trouble with studies of this kind is that, while they establish that open placebo is more effective than no treatment, they do not compare it against the effectiveness of deceptive placebo, which may be much greater. Also, we have some experimental evidence that may lead us to suspect that deceptive placebo is much more effective: trials have shown that peppermint oil, Chinese herbs, hypnotherapy, and fecal bacteria, among many other diverse substances, each works much better than (open) placebo as a treatment for IBS (Bensoussan et al. 1998; Enck et al. 2008; Galovski and Blanchard 1998; Pittler and Ernst 1998). Given the enormous diversity in the chemical or psychological function of these treatments, it seems overwhelmingly likely that at least one of them is nothing more than a deceptive placebo.

The trouble is that, since current clinical research ethics guidelines prohibit the deception of patients, researchers are unable to compare the effectiveness of deceptive placebo with open placebo. Other than Park and Covi's flawed 1965 study, we have no evidence suggesting that such open placebos work anything like as well as deceptive placebos, and none is likely to be forthcoming unless research guidelines are changed.

If further evidence does appear, it may show that open placebos can be as effective as deceptive placebo—that the placebo effect can be of full benefit even when a patient consciously believes there is no commonality between the placebo and their past pharmacological treatments. Until then, given the paucity of evidence to that effect, we should assume what is more plausible: that the effect of open placebo is much more limited than that of deceptive placebo. We ought to assume that, in order for a placebo treatment to provide maximum benefit, the patient must *falsely* believe that he will get better through the action of some pharmacological agent.

Although we cannot settle the matter with empirical evidence, a categorical argument is often used to support the claim that deception is *not* required in the use of placebos: the placebo effect can be utilized even without deceptively giving an inert treatment. Part of the benefit of regular, non-deceptive therapies is that they employ the placebo effect, as Dan Moerman suggests in this volume (see Chapter 7). The placebo effect is also employed in the course of a clinical consultation, when a doctor engages with the patient and shows genuine concern. This effect can be increased by maximizing the patient's unconscious expectation of benefit when prescribing an active medication, either by verbal means or by using non-verbal cues (see Chapter 7). Deception is not required in order to harness the placebo effect in these ways.

However, we should be careful about how far we stretch this point; for one thing, there are many cases in which no efficacious medicine can be given, as I explore further in this chapter. In these cases, doctors may be tempted to give ineffective but pharmacologically active medications in the hope that this avoids deception while eliciting a placebo response (Kolber 2008). Molly might have given Eric aspirin, for example, thinking that she could tell him he was receiving a medicine without deceiving him, but this would be a mistake. Even though aspirin is a pharmacologically active medicine, if Molly believes it will have no beneficial pharmacological effect on Eric's ailment, it is a placebo, a deceptive placebo if she leads him to falsely believe that he is getting a therapy with a significant pharmacological action. If the doctor wants to harness the placebo effect using pills or creams when it is not possible to give a significantly effective treatment, deception will always be necessary.

On a dogmatic reading of the rule against deceiving patients, this makes the effective and ethical use of placebos in the clinic impossible. However, I will argue, placebos represent a special case for clinical deception: a case in which it is at least possible to deceive patients without harming them or diminishing their autonomy. Because of this, doctors should be permitted to consider using placebo medications, even if it is true that bedside manner alone could elicit a beneficial placebo effect.

4.2.2 Can the deceptive placebo be ethically justified?

The prima facie presumption in medical ethics is that doctors should never deceive their patients in any situation. As the American Medical Association puts it, "A physician shall . . . be honest in all professional interactions, and strive to report physicians . . . engaging in fraud or deception, to appropriate entities" (2001). Jackson has argued that deception can be ethical so long as it does not involve actual lying (1991), and Takarangi and Loftus suggest in this volume that deceptive techniques could be carefully used in the clinic to directly benefit patients (see Chapter 12). However, the orthodox view is certainly that doctors have a duty neither to lie to, nor deceive their patients; that deception is to be avoided in its own right as something that is harmful to patients and contrary to the goals of medicine in general.

The reasoning behind this orthodox view proceeds roughly as follows: deception, if uncovered, undermines trust between the patient and doctor and may distress the patient. Deception can limit a patient's autonomy by preventing him from making informed medical decisions. Deception also diminishes the transparency of the medical consultation process, creating opportunities for unethical doctors to abuse the patient in other ways.

However, medical practice generates a wide range of scenarios in which deception may be, on balance, beneficial to the patient, not only in the case of placebo prescription but also, more frequently, in cases where a diagnosis is made that would be exceedingly distressing to a patient.

As Daniel Sokol has pointed out, the demands of compassion can sometimes overwhelm the presumption against deceiving patients (2007). If a clinical deception can be considered compassionate—that is, if it can reliably be expected to reduce anxiety or stress, if the deception is likely to succeed, and if these goals cannot be met without deception—then that deception may be morally justified.

There certainly may be cases where placebo deception is justified on the grounds that it is sufficiently compassionate relative to the moral costs of deceiving patients. However, I do not wish to advance an "all things considered" defense of placebo deception. Instead, I wish to argue that, so long as it is limited in the right way, placebo deception is a special case in which the usual presumption against the deception of patients ought to be suspended.

4.2.3 Placebo deception as a special case

When a doctor gives us a placebo, we are deceived into believing something that will become true the moment it is believed—that we will feel better. Placebo is just one of a range of cases that bear this property. The most straightforward is the case in which one person tries to *encourage* another person to perform well at some task, despite having misgivings about that person's actual performance. Suppose I am coaching a gymnast who is very weak at the balance beam, and I have come to believe that her problem is a lack of confidence, I tell her (falsely) that I believe she can perform her routine without falling off. Because she sees me as an expert judge, she is thus deceived and, as a result, gains confidence and performs exceedingly well. My deception creates in her a *self-fulfilling* belief.

Indeed, encouragement is a major component of every normal medical treatment; the American Medical Association even recommends that encouragement can stand in place of the deceptive use of placebo (American Medical Association's Council on Ethical and Judicial Affairs 2006–2007). However, as

Adam Kolber has pointed out, when a doctor encourages a patient whose condition is unlikely to improve, that is in one sense just as deceptive as prescribing a placebo (2008).

Optimistic, positive illusions are indicative of good mental health (Taylor and Brown 1988). If I falsely believe that my life will go well, that tends to make it true that my life will go well. Conversely, if I am gripped by a realistic but depressive pessimism, that pessimistic outlook tends to be self-fulfilling as well. Our general beliefs about how life will go are thus *self-fulfilling* too. As Blease has observed, when we use cognitive behavioral therapy to treat people for depression, we ask them to systematically eliminate depressive thoughts even if those thoughts are realistic or honest (2011). Also, when my therapist tries to make me believe something that she believes to be false, she deceives me for my own good.

As I described earlier, one cannot willfully convince oneself to believe in the benefits of a known inert substance. In the case of placebo prescription, as in the cases of cognitive behavioral therapy for depression or encouragement toward patients with a poor prognosis, the doctor *deceives* the patient into one false belief in order to *persuade* him into holding a true belief. This property makes it possible for the deceptive use of placebos to be carried out within the ethical boundaries of medical practice.

In such cases, the doctor's ends justify her deceptive means, provided the following conditions are met: first, the false belief must be required in order to gain the true belief—otherwise, honesty could achieve the same ends. Second, the true belief must be genuinely beneficial to the patient. Finally, this benefit must be assessed by the patient, in terms of his own endorsed ends, rather than on some objective basis by the doctor. For example, my doctor may think that it would benefit me to be vaccinated against measles, but that would not justify her vaccinating me without my knowledge, unless I have asked to be vaccinated, either explicitly or implicitly (say, by visiting a vaccination booth and rolling up my sleeve).

It is important to note that this third requirement will normally be upheld in the case of placebo prescription, provided that the patient has voluntarily sought the assistance of the doctor regarding the alleviation of some set of symptoms, and provided that the doctor assures the patient that it is only those symptoms that will be alleviated. When a patient comes to the doctor complaining of some malady, we can reasonably infer that they want their symptoms to be treated.

It is certainly true that deception prevents a patient from giving fully *informed* consent. Sometimes, it is objected that the doctor acts paternalistically in conferring a benefit upon the patient without his consent, whether the patient in fact desires that benefit or not. The American Medical Association's Council on

Ethical and Judicial Affairs, for example, holds the view that since patients cannot be fully informed regarding deceptive placebo treatments, these treatments will always be paternalistic and hence unethical (Shah and Goold 2009). However, this objection reveals an exceedingly dogmatic and inflexible understanding of the nature of the relationships between paternalism and consent.

A patient is only treated paternalistically if the doctor confers on him a benefit that the patient did not request. Paternalism frustrates the stated goals of the patient in order to promote some other goal that the doctor has judged more important. However, if the patient, either explicitly or implicitly, demands that his symptoms be alleviated, then there is no way that it can be paternalistic for the doctor to try to meet these goals. Along similar lines, if an addict asks that his friend confiscate his drugs, it cannot be paternalistic to confiscate them. In light of the addict's request, his friend respects his autonomy in taking the drugs, rather than violating it.

It is true that the patient has not given consent (either implicit or explicit) to be deceived about the mechanism of his treatment. He has also not explicitly consented to be given placebo. In this sense, a deceptive treatment violates the doctrine of informed consent. However, does this matter? Once a doctor receives a patient's consent to treat some ailment, she is not required to obtain separate consent for each step of the treatment process. So long as none of the steps involves any significant cost or harm to the patient, she may execute the treatment however she sees fit. It is not paternalistic for a doctor to unilaterally select an electronic rather than alcohol-based thermometer, or to choose one brand of aspirin over another. We do not require patients to explicitly consent to have their temperature measured with a digital thermometer, because it is not reasonable to expect that their goals will be frustrated if the doctor unilaterally decides to use one.

Choices of this kind cannot frustrate the aims of the patient or cause harm. By the same token, if the doctor decides to advance the patient's stated interests by leading him into a false belief about the nature of his treatment, she does not frustrate his goals or make him any worse off.

4.3 **Constraints on the deceptive use of placebos**

There is an exception to this defense, however, whenever there is a real medical alternative to the placebo. If there is a meaningful choice that the patient might make between one therapy and another, the deceptive prescription of a placebo frustrates the patient's ability to make this choice. In such cases, it is certainly paternalistic for the doctor to use deception to force the patient to accept one reasonable option (the placebo) at the expense of another.

It is therefore a strict moral requirement that placebos are only ever prescribed deceptively when there is no alternative treatment that a reasonable patient might choose. If doctors adhere to this requirement, the patient cannot be a victim of paternalism and his autonomy will be preserved. It also guarantees that the patient does not miss out on optimal medical care.

This requirement places a serious constraint on the ethical use of placebos. To take one obvious example, a doctor should never prescribe a placebo for a harmless headache if analgesics that the patient might reasonably prefer are available. Doctors must be limited to prescribing a placebo when the symptom to be treated is otherwise untreatable.

It is not all bad news for the placebo-prescribing doctor, however. Placebos can still be used to treat untreatable symptoms of treatable ailments. A patient with a treatable ear infection causing untreatable nausea, for example, could be given antibiotics for the infection and placebo for the nausea. A patient with untreatable viral conjunctivitis could be told he would receive nothing for the virus, but placebo for his itchy, uncomfortable eyes.

This is the first and most important of a number of important considerations that must constrain the prescription of placebos if they are to be employed in an ethically defensible way. In the next section, I consider the other major constraints on placebo prescription.

4.3.1 Other moral limits on placebo deception

There remain four reasonable objections frequently made against the deceptive use of placebos, and these objections circumscribe the ethical limits of placebo prescription.

The first set of objections relates to cases of misdiagnosis. Suppose Hanna has misdiagnosed Ian, thinking that he has untreatable viral conjunctivitis when he actually has a form of bacterial conjunctivitis that can be treated with antibiotics. When a doctor sends a patient away with placebos, the patient may wrongly believe that his doctor understands his condition. He may be less likely to seek a second opinion from a more competent doctor, even if his condition worsens. He may also unwittingly mislead the second doctor about the "medications" he is currently taking (American Medical Association 2001). Thus, the doctor's misdiagnosis may mean that he misses out on an effective therapy, and her deception can make it much harder for him to obtain that therapy than the misdiagnosis would on its own.

Now, it is important to note that in the case I described at the outset, Ian is only told to expect relief of discomfort; he is not told to expect the underlying symptoms or disease to be cured. Because of this, if his condition worsens, he will not be prevented from seeking a second consultation or a second opinion from a different doctor. In this respect, Ian is no worse off than any other patient whose doctor has made the wrong diagnosis.

For some illnesses, however, the divide between symptoms and disease will be far less clear than it is in the case of Hanna and Ian. In these cases, it may be wiser not to use the placebos at all.

The second set of objections concerns cases where the consulting doctor is unable to make any firm diagnosis—perhaps the most common case where a doctor might be tempted to prescribe a placebo. In these cases, it is still true that no active treatment can be ethically prescribed, but it might not be true that no active treatment is available to treat the underlying, undiagnosed ailment. In these cases, a similar objection appears: placebo prescription requires the doctor to mislead the patient into believing that a diagnosis has been made. If a patient is given a placebo, he will be much less likely to revisit his doctor if new symptoms arise, which might enable a positive diagnosis (Powell and Bailey 2009).

These cases are more ethically complex than situations in which the malady is understood but no treatment is available. However, even in such circumstances, there is still a way to prescribe a placebo. The doctor can protect the patient's ability to obtain the best medical care by saying something like this: "I do not have enough information to diagnose your illness, but here are some pills to help to alleviate your discomfort. If you develop any new symptoms, please come for a follow-up examination." Pain, discomfort, nausea, anxiety, and similar symptoms cannot be misdiagnosed or not diagnosable. If the patient reports feeling pain, then the pain is a candidate for treatment by placebo. Of course, if the patient's only symptoms are those that may be alleviated by placebo, such as headache, nausea, or anxiety, then this strategy will interfere with the diagnosis of the patient, creating a risk that a positive diagnosis will be delayed or prevented. In such cases, the doctor should avoid using a placebo.

The third set of objections concerns the abuse of placebo prescription by unethical doctors. Doctors may be tempted to use placebos to rid themselves of troublesome patients, or to increase the number of patients they can treat. This worry is explicitly mentioned in the American Medical Association's decision prohibiting the use of placebo (American Medical Association's Council on Ethical and Judicial Affairs 2006–2007). In these cases, it is thoroughly unethical for the doctor to prescribe a placebo.

As I have already argued, part of the reason why placebo prescription is a special type of deception is that the patient is deceived for his own ends, which he declares either explicitly or implicitly when he visits the doctor and asks to be treated. However, in cases where the doctor wants to get rid of the patient for the sake of efficiency or convenience, the doctor's ends differ from the ends of the patient.

If the doctor deceives the patient for reasons that are at odds with the patient's demonstrated goals, then the deception becomes coercive. Onora O'Neill puts it this way: "Victims may want the same ends as their coercers; but that is not the same as sharing those ends. One who is coerced, even if pointlessly, is not pursuing, nor therefore sharing, ends at all" (1985). If the doctor leads the patient to walk away happily with some inert substance, the patient is not sharing the doctor's goal: that the patient leaves the clinic and goes home. The doctor has coerced her patient into leaving without being treated, satisfying her own goals but not the patient's.

Another reasonable objection against the clinical placebo is that, if the use of placebo becomes too widespread, its effectiveness will diminish, since patients will develop less of an association between taking medicines and benefiting from their pharmacological actions. If this were true, then the widespread use of placebos would also diminish the benefit of *active* medications, which, after all, employ the placebo effect as part of their mechanism.

In a similar vein, there may be objections that the widespread use of placebos would undermine the background level of trust between patients and doctors *in every consultation*, leading patients to suspect that every medicine is inert, even if they agree that it is sometimes appropriate for doctors to prescribe inert medications. This could make it harder to deceive patients and, again, could undermine the effectiveness of active medications as well as placebos.

Whether or not any of these threats are real is a largely empirical question—a question that, like all the other empirical questions surrounding placebo use, will be very difficult to investigate within current research ethics guidelines. However, it is worth pointing out that placebos will never be all that widely used if they are used only within the constraints I have outlined here. Placebos will be a treatment *option* that is used only when better options are unavailable. We can mitigate these risks even more if we are careful to avoid practical pitfalls in our methods of placebo prescription. For example, doctors should be discouraged from "debriefing" patients once their condition improves, revealing their use of deceptive placebo.

4.4 **Dealing with the discovery of deception**

There is one more objection to the use of deceptive placebos that imposes a constraint on how they are used: namely, that the use of placebos may undermine the important relationship of trust between doctors and their patients (Kanaan 2009). Patients may lose faith in their doctors if they come to feel they are being wrongfully deceived, and this will be much more detrimental than the "background" erosion of trust I have discussed previously.

Now, the doctor's decision to deceptively prescribe placebo is a special case, which is ethically defensible, so it is not certain that trust will be eroded if placebo deception is uncovered by the patient. If a patient discovers that a placebo has been used, the doctor can offer a robust moral justification for her actions. However, there is no ethical justification for doctors to engage in non-placebo deceptions, and any additional deceptions must be avoided.

Unfortunately, these kinds of inessential deceptions can quickly creep in if a patient asks directly whether or not they are receiving a placebo. Suppose, for example, that the patient makes a specific enquiry about the nature of his treatment after the doctor has provided a placebo. Or suppose he asks the name of his treatment. Most patients have no interest in the exact pharmacological mechanism of their treatment, but some inevitably do ask such questions. What is the doctor to do in these cases?

Imagine Eric asks Molly about the active ingredient in the cream he has been given. Molly is faced here with a choice: she can either admit that the cream is inert, or she can create a new deception and tell Eric that the cream contains (for example) a corticosteroid. If Eric tells another doctor that he is using a corticosteroid, she may refuse to prescribe Eric the optimal treatment for some other ailment.

Now, Molly could avoid this outcome by telling Eric, truthfully, that the cream contains an active ingredient, witch hazel, which is commonly used to treat other skin-related ailments. In doing this, she would avoid lying, but succeed in deceiving Eric into holding the belief that the treatment is pharmacologically active and indicated for his symptoms. If he visits another doctor, that doctor will realize that Eric has been given a placebo. While this is better than directly lying to the patient, there is another important objection: even if Molly never lies about what the cream contained, if Eric discovers that the cream is not indicated for his neuropathic itch, he will know that Molly further deceived him in order to protect her original placebo deception.

Doctors need to be able to recognize the point where further deception would not fall under the moral umbrella of placebo deception. The initial deception involved in placebo prescription is permissible because it furthers the patient's stated aims, but it is not clear that subsequent supporting deceptions advance the patient's aims at all; they merely serve to cover the doctor's tracks. As I argued earlier, if a deception serves the doctor's aims and not the patient's, it is coercive. Molly should not be so desperate to defend her initial deception that she engages in additional coercive, non-beneficial deceptions. She should tell Eric something like this: "I had prescribed you a placebo, but now that you know about it there will be no beneficial placebo effect. We'll have to rely on your natural capacity for healing instead, although I do not expect your symptoms to improve." Patients may be embarrassed or angry to discover that their doctors have deceived them, so these situations ought to be avoided as far as possible. While the patient may prefer to avoid embarrassment, this is not an aim he expresses in seeking out a doctor, and it will be a case of unethical paternalism if he is protected from an uncomfortable confrontation for the sake of his own tranquility.

4.5 **Placebos for depression**

Perhaps my arguments so far have created the impression that placebos can only be used in rare clinical scenarios. It is true that the constraints I have mentioned greatly limit the range of cases in which a doctor could prescribe a placebo to a patient, but the ethical hurdles can be surmounted in one of the most familiar clinical presentations: the depressed patient.

Kirsch's chapter in this volume (Chapter 2) suggests both that modern antidepressants are exceedingly effective and that their effectiveness is entirely grounded in the placebo effect. If this is correct, then there is a multi-billion dollar industry in the production and prescription of placebos—and while the clinicians in question certainly do not intend to prescribe placebos, the unintentional nature of their actions makes no practical difference to the patients.

If we conceive of depression as a symptom rather than a disease, a doctor will satisfy all the ethical requirements I have given for the deceptive use of placebo when she gives a placebo to a depressed patient. I said that placebos should only be given when there is no reasonable alternative, and if Kirsch's results are correct (see Chapter 2), then all the competing pharmacological treatments should be considered placebos.[2] I also said that a placebo should be presented as an agent of symptomatic relief rather than as a cure, and I see no reason why placebo could not be prescribed in this way to a depressed patient. A doctor might say: "I do not know why you are depressed—modern medicine does not understand depression very well. It could be that you have a chemical imbalance or it could be due to stress in your life. Trials have found that 60% of patients feel significantly better when they take an antidepressant, so that is what I am prescribing for you. If your depression gets worse, or if you develop new symptoms, come see me again."

Depression is a common ailment that places a very heavy burden on our society. Currently, assuming Kirsch is correct, doctors prescribe placebos for this ailment: expensive placebos with serious unwanted side-effects. We also prescribe these placebos in a way that entirely ignores all the moral limitations I have described—we give patients antidepressants when we could easily send them to therapy or prescribe exercise, we tell patients we are treating the ailment rather than the symptoms, and we overuse the placebo in a way which is probably diminishing its effectiveness. However, prescribed correctly, depression provides the clearest case for allowing doctors to intentionally and responsibly prescribe placebos in the clinic.

4.6 **The ethics of charging money for inert therapies**

Placebo treatments have repeatedly been shown to be more powerful when larger prices are imposed on the patients who pay for them (Waber et al. 2008). When people perceive more value in something simply because it has a higher price, it is hard to shake the feeling that they have been duped. Thus, it is sometimes suggested that there is something unethical about expecting patients to pay for inert medications. This objection, however, does not hold up under close scrutiny, at least when it comes to placebo treatments.

Consider first that even active medications have a large placebo component. This is illustrated very clearly by the recent study of Bingel et al. (2011) which showed that the effectiveness of a powerful opiate analgesic was reduced by more than 50% when the patient was unaware it had been administered, and subsequently reduced by nearly 100% when the patient was (falsely) informed that the analgesic had been withdrawn. If a drug's action turns out to be 50% placebo, or 80% placebo, we do not insist that the vendors of these drugs reduce their prices by a corresponding amount.

Consider too that we frequently prescribe medications for which the mechanism is poorly understood, or not understood at all—at best, we have some evidence that these medicines provide benefit compared to an openly prescribed research placebo, but no evidence for what that benefit is or why the medicine provides it. Thus, there is no factual basis for the suggestion that we are normally confined to selling medicines that are known to have a specific pharmacological action. Many drugs on the market could (for all we know) have an entirely psychological mechanism.

In this light, it should be clear that we could only object to the sale of placebo treatments if we thought that placebo benefits were in some sense false benefits. However, that cannot be correct, since placebos provide symptomatic relief—something for which patients will willingly and happily pay.

4.7 **Conclusions**

The ethical use of deceptive placebos requires doctors to walk a fine line, both medically and morally. They must first ensure that the placebo is genuinely the only reasonable treatment available for the patient's symptoms. They must make it very clear to the patient that they are only treating the felt symptoms of the ailment, and not the underlying complaint. Most importantly, they must ensure that their ends in deceiving the patient are always shared by the patient, in order that their use of placebo will not be paternalistic and coercive.

Meeting all these needs simultaneously is a demanding task but I doubt that it is overly demanding for skilled doctors. The benefits, meanwhile, are significant: there are a large number of cases in which no treatment can be offered or in which no diagnosis can be made. Provided that placebos are as effective at treating symptoms like pain and nausea as I have assumed that they are, the medical and moral difficulties involved in their ethical use are costs worth bearing. We should allow doctors to use placebos, within appropriate ethical constraints.

Acknowledgement

This chapter was originally published as: Bennett Foddy, The ethical placebo, *The Journal of Mind–Body Regulation*, 1 (2), pp. 53–62, © The Authors, 2011.

Notes

1 Harmful "nocebo" effects are sometimes observed in a research setting, where patients have no positive expectation that the treatment will work. As I have argued elsewhere, these effects are likely to be very rare in a clinical setting.
2 Perhaps a depressed patient could more fruitfully be prescribed exercise or meditation than placebo. Even if that is true, there will be very many cases where this is not feasible, either because the depressed patient is already getting regular exercise or because they are unable to exercise.

References

American Medical Association's Council on Ethical and Judicial Affairs (2006–2007). *Code of medical ethics: current opinions with annotations, 2006–2007*. Chicago, IL: American Medical Association.

American Medical Association (2001). *Principles of medical ethics*. Available at: http://www.ama-assn.org/ama/pub/physician-resources/medical-ethics/code-medical-ethics/principles-medical-ethics.page.

Benedetti, F. (2006). Placebo analgesia. *Neurological Sciences*, **27**, S100–102.

Bensoussan, A., Talley, N. J., Hing, M., Menzies, R., Guo, A., and Ngu, M. (1998). Treatment of irritable bowel syndrome with Chinese herbal medicine—a randomized controlled trial. *Journal of the American Medical Association*, **280**(18), 1585–1589.

Bingel, U., Wanigasekera, V., Wiech, K., et al. (2011). The effect of treatment expectation on drug efficacy: imaging the analgesic benefit of the opioid Remifentanil. *Science Translational Medicine*, **3**(70), 70ra14. DOI: 10.1126/scitranslmed.3001244

Blease, C. (2011). Deception as treatment: the case of depression. *Journal of Medical Ethics*, **37**(1), 13–16. DOI: 10.1136/Jme.2010.039313

Colloca, L. and Benedetti, F. (2006). How prior experience shapes placebo analgesia. *Pain*, **124**(1–2), 126–133. DOI: 10.1016/J.Pain.2006.04.005

Enck, P., Zimmermann, K., Menke, G., Muller-Lissner, S., Martens, U., and Klosterhal-fen, S. (2008). A mixture of Escherichia coli (DSM 17252) and Enterococcus faecalis (DSM 16440) for treatment of the irritable bowel syndrome—a randomized controlled trial with primary care physicians. *Neurogastroenterology and Motility*, **20**(10), 1103–1109. DOI: 10.1111/J.1365–2982.2008.01156.X

Foddy, B. (2009). A duty to deceive: placebos in clinical practice. *American Journal of Bioethics*, **9**(12), 4–12. DOI: 10.1080/15265160903318350

Galovski, T. E. and Blanchard, E. B. (1998). The treatment of irritable bowel syndrome with hypnotherapy. *Applied Psychophysiology and Biofeedback*, **23**(4), 219–232.

Gibbard, A. (1990). *Wise choices, apt feelings, a theory of normative judgment*. Cambridge, Massachusetts: Harvard University Press.

Jackson, J. (1991). Telling the truth. *Journal of Medical Ethics*, **17**(1), 5–9.

Kanaan, R. (2009). When doctors deceive. *American Journal of Bioethics*, **9**(12), 29–30. DOI: 10.1080/15265160903234102

Kaptchuk, T. J., Friedlander, E., Kelley, J. M., et al. (2010). Placebos without deception: a randomized controlled trial in irritable bowel syndrome. *PLoS One*, **5**(12). DOI: 10.1371/journal.pone.0015591

Klein, D. F. (1994). Identified placebo treatment. *Neuropsychopharmacology*, **10**(4), 271–272.

Kolber, A. (2008). A limited defense of clinical placebo deception. *Yale Law and Policy Review*, **75**, 75–134.

O'Neill, O. (1985). Between consenting adults. *Philosophy and Public Affairs*, **14**(3), 252–277.

Park, L. C. and Covi, L. (1965). Nonblind placebo trial: an exploration of neurotic patients' responses to placebo when its inert content is disclosed. *Archives of General Psychiatry*, **12**(4), 336–345.

Pittler, M. H. and Ernst, E. (1998). Peppermint oil for irritable bowel syndrome: a critical review and meta-analysis. *American Journal of Gastroenterology*, **93**(7), 1131–1135.

Powell, T. and Bailey, J. (2009). Against placebos. *American Journal of Bioethics*, **9**(12), 23–25. DOI: 10.1080/15265160903244234

Primoratz, I. (1984). Lying and the methods of ethics. *International Studies in Philosophy*, **16**(3), 35–57.

Shah, K. R. and Goold, S. D. (2009). The primacy of autonomy, honesty, and disclosure—Council on Ethical and Judicial Affairs' placebo opinions. *American Journal of Bioethics*, **9**(12), 15–17. DOI: 10.1080/15265160903316339

Sokol, D. K. (2007). Can deceiving patients be morally acceptable? *British Medical Journal*, **334**(7601), 984–986.

Taylor, S. E. and Brown, J. D. (1988). Illusion and well-being—a social psychological perspective on mental health. *Psychological Bulletin*, **103**(2), 193–210.

van Laarhoven, A. I. M., Vogelaar, M. L., Wilder-Smith, et al. (2011). Induction of nocebo and placebo effects on itch and pain by verbal suggestions. *Pain*, **152**(7), 1486–1494. DOI: 10.1016/J.Pain.2011.01.043

Waber, R. L., Shiv, B., Carmon, Z., and Ariely, D. (2008). Commercial features of placebo and therapeutic efficacy. *Journal of the American Medical Association*, **299**(9), 1016–1017.

Wear, S. (1998). *Informed consent: patient autonomy and clinician beneficence within health care* (2nd edn.). Washington, DC: Georgetown University Press.

Chapter 5

Trust and the placebo effect

Marie Prévost, Anna Zuckerman,
and Ian Gold

5.1 The meaning of placebos

Placebos have likely been around for as long as there have been people and, as
Shapiro and Shapiro (1997) remark, the history of pre-modern medicine is the
history of placebos. There is little controversy that placebo effects exist. However, what this effect is remains controversial. The placebo effect involves
expectancy—a cognitive process reflecting what the patient expects from a
treatment (Kirsch 1985, 2004). Placebo effects are also conditioning effects; the
habit of experiencing a positive outcome from treatment trains one to expect
positive outcomes from all treatments (Wickramasekera 1980). Placebo effects
are thus a component of all interactions that attempt to ameliorate disease or
distress.

Above all, however, placebos seem to exert their effects in virtue of the meanings they have; the meanings patients attach to things, concepts, and people
have healing effects (Kirmayer 1993). As Moerman and Jonas (2002) put it, a
placebo effect is "the physiologic or psychological effect of meaning in the treatment of illness" (see Chapter 7). Indeed, apart from being brought about by
"medication" and sham surgery such as a simple skin incision (Cobb et al. 1959;
Dimond et al. 1960), placebos effects have been shown to depend on such things
as the color of a pill (Blackwel et al. 1972; deCraen et al. 1996), the brand of a
medication (Branthwaite and Cooper 1981), the length of treatment (Irvine
et al. 1999), the description of a treatment (Amigo et al. 1993; Desharnais
et al. 1993; Thomas 1987), the attitude of the physician (Di Blasi et al. 2001), and
the color of the physician's clothes (Blumhagen 1979).

It is widely accepted that the relationship between doctor and patient is an
important contributor to the meaning of the healing environment (Di Blasi
et al. 2001; Harrington 1997). The doctor–patient relationship, however, is
complex, textured, and polysemous. It depends, of course, on the personalities
involved, but it derives its meaning no less from the cultural context in which it

occurs. A deep understanding of the placebo effect, and its judicious use in the clinic, requires that we are able to isolate the aspects of meaning in the doctor–patient relation that are conducive to healing.

It is commonplace that trusting your doctor is essential, but little attention has been given to the question of whether trust makes a real difference to clinical outcomes. That is to say, is trust desirable for emotional or ethical reasons alone, or could the presence of trust in the doctor–patient relationship contribute to healing? Barrett and colleagues (2006, p. 191) recommend that clinicians "develop relationships of trust, compassion and empathy," and Kirsch (see Chapter 2) suggests that trust is "one of the most important clinical tools that clinicians have at their disposal." Our aims in this chapter are to take some first steps in developing the hypothesis that trust in the doctor–patient relationship may be a contributor to the placebo effect and thus to healing, and to motivate the study of trust in medical interactions. In this direction, recent work has begun to explore the neurobiological underpinnings of relationships of trust. If trust plays a role in the doctor–patient relationship, the neurobiology of trust may illuminate the biological mechanisms through which placebos exert their effects.

5.2 **"Trust me, I'm a doctor"**

There is wide agreement that it is important for physicians to build a trusting relationship with their patients. In ancient times, doctors were careful to adopt "a manner and bearing that would instill trust and respect"—including, notably, adopting the Hippocratic Oath—although this had more to do with overcoming the prevalent suspicion that doctors were quacks than with a moral concern for their patients (Frede 1987). The same sentiment, with ethical motivations, continues to be articulated by those concerned with the art of medicine:

> To me the most important thing in a relationship is that the heart of the relationship is a moral enterprise that occurs between not only the doctor and his patient, but the lawyer and his client, the minister and his confessor and the teacher and his student. All of these relationships have a dependent person who needs help, who goes to another person who professes to be able to help. They enter into a fiduciary relationship. (Colgan 2009)

Evidence that trust is not only a pragmatic or moral value in medicine but of clinical benefit, however, is sparse (Pearson and Raeke 2000). Armstrong and colleagues (2006) propose that trust in the healthcare system and in one's physician are the major predictors of adherence to treatment, healthcare utilization, healthcare quality, and health behavior. Indeed, patients' satisfaction, acceptance of medication, adherence to treatment, and self-reported health improvements are associated with their trust in their doctor (Altice et al. 2001; Rotenberg et al. 2008; Safran et al. 1998). Trust has also been associated with better health status (Hibbard 1985) and better self-reported health as far as eight years after the first evaluation (Barefoot et al. 1998). On the other hand, distrust in the healthcare system, but not with the primary physician, is associated with self-reported poor health (Armstrong et al. 2006).

5.3 **Trust and depression**

One indirect source of evidence about the possible health benefits of trust comes from the study of depression. Low depression scores are observed in children who trust their parents (Sakai 2010) or who are generally more trusting (Lester and Gatto 1990). Similarly, children who trust their neighborhood have an absence of emotional disorders (Meltzer et al. 2007). Successful treatment of depression by means of cognitive therapy requires that patients trust their therapist's views over their own beliefs and feelings (Beck et al. 1979). As patients tend to have a pessimistic view of their life and future, they believe their depression will not resolve. It is thus crucial that they fully trust their therapist's more optimistic view. Studies show that people who are generally more trusting have lower depression scores (Kouvonen et al. 2008; Lester and Gatto 1990; Muris et al. 2001) and, more specifically, that patients who trust their doctor have lower depression scores than those who have low or no trust in their doctor (Piette et al. 2005). Indeed, being able to trust a health professional to act in one's best interest is the most important feature of medical care reported by depressed patients (Cooper et al. 2000). Grotberg (1999) even includes trust as one of the five ingredients needed to build resilience and help face life's adversities.

As depression is a chronic illness, patients are more likely to be involved in a long-term relationship with their doctor. There is evidence that the length of the doctor–patient relationship is associated with trust in the doctor (Baker et al. 2003; Mainous et al. 2001; Parchman and Burge 2004) and that the longer a visit to the doctor, the more trust a patient places in their doctor (Fiscella et al. 2004). Weiss and Blustein (1996) showed that the longer the doctor–patient relationship, the lower the number of patient hospitalizations. While acknowledging that Weiss and Blustein's findings could reflect an effect of efficient prevention and follow-up, it is also possible that the trust established exerts a beneficial effect on health. Depressed patients are thus more likely to trust their doctor and assign a benevolent meaning to their intentions. Indeed, recent findings suggest that about 80% of the response to antidepressants is a placebo response (Kirsch et al. 2008).

5.4 **Toward a science of trust in medicine**

We have already noted that evidence of a relationship between trust and health benefits is sparse. This is in part because trust is assessed in different contexts by means of different scales based on different definitions of the term. In addition, diverse notions of trust are sometimes conflated. For example, trust in the competence of a doctor is not always distinguished from trust in their benevolence. This conceptual confusion is a symptom of a pervasive problem in research on trust. Although we all have an intuitive understanding of what trust is, there is in fact a large range of distinguishable concepts of trust (Castelfranchi and Falcone 2010; Cook 2001; Hardin 2002; Mcknight et al. 1998; Rotenberg et al. 2008) We trust our bank to protect our money, our colleagues to do their work, our friends to be there when we need them, our partners to be loyal. Trust is required both to lend a friend money for lunch and for governments to provide a trillion dollars to stave off economic disaster. Though related, it is very unlikely that these notions of trust are the same.

The diversity of the common-sense concepts of trust is reflected in trust research. For evolutionary theorists, trust is a "propensity to cooperate in the absence of behavioural indicators" (Macy 1996). For economists, it reflects the belief in, and the willingness to depend on, another party (Mcknight et al. 1998). For moral philosophers or sociologists, it may be the acceptance of "vulnerability to another's possible, but not expected, ill will (or lack of good will) toward one" (Baier 1986) or the willingness to take a risk in a social interaction (Mayer et al. 1995). In psychological models, trust is construed as depending on a large range of factors including whether the trustee is a person or an institution, and—if a person—their reliability, honesty, and various aspects of their behavior, among other things (Rotenberg et al. 2008).

Castaldo (2002) evaluated 273 terms related to trust using publications from the 1960s to the 1990s in the fields of management, marketing, psychology, and sociology, and identified seventy-two distinct definitions of trust. Given that some significant fields were omitted in this study (economics and political theory in particular), it would not be surprising if an extension of Castaldo's analysis would produce many more. Castelfranchi and Falcone (2010) remark that:

> There is not yet a shared or prevailing, and clear and convincing notion of trust . . . On the contrary, most authors working on trust provide their own definition, which frequently is not really general but rather tailored for a specific domain . . . The consequence is that there is very little overlapping among the numerous definitions of trust, while a strong common conceptual kernel for characterizing the general notion has yet to emerge.

A rather blunt conclusion seems to be warranted: a field characterized by a central concept that can be defined in at least seventy-two distinct ways has not yet found its conceptual bearings.

If a scientific investigation of a potential role for trust in medicine is to be carried out, the concepts of trust that may be apposite will have to be distinguished. Of course, these concepts can define other relationships that are similar to the patient–doctor one, like the food provider relationship with the consumer, and that similarly influence placebo effects, like those at stake in diets (see Chapter 11). Consider, as an illustration, two distinct concepts of trust that are likely to be at play in the doctor–patient interaction. People trust their doctors in the sense that they believe they are competent. Call this notion of trust "reliance" (Baier 1986). Patients rely on their doctors in the sense that they expect them to behave in a way that will manifest their medical knowledge to the benefit of the patient. One could rely on an artificial intelligence system capable of making diagnoses in the same way.

In contrast, people also trust their doctors to have their patients' best interests at heart—to spend as much time with them as good medical practice warrants, to prescribe medication based on patients' needs rather than the interests of pharmaceutical companies, and so on. Call this "dependence." Dependence is different from reliance to the extent that dependence, but not reliance, is contingent in some way on the state of mind of the person on whom one depends. A patient thus relies on their doctor when they believe that the doctor will display clinical competence whatever their reasons or motives for action. In contrast, it is a necessary condition of dependence that the doctor deploys their medical knowledge for the right sort of reason. The intentions of the trustee are thus crucial to dependence (Rosseau and Camerer 1998). This is what is meant by the claim that doctors have patients' best interests at heart. As Baier puts it (1986, p. 234), depending on someone "seems to be reliance on their good will toward one, as distinct from their dependable habits, or only on their dependably exhibited fear, anger, or other motives compatible with ill will toward one, or on motives not directed on one at all." Reliability and dependence are, therefore, clearly separable: competent doctors can be mercenary, and quacks can be magnanimous.

A study setting out to evaluate the possibility of a relationship between a placebo effect and trust in medical practice, therefore, would have to distinguish (among many other things) between reliance and dependence as two distinct components of the doctor–patient relationship. A possible experiment could, for example, compare the placebo effects generated by a diagnosis given by an artificial intelligence system and one given by an experienced and familiar diagnostician; reliance is presumably present in both conditions, but dependence is represented only in the latter. The "open-hidden paradigm" (Levine and Gordon 1984) makes use of something close to this condition. In one condition, a doctor administers a drug (open), and in a second condition, a computer administers the drug (hidden) without patients' awareness. The open condition is associated with better clinical outcomes than the hidden condition. In an extension of this paradigm, one condition would have a patient aware that they were being administered a drug by a computer, and in a second condition would know that the doctor was administering it. A second experiment might compare the effects of being given medical treatment by two competent doctors, one of whom is believed to be benevolent and another of whom is believed to be exclusively self-interested. Here again, reliance is separated out from dependence. Finally, one could set the phenomena known to modulate the placebo effect against the putative effect of trust in an effort to establish their relative powers. A placebo in the form of an injection, for example, is known to be more effective than one given in the form of a pill (Traut and Passarelli 1957). What will be the outcome of a pill given by a doctor on whom one relies, compared to an injection given by one who is unreliable? Also, what will be the outcome with a doctor on whom one not only relies but depends?

Reliance and dependence are two of the possible relationships that characterize doctor–patient interactions, but it is unlikely that they exhaust all the options. For example, integrity might be a strong determinant of trust in other systems, such as politics, where competence and expertise (and by extension, reliance) seem to have less weight (see Chapter 14). A systematic study of the effect of trust on healing will therefore have to begin with the conceptual work of distinguishing other notions of trust that may be relevant and designing experimental paradigms to isolate their effects.

5.5 The biology of trust

As we suggest in the previous section, one important motivation for investigating the role of trust in medical interactions is the advances being made in understanding the biological bases of states of trust, in particular, the effects of the brain-produced hormone, oxytocin. Oxytocin appears to be a major biological marker of pro-social attitudes and, over the past decade, a series of papers has consistently linked the extent of trust in economic exchanges with oxytocin levels (Baumgartner et al. 2008; Declerck et al. 2010; Kosfeld et al. 2005; Zak et al. 2005, 2007). People have also been found to be more trusting with personal information when receiving intra-nasal oxytocin than when receiving a placebo (Mikolajczak et al. 2010).

Crucially, oxytocin also seems to be able to modulate the immune system. Healthy men given a bacterial endotoxin and intravenous oxytocin show significantly lower levels of plasma immune markers than participants receiving the bacterial endotoxin alone (Clodi et al. 2008). In addition, intra-nasal administration of oxytocin diminishes endogenous levels of stress markers in procedures inducing social stress (Ditzen et al. 2009; Heinrichs et al. 2003) and self-report measures of anxiety (Heinrichs et al. 2003). Evidence of the protective effects of oxytocin is even clearer in the animal literature. Oxytocin treatment in rats reduces the damage to burned skin compared to no treatment (Iseri et al. 2010); oxytocin has an anti-ulcer effect (Asad et al. 2001); it enhances the survival of damaged tissue (Petersson et al. 2001); and it reduces edema in the paw (Petersson et al. 2001).

The dual role of oxytocin in states of trust and in the enhancement of immune function provides the beginnings of a hypothetical mechanism of action for some placebo effects. While there is no direct evidence of this mechanism at work, there are some suggestive findings. In animals, continuous stroking enhances circulating levels of oxytocin (Carter 2006; Lund et al. 2002; Odendaal and Meintjes 2003). Furthermore, while there is no significant increase of oxytocin in humans following physical contact of strangers or familiar others (Grewen et al. 2005; Turner et al. 1999; Wikstrom et al. 2003), a history of frequent hugs from a partner has been associated with higher basal levels of oxytocin (Light et al. 2005). Most interestingly, when people are massaged and then act as a financial trustee, the increase in their circulating oxytocin level is proportional to the extent of the trust placed in them as well as the amount of money they return to the "investor" (Morhenn et al. 2008). These findings thus lead to the speculation that palpation (or indeed the laying on of hands by a faith healer) accompanied by trust may activate oxytocin.

It has been suggested that the positive effects of touch on the physiology of mammals is mediated by other agents such as serotonin (Field 1998), which also diminishes social stress reactivity (Hanley and Van de Kar 2003). Given the wide range of neural systems with which oxytocin interacts (Argiolas and Gessa 1991), other hormones and peptides are likely to be involved in an effect on health. Exploring the function of oxytocin in the context of trust, as well as the biological systems with which oxytocin interacts, may enable us to map some of the neural circuitry underlying the placebo effect.

5.6 Concluding remarks: from placebos to politics

There is (we are regularly told) a crisis of trust. We no longer trust because our trust has too often been betrayed. Nowhere is the crisis clearer than in biomedicine. As a result, the picture of the benevolent, paternalistic doctor in whom one places one's trust has been supplanted by a picture of the patient as fully autonomous and the doctor as a provider of medical information on the basis of which the patient makes a free decision about their medical care.

At the center of this conception of the doctor–patient relationship is the idea of informed consent in clinical encounters. The notion of informed consent was first articulated in the context of medical experimentation. Among the atrocities perpetrated by the Nazis were experiments conducted on concentration camp inmates, and reflection on those acts (beginning with the Nuremberg Code) laid the foundation for an account of the experimental subject—and, by extension, the medical patient—as one who must give informed consent to medical procedures. As a result, informed consent to medical experimentation and intervention has become a necessary condition of all medical encounters. It is no longer acceptable for a doctor to act paternalistically, on the basis of judgments about what is in the patient's best interests. "Trust me, I'm a doctor" is a phrase that can now only be uttered ironically.

However, the concept of informed consent is plagued by conceptual problems. As Manson and O'Neill (2007) argue, the idea of communicating fully and unambiguously all of the relevant information concerning a medical intervention may be incoherent even when a patient is fully competent and cognitively capable of understanding what is being conveyed. Among other problems, there will always be areas of potential ambiguity that cannot be anticipated by the physician. A patient told that he is being prescribed electroconvulsive therapy for depression may react differently than he would to being told he will receive shock therapy, even though shock therapy and electroconvulsive therapy are the same (see Manson and O'Neill 2007, p.13). Further, it is unreasonable to require that doctors disclose every possible consequence or aspect of a medical intervention as part of the process of informed consent. An anesthetic used in the course of surgery need not be described as a narcotic in order for its use to be permissible. More practically, as medical treatments become more complex, it is unreasonable to expect that even the best-educated layman will be able to understand what is being proposed. Gene therapy, for example, may come to be the best treatment for some forms of cancer, but it would be absurd to argue that it could only be offered to molecular biologists on the grounds that only they could be fully informed about what it involved. Finally, it would be unethical to withhold medical treatment from patients who were cognitively impaired or otherwise not in a position to make a decision about receiving medical treatment.

Manson and O'Neill (2007) argue that while informed consent should not be abandoned as a standard for medical practice, it cannot stand as the sole protector of the rights of patients. Trust must be present as well. While blind trust in anyone, including one's doctor, makes no sense, we need not give or withhold trust blindly. In any case, it is impossible to do away with trust even if we wanted to. The medical system, for example, attempts to maintain appropriate ethical standards by ensuring accountability for wrongdoing. One can therefore expect good behavior from a doctor not because one trusts him but because the doctor understands the consequences of misbehavior. However, accountability does not eliminate the need for trust; it only pushes it back. Mechanisms of accountability:

> [I]nvite us to transfer trust from the primary agents who provide some good or service (nursing care, a DNA test, a blood test) to those who devise or impose second-order systems for holding those primary providers to account . . . Those who rely on systems of accountability in effect place their trust in second-order systems for controlling and securing the reliable performance of primary tasks, and in those who devise and revise such systems of accountability. Pushing trust one stage, or several stages, back does not eliminate the need to place or refuse trust, and to do so intelligently. (Manson and O'Neill 2007, p. 163)

Given that trust is indispensible in medical care, when it is given "intelligently," it may provide a better model for thinking about the relationship between doctor and patient. Even the ethical concern that the deception used when prescribing placebos will harm the relationship of trust might not be justified, as Foddy argues earlier in this volume (see Chapter 4). If I have good reason to trust my doctor—not blindly, but on the basis of information about the doctor, and the judgment I make from my acquaintance with him/her—then the inevitable gap between the information I have and the information I would need to offer a fully informed consent can be bridged. The uncovered deception might not damage the doctor–patient relationship if the patient acknowledges that his doctor's decision is based on both expertise and good intentions. Only total trust allows this implicit agreement that the doctor's decision, including the decision to deceive, is the best one in the present context. As Manson and O'Neill (2007, p. 159) put it, "[t]rust matters, in biomedicine as elsewhere, because individuals have limited epistemic and practical capacities."

This is not the place for a systematic evaluation of the ethics of medical practice, but the idea that trust may be an indispensible feature of the doctor–patient interaction provides a locus for the meeting of the ethics of medical practice and the art of the effective clinician. If it is the case that a relationship of trust between doctor and patient can exert a beneficial effect on the health of the patient, then the attempt of biomedical ethics to do away with the concept of trust may not only be conceptually incoherent and practically impossible but clinically inadvisable. Trusting your doctor may be good for your health. Also, ironically, intelligently placing trust in one's doctor may be one method available to the patient for taking their health into their own hands.

Acknowledgement

This chapter was originally published as: Marie Prévost, Anna Zuckerman, and Ian Gold, Trust in placebos, *The Journal of Mind–Body Regulation*, 1 (3), pp. 138–142, © The Authors, 2011.

References

Altice, F. L., Mostashari, F., and Friedland, G. H. (2001). Trust and the acceptance of and adherence to antiretroviral therapy. *Journal of Acquired Immune Deficiency Syndromes*, **28**(1), 47–58.

Amigo, I., Fernandez, A., and Gonzalez, A. (1993). The effect of verbal instruction on blood pressure measurement. *Journal of Hypertension*, **11**(3), 293–296.

Argiolas, A. and Gessa, G. L. (1991). Central functions of oxytocin [review]. *Neuroscience & Biobehavorial Reviews*, **15**(2), 217–231.

Armstrong, K., Rose, A., Peters, N., Long, J. A., McMurphy, S., and Shea, J. A. (2006). Distrust of the health care system and self-reported health in the United States. *Journal of General Internal Medicine*, **21**(4), 292–297. DOI: 10.1111/j.1525-1497.2006.00396x

Asad, M., Shewade, D. G., Koumaravelou, K., Abraham, B. K., Vasu, S., and Ramaswamy, S. (2001). Gastric antisecretory and antiulcer activity of oxytocin in rats and guinea pigs. *Life Science*, **70**(1), 17–24.

Baier, A. (1986). Trust and antitrust. *Ethics*, **96**(2), 231–260.

Baker, R., Mainous, A. G., Gray, D. P., and Love, M. M. (2003). Exploration of the relationship between continuity, trust in regular doctors and patient satisfaction with consultations with family doctors. *Scandinavian Journal of Primary Health Care*, **21**(1), 27–32.

Barefoot, J. C., Maynard, K. E., Beckham, J. C., Brummett, B. H., Hooker, K., and Siegler, I. C. (1998). Trust, health, and longevity. *Journal of Behavioral Medicine*, **21**(6), 517–526.

Barrett, B., Muller, D., Rakel, D., Rabago, D., Marchand, L., and Scheder, J. C. (2006). Placebo, meaning, and health. *Perspectives in Biology and Medicine*, **49**(2), 178–198.

Baumgartner, T., Heinrichs, M., Vonlanthen, A., Fischbacher, U., and Fehr, E. (2008). Oxytocin shapes the neural circuitry of trust and trust adaptation in humans. *Neuron*, **58**(4), 639–650. DOI: 10.1016/J.Neuron.2008.04.009

Beck, A. T., Rush, A. J., Shaw, B. F., and Emery, G. (1979). Cognitive theory of depression. New York: Guilford Press.

Blackwel, B., Bloomfie, S., and Buncher, C. R. (1972). Demonstration to medical students of placebo responses and non-drug factors. *Lancet*, **1**(7763), 1279–1282.

Blumhagen, D. W. (1979). Doctors white coat—image of the physician in modern America. *Annals of Internal Medicine*, **91**(1), 111–116.

Branthwaite, A. and Cooper, P. (1981). Analgesic effects of branding in treatment of headaches. *British Medical Journal*, **282**(6276), 1576–1578.

Carter, C. S. (2006). Biological perspectives on social attachment and bonding. In: C. S. Carter (Ed.), *Attachment and bonding: a new synthesis* (ed. C. S. Carter). Cambridge, MA: MIT Press, pp. 85–100.

Castaldo, S. (2002). Fiducia e relazioni di mercato. Bologna: Il Mulino.

Castelfranchi, C. and Falcone, R. (2010). *Trust theory: a socio-cognitive and computational model.* Sussex, UK: Chichester Wiley.

Clodi, M., Vila, G., Geyeregger, R., et al. (2008). Oxytocin alleviates the neuroendocrine and cytokineresponse to bacterial endotoxin in healthy men. *American Journal of Physiology, Endocrinology and Metabolism,* **295**(3), E686–E691.

Cobb, L. A., Thomas, G. I., Dillard, D. H., Merendino, K. A., and Bruce, R. A. (1959). An evaluation of internal-mammary-artery ligation by a double-blind technic. *New England Journal of Medicine,* **260**(22), 1115–1118.

Colgan, R. (2009). *Advice to the young physician: on the art of medicine.* New York: Springer.

Cook, K. (2001). *Trust in society.* New York: Russell Sage Foundation Series on Trust.

Cooper, L. A., Brown, C., Vu, H. T., et al. (2000). Primary care patients' opinions regarding the importance of various aspects of care for depression. *General Hospital Psychiatry,* **22**(3), 163–173.

Declerck, C. H., Boone, C., and Kiyonari, T. (2010). Oxytocin and cooperation under conditions of uncertainty: the modulating role of incentives and social information. *Hormones and Behavior,* **57**(3), 368–374. DOI: 10.1016/J.Yhbeh.2010.01.006

deCraen, A. J. M., Roos, P. J., deVries, A. L., and Kleijnen, J. (1996). Effect of colour of drugs: systematic review of perceived effect of drugs and of their effectiveness. *British Medical Journal,* **313**(7072), 1624–1626.

Desharnais, R., Jobin, J., Cote, C., Levesque, L., and Godin, G. (1993). Aerobic exercise and the placebo effect—a controlled study. *Psychosomatic Medicine,* **55**(2), 149–154.

Di Blasi, Z., Harkness, E., Ernst, E., Georgiou, A., and Kleijnen, J. (2001). Influence of context effects on health outcomes: a systematic review. *Lancet,* **357**(9258), 757–762.

Dimond, E. G., Kittle, C. F., and Crockett, J. E. (1960). Comparison of internal mammary artery ligation and sham operation for angina pectoris. *American Journal of Cardiology,* **5**(4), 483–486.

Ditzen, B., Schaer, M., Gabriel, B., Bodenmann, G., Ehlert, U., and Heinrichs, M. (2009). Intranasal oxytocin increases positive communication and reduces cortisol levels during couple conflict. *Biological Psychiatry,* **65**(9), 728–731. DOI: 10.1016/J. Biopsych.2008.10.011

Field, T. M. (1998). Massage therapy effects. *American Psychologist,* **53**(12), 1271–1281.

Fiscella, K., Meldrum, S., Franks, P., et al. (2004). Patient trust—is it related to patient-centered behavior of primary care physicians? *Medical Care,* **42**(11), 1049–1055.

Frede, M. (1987). *Philosophy and medicine in antiquity. Essays in ancient philosophy.* Minneapolis, MN: University of Minnesota Press.

Grewen, K. M., Girdler, S. S., Amico, J., and Light, K. C. (2005). Effects of partner support on resting oxytocin, cortisol, norepinephrine, and blood pressure before and after warm partner contact. *Psychosomatic Medicine,* **67**(4), 531–538. DOI: 10.1097/01.Psy.0000170341.88395.47

Grotberg, E. H. (1999). *Tapping your inner strength: how to find the resilience to deal with anything.* Oakland, CA: New Harbinger.

Hanley, N. R. S. and Van de Kar, L. D. (2003). Serotonin and the neuroendocrine regulation of the hypothalamic–pituitary–adrenal axis in health and disease. *Vitamins and Hormones—Advances in Research and Applications,* **66**, 189–255.

Hardin, R. (2002). *Trust and trustworthiness.* New York: Russell Sage Foundation Series on Trust.

Harrington, A. (1997). *The placebo effect*. London: Harvard University Press.

Heinrichs, M., Baumgartner, T., Kirschbaum, C., and Ehlert, U. (2003). Social support and oxytocin interact to suppress cortisol and subjective responses to psychosocial stress. *Biological Psychiatry*, 54(12), 1389–1398. DOI: 10.1016/S0006-3223(03)00465-7

Hibbard, J. H. (1985). Social ties and health status: an examination of moderating factors. *Health Education Quarterly*, 12(1), 23–34.

Irvine, J., Baker, B., Smith, J., et al. (1999). Poor adherence to placebo or amiodarone therapy predicts mortality: results from the CAMIAT study. Canadian Amiodarone Myocardial Infarction Arrhythmia Trial. *Psychosomatic Medicine*, 61(4), 566–575.

Iseri, S. O., Dusunceli, F., Erzik, C., Uslu, B., Arbak, S., and Yegen, B. C. (2010). Oxytocin or social housing alleviates local burn injury in rats. *Journal of Surgical Research*, 162(1), 122–131. DOI: 10.1016/j.jss.2009.02.018

Kirmayer, L. J. (1993). Healing and the invention of metaphor: the effectiveness of symbols revisited. *Culture, Medicine and Psychiatry*, 17(2), 161–195.

Kirsch, I. (1985). Response expectancy as a determinant of experience and behavior. *American Psychologist*, 40(11), 1189–1202.

Kirsch, I. (2004). Conditioning, expectancy, and the placebo effect: comment on Stewart-Williams and Podd (2004). *Psychological Bulletin*, 130(2), 341–343. DOI: 10.1037/0033-2909.130.2.341

Kirsch, I., Deacon, B. J., Huedo-Medina, T. B., Scoboria, A., Moore, T. J., and Johnson, B. T. (2008). Initial severity and antidepressant benefits: a meta-analysis of data submitted to the Food and Drug Administration. *PLoS Medicine*, 5(2), 260–268. DOI: 10.1371/Journal.Pmed.0050045

Kosfeld, M., Heinrichs, M., Zak, P. J., Fischbacher, U., and Fehr, E. (2005). Oxytocin increases trust in humans. *Nature*, 435(7042), 673–676. DOI: 10.1038/Nature03701

Kouvonen, A., Oksanen, T., Vahtera, J., et al. (2008). Low workplace social capital as a predictor of depression—the Finnish public sector study. *American Journal of Epidemiology*, 167(10), 1143–1151. DOI: 10.1093/Aje/Kwn067

Lester, D. and Gatto, J. L. (1990). Interpersonal trust, depression, and suicidal ideation in teenagers. *Psychological Reports*, 67(3), 786–786.

Levine, J. D. and Gordon, N. C. (1984). Influence of the method of drug administration on analgesic response. *Nature*, 312(5996), 755–756.

Light, K. C., Grewen, K. M., and Amico, J. A. (2005). More frequent partner hugs and higher oxytocin levels are linked to lower blood pressure and heart rate in premenopausal women. *Biological Psychology*, 69(1), 5–21. DOI: 10.1016/J.Biopsycho.2004.11.002

Lund, I., Yu, L. C., Uvnas-Moberg, K., et al. (2002). Repeated massage-like stimulation induces long-term effects on nociception: contribution of oxytocinergic mechanisms (retracted article: see vol. 29, p. 868, 2009). *European Journal of Neuroscience*, 16(2), 330–338. DOI: 10.1046/J.1460-9568.2002.02087.X

Macy, M. (1996). Natural selection and social learning in prisoner's dilemma—coadaptation with genetic algorithms and artificial neural networks. *Sociological Methods & Research*, 25(1), 103–137.

Mainous, A. G., III, Baker, R., Love, M. M., Gray, D. P., and Gill, J. M. (2001). Continuity of care and trust in one's physician: evidence from primary care in the United States and the United Kingdom. *Family Medicine*, 33(1), 22–27.

Manson, N. C., and O'Neill, O. (2007). *Rethinking informed consent in bioethics*. New York: Cambridge University Press.

Mayer, R. C., Davis, J. H., and Schoorman, F. D. (1995). An integrative model of organizational trust. *Academy of Management Review*, **20**(3), 709–734.

Mcknight, D. H., Cummings, L. L., and Chervany, N. L. (1998). Initial trust formation in new organizational relationships. *Academy of Management Review*, **23**(3), 473–490.

Meltzer, H., Vostanis, P., Goodman, R., and Ford, T. (2007). Children's perceptions of neighbourhood trustworthiness and safety and their mental health. *Journal of Child Psychology and Psychiatry*, **48**(12), 1208–1213. DOI: 10.1111/J.1469-7610.2007.01800.X

Mikolajczak, M., Pinon, N., Lane, A., de Timary, P., and Luminet, O. (2010). Oxytocin not only increases when money is at stake, but also when confidential information is in the balance. *Biological Psychology*, **85**(1), 182–184.

Moerman, D. E. and Jonas, W. B. (2002). Deconstructing the placebo effect and finding the meaning response. *Annals of Internal Medicine*, **136**(6), 471–476.

Morhenn V.B., Park J.W., Piper E., and Zak P.J. (2008). Monetary sacrifice among strangers is mediated by endogenous oxytocin release after physical contact. *Evolution and Human Behavior*, **29**(6), 375–383.

Muris, P., Meesters, C., van Melick, M., and Zwambag, L. (2001). Self-reported attachment style, attachment quality, and symptoms of anxiety and depression in young adolescents. *Personality and Individual Differences*, **30**(5), 809–818.

Odendaal, J. S. J. and Meintjes, R. A. (2003). Neurophysiological correlates of affiliative behaviour between humans and dogs. *Veterinary Journal*, **165**(3), 296–301. DOI: 10.1016/S1090-0233(02)00237-X

Parchman, M. L. and Burge, S. K. (2004). The patient–physician relationship, primary care attributes, and preventive services. *Family Medicine*, **36**(1), 22–27.

Pearson, S. D. and Raeke, L. H. (2000). Patients' trust in physicians: many theories, few measures, and little data. *Journal of General Internal Medicine*, **15**(7), 509–513.

Petersson, M., Wiberg, U., Lundeberg, T., and Uvnas-Moberg, K. (2001). Oxytocin decreases carrageenan induced inflammation in rats. *Peptides*, **22**(9), 1479–1484.

Piette, J. D., Heisler, M., Krein, S., and Kerr, E. A. (2005). The role of patient–physician trust in moderating medication non-adherence due to cost pressures. *Archives of Internal Medicine*, **165**(15), 1749–1755.

Rosseau, D. M. and Camerer, C. (1998). Not so different after all: a cross-discipline view of trust. *The Academy of Management Review Journal*, **23**(3), 393–404.

Rotenberg, K. J., Cunningham, J., Hayton, N., et al. (2008). Development of a children's trust in general physicians scale. *Child: Care, Health and Development*, **34**(6), 748–756. DOI: 10.1111/j.1365-2214.2008.00872.x

Safran, D. G., Taira, D. A., Rogers, W. H., Kosinski, M., Ware, J. E., and Tarlov, A. R. (1998). Linking primary care performance to outcomes of care. *Journal of Family Practice*, **47**(3), 213–220.

Sakai, A. (2010). Children's sense of trust in significant others: genetic versus environmental contributions and buffer to life stressors. In: *Interpersonal trust during childhood and adolescence* (ed. K. J. Rotenberg). London: Cambridge University Press.

Shapiro, A. K., and Shapiro, E. (1997). *The powerful placebo: from ancient priest to modern physician*. Baltimore, MD: JHU Press.

Thomas, K. B. (1987). General practice consultations—is there any point in being positive. *British Medical Journal*, **294**(6581), 1200–1202.

Traut, E. F. and Passarelli, E. W. (1957). Placebos in the treatment of rheumatoid arthritis and other rheumatic conditions. *Annals of the Rheumatic Diseases*, **16**(1), 18–22.

Turner, R. A., Altemus, M., Enos, T., Cooper, B., and McGuinness, T. (1999). Preliminary research on plasma oxytocin in normal cycling women: investigating emotion and interpersonal distress. *Psychiatry: Interpersonal and Biological Processes*, **62**(2), 97–113.

Weiss, L. J. and Blustein, J. (1996). Faithful patients: the effect of long-term physician–patient relationships on the costs and use of health care by older Americans. *American Journal of Public Health*, **86**(12), 1742–1747.

Wickramasekera, I. (1980). A conditioned-response model of the placebo effect—predictions from the model. *Biofeedback and Self-Regulation*, **5**(1), 5–18.

Wikstrom, S., Gunnarsson, T., and Nordin, C. (2003). Tactile stimulus and neurohormonal response: a pilot study. *International Journal of Neuroscience*, **113**(6), 787–793. DOI: 10.1080/00207450390200954

Zak, P. J., Kurzban, R., and Matzner, W. T. (2005). Oxytocin is associated with human trustworthiness. *Hormones and Behavior*, **48**(5), 522–527. DOI: 10.1016/J. Yhbeh.2005.07.009

Zak, P. J., Stanton, A. A., and Ahmadi, S. (2007). Oxytocin increases generosity in humans. *PLoS One*, **2**(11). DOI: 10.1371/journal.pone.0001128

Chapter 6

Placebo science in medical education

Natasha K. J. Campbell and Amir Raz

6.1 Introduction

In 1969, the social scientist William McGuire described the three stages of what he called the life history of an artifact (McGuire 1969). In the first stage, the artifact is ignored. In the second, it is controlled for its presumed contaminating effects. Finally, it is studied as a phenomenon in its own right. Placebo effects conform to this description, and the study of placebos and their effects (placebo science) reveals that both are central to medicine of the past, present, and future. Although researchers, scientists, and academics currently explore placebo science as a unique topic, it is seldom alluded to in the formal study of medicine. Considering the history of placebos, the absence of direct medical education in this field is surprising.

In many ways, the history of medicine is a history of placebos (Shapiro and Shapiro 1997). For millennia, people viewed disease as the result of supernatural forces and healers treated patients with whatever remedy seemed suitable, from tortoise shells and herbs to prayer and blood-letting (Bausell 2007). With biochemically viable therapies few and far between, healing practices involved the widespread use of placebos, relying heavily on placebo effects and related phenomena. The first systematic physician and empiricist, Hippocrates, posited that natural processes caused disease, rather than gods or magic. He proposed the compelling humoral theory that health follows a balance between humors (earth, air, fire, and water), whereas disease follows their imbalance. This theory was emphasized by generations of succeeding physicians, including Galen (Phillips 1987).

Despite guiding medicine for over two thousand years, these precepts remained unproven and the vast majority of treatments remained ineffective beyond their placebogenic qualities. Placebo-like therapies, in fact, remained popular well into the seventeenth and eighteenth centuries. For example, the first edition of the *London pharmacopoeia*, published in 1618, included remedies such as powders from precious stones, fox lungs, and oil of bricks. Although pharmacopeias continued to drop debatable remedies throughout the eighteenth century, the 1764 *London pharmacopoeia* retained mithridate, bezoars, and crabs' eyes, among other treatments (Shapiro and Shapiro 1997). Unbeknownst to prescribers and users, however, the role of placebos began a new course during the eighteenth century.

As Stewart Justman describes in Chapter 9, Benjamin Franklin's disproval of mesmerism represents one of the earliest accounts of placebo treatments used as an experimental control. The widespread adoption of randomized controlled trials, however, did not catch on until after World War II, when a physician, Henry Beecher, noted that patients improved—sometimes dramatically—in placebo control groups (Beecher 1955). Rather than stimulating interest in placebos as treatment, the report consolidated the role of placebos as an experimental control to determine the efficacy of medical treatments. During the latter half of the nineteenth century, therefore, as the value of a well-designed, controlled therapeutic trial came to light, the field of medicine began rejecting "ineffective" remedies and neglecting "mere" placebo effects. Indeed, the development of placebo-controlled clinical trials alongside unprecedented advancements in medical science and technology provided physicians with effective therapies for an increasing number of conditions, propelling conventional medicine into dominance across North American hospitals, clinics, and medical schools. Using this controlled methodology, twentieth-century medicine introduced an increasing number of analgesic, anesthetic, antibiotic, immunological, hormone, hypertensive, cardiac, and other drugs with a high degree of specificity, sensitivity, and predictability. To this day, randomized, double-blind, placebo-controlled studies comprise the "gold standard" for drug evaluation.

Placebos emerged as a primary topic of study as scientists began to successfully investigate the neurobiological mechanisms underlying placebo effects in controlled trials. In the late 1970s, a seminal study demonstrated that placebo analgesia was blocked by the opioid antagonist naloxone (Levine et al. 1978). In other words, blocking the same receptors that respond to morphine would also block the powerful painkilling effects of placebos, indicating the involvement of endogenous opioids. In light of more recent pharmacological and neuroimaging studies, multiple neurotransmitter systems—including dopamine, cholecystokinin, opioids, and cannabinoids—are now implicated in different types of placebo analgesia (Benedetti et al. 2005, 2011; Scott et al. 2007). As interest and insight about the subject grew, scientists discovered and defined nuances between various types of placebos, placebo effects, and placebo responses.

6.2 **What are placebo effects?**

The definitions of placebo, placebo effect, and placebo response continue to be a source of debate among practitioners, scholars, and researchers alike. In light of randomized controlled trials, the placebo *response* is defined as the response to treatment observed in the sham treatment group. The placebo *effect*, on the other hand, is what can be observed after controlling for confounding elements such as spontaneous remission, the natural course of the disease, or regression to the mean. More broadly, the placebo effect is an improvement in health or behavior which engulfs a biopsychosocial phenomenon attributable to the placebo and treatment context (Kirsch 2003).

On the psychosocial end of the placebo effect spectrum, alternative nomenclature appears. As described by Dan Moerman (see Chapter 7), for example, "the meaning effect" is a similar notion that draws on anthropology and pertains to the meaning attached to the treatment, as well as the setting and the context surrounding the medical encounter (Moerman 2002). The concept sheds light on the reasons why, for instance, four placebos work better than two (De Craen et al. 1999), and why placebo injections work better than placebo pills (Chaput De Saintonge and Herxheimer 1994). On the psychobiological end of the spectrum, researchers highlight the central role of expectation, suggestion, and conditioning in placebo-related phenomena (Benedetti et al. 2003). Furthermore, while many physicians exclusively associate placebo effects with biochemically inert therapies or complementary and alternative medicine, the placebo effect may include active substances. In other words, the placebos are not limited to sugar pills or saline injections. The placebo literature, for example, draws a line between "pure" (biologically inert) and "impure" placebos (biologically active, but activity unrelated to the treated condition). Impure placebos may comprise of, for example, vitamins for chronic insomnia (Ernst 2001). New studies, moreover, demonstrate that the non-indicated use of active drugs is more frequent than the use of "pure" placebos (Kermen et al. 2010; Meissner et al. 2011) among physicians.

Regardless of the terminology employed, all medical treatment consists of a unique biopsychosocial context which affects the therapeutic outcome, and it is this premise which imbues the placebo effect with its power. Unfortunately, the medical education community remains largely unaware of these findings from placebo science.

6.3 **A (brief) recent history of medical education in North America**

With the advent of effective evidence-based medications such as antibiotic treatments, clinical care and medical education began shifting from patient- to disease-centered medicine, leaving out many "traditional" skills and placing a stronger emphasis on scientific medicine. The discovery of penicillin marked the first time that doctors had an efficacious treatment for bacterial infections. Unfortunately, not all ills responded to this mechanistic approach. Medicine subsequently diverged; conventional medicine focused on the merits of the scientific method and the mechanistic treatment of curable diseases, while alternative medical systems (often termed collectively as complementary and alternative medicine, CAM[1]) focused on the traditional healer–patient relationship (Buckman and Sabbagh 1993).

Toward the end of the twentieth century, the Flexnerian system of medical education (Flexner 1910), which advocates one to two years of preclinical basic sciences and two to three years of clinical training, prevailed as the primary educational model in medical schools. However, this method was heavily criticized and several reports recommended that medical curricula include courses that emphasized compassion, communication, and social aspects of health and disease (see Amin and Eng 2003 for a review). In 1969, McMaster University in Hamilton, Canada, introduced a novel problem-based learning method that emphasized integration by breaking down the boundary between human body systems and subjects. Until then, medical school courses were universally organized according to specific body systems or functions (e.g., cardiology). Nevertheless, despite additional calls for a biopsychosocial approach to teaching (Engel 1977, 1997), many medical programs across North America maintain a dominant biomedical perspective oriented towards specialization (Weatherall 2006; Hodges et al. 2011).

Although some medical schools in North America teach aspects of mind–body regulation (e.g., classes devoted to CAM), few specifically offer courses on placebo science. The Georgetown University School of Medicine, for example, introduced a mandatory mind–body medicine program to its curriculum as a result of a grant from the National Institute of Health's National Center for Complementary and Alternative Medicine in 2003. Whereas many of the topics covered in the program (e.g., acupuncture, meditation) share the common denominator of promoting well-being, it is with placebo science that researchers are able to study these topics scientifically. For many physicians, this science of placebos remains shrouded in mystery—hard to believe given the widespread yet ethically debated use of placebos in medicine today.

6.4 Why medical students should learn placebo science: potential benefits and risks of placebos in the clinic

Placebo science supports both positive and negative therapeutic outcomes following the provision of inactive treatment within the clinical context. The strongest evidence for both placebo-derived clinical benefit and harm stems from research on deceptive or blinded placebos. Although the applicability of such prescriptions is limited in the clinic, learning how, when, and why they work reveals the powerful therapeutic power of communication and expectation, insights students can translate directly into practice as doctors. Meta-analyses of placebo response rates in randomized clinical trials reveal not only that presumably somatic conditions can respond to placebos (e.g., asthma and back pain) but also that trusted medical interventions may owe their effectiveness almost entirely to placebo effects (e.g., antidepressants and arthroscopic knee surgery).

In addition to reinforcing the role of non-drug effects in health, emerging research with non-deceptive placebos supports their use as a viable therapeutic tool. For example, irritable bowel syndrome (IBS) is a functional bowel disorder that causes chronic abdominal pain and discomfort, but has no detectable organic cause, no reliable diagnostic test, and no known cure. Approximately 30–50% of all patients do not respond to conventional treatment (Jarcho et al. 2008) but many non-responders appear to benefit from a variety of alternative therapies (Bensoussan et al. 1998; Pittler and Ernst 1998; Poynard et al. 1994). Exploring the potential of non-deceptive placebos in IBS, an innovative open-label clinical trial demonstrated clinically meaningful symptom relief among patients taking placebos relative to patients who received no pills but identical care (Kaptchuk et al. 2010). Without deceiving patients, the researchers told participants they would receive placebo pills and emphasized that:

1 the placebo effect is powerful;
2 the body can automatically respond to taking placebos as a result of classical conditioning;
3 fostering a positive but realistic expectancy is helpful;
4 adherence to the medical ritual of pill taking is critical.

Using a similar trial design, additional research demonstrates that open-label placebos may benefit patients with a major depressive disorder (Kelley et al. 2012).

Whereas placebos lead to positive therapeutic effects, nocebos represent their negative counterpart. Nocebo effects encompass a phenomenon whereby negative treatment expectations lead to adverse outcomes (Colloca and Finniss 2012). In clinical practice, the manner in which information about treatment side-effects is presented to patients (for example, by listing potential side-effects to obtain informed consent) can predispose patients to experiencing these very same symptoms. One influential study demonstrated that listing "headache" as a side-effect of lumbar puncture treatment, compared to providing no such suggestion, significantly increased the likelihood of post-operative headaches

(Daniels and Sallie 1981). Conversely, physicians may manipulate clinical outcomes by positively framing the effects of certain interventions, thereby reducing nocebo effects. When psychiatrists prescribe antidepressants (see Chapter 3), they use language about dosing to shape patient expectations of and responses to potential side-effects. A study examining the effects of positive framing regarding an anesthetic injection during labor provides another example: telling patients "We are going to give you a local anesthetic that will numb the area and you will be comfortable during the procedure" as opposed to "You are going to feel a big bee sting; this is the worst part of the procedure" resulted in significantly lower pain scores (Varelmann et al. 2010).

Placebo science bridges the gap between the art of healing and the science of medicine. A prominent medical historian argues that physicians are walking placebos (Harrington 1997). To some healthcare professionals, however, the concept of a placebo merely intimates variations on the theme of "noise" or "nothing," and the concept of a "walking placebo" seems insulting. On the contrary, one can be both a scientific physician and a walking placebo; that is, a physician's bedside manner and personality can be as scientifically informed and astute as their knowledge of, for instance, the treatment of respiratory infections. Through this perspective, we frame the distinction between *curing* and *healing*: physicians can cure abnormalities of the body and heal the problems that arise from a patient's subjective experience of those abnormalities (Boudreau et al. 2007). Palliative medicine—wherein healthcare practitioners focus on relieving and preventing the suffering of patients—exemplifies a conventional field of medicine where emotional, social, and psychological factors are of primary importance. These principles, however, apply to any form of medical care. In any specialty, physicians have the ability to change expectancy, experience, and outcome by capitalizing on certain conditioned social cues (Jonas 2011) and choosing words wisely (Colloca and Miller 2011), in order to create an optimal healing environment. Therefore, to maximize patient benefit and minimize risk, physicians must be aware of their own potential to induce both placebo and nocebo effects, regardless of the interventions they prescribe.

6.5 **Ethical and philosophical considerations**

Whereas learning about placebo science offers insights that medical students can apply directly as doctors, the subject of placebos raises a number of ethical and philosophical questions that are difficult to address within a busy training curriculum yet fundamental to socially responsible medicine. The continuing debate over the merits of placebo- versus active-controlled trials, for example, speaks not only to the juxtaposed obligation to treat and need to identify effective treatments but to the ways in which a medicine's effectiveness is measured, interpreted, and regulated. The use of placebo interventions in clinical care presents different yet similarly far-reaching implications to medical practice, from individual doctor–patient relationships to public perceptions and trust of the medical community/establishment. Rarely, if ever, is the debate one-sided, whether discussing issues of deception, standards of evidence, or an over-medicated public. Bennett Foddy's position on the deceptive use of placebos in the clinic (see Chapter 4) is at once aggressively challenged (Brody 2009; Kolber 2009; Shah and Goold 2009) yet reflective of widespread practice, where many physicians prescribe placebos to patients using varying degrees of deception (Fässler et al. 2010).

Philosophically, the topic of placebo challenges several widely held assumptions, most notably the dominance of bottom–up over top–down regulation of processes mediating health and disease. Central to this volume, the story of antidepressants casts doubt on the assumed integrity of big pharma and regulatory agencies, not to mention the way we conduct clinical research or distinguish between effective and ineffective treatments. That openly administered placebos can still elicit clinical improvement, even if only subjectively, is not only counterintuitive but a doorway to novel clinical approaches and research questions.

6.6 The current state of placebo science knowledge

6.6.1 Physicians

Recent studies report that many North American physicians use placebos in clinical practice (Raz et al. 2011; Sherman and Hickner 2008), mirroring similar trends in New Zealand, Europe, and Israel. A systematic review of twenty-two studies from twelve different countries found that between 17% and 80% of physicians reported administering a placebo at some point in their professional career, with many doing so on a regular basis (Fässler et al. 2010). Regardless of geography, the use of placebos and placebo-like interventions outside of randomized control trials is widespread. However, Western medical thinking generally leads students to frown upon using placebos clinically, under the appellation of "bad professional form." Ethical guidelines and professional codes in the United States and Britain likely fuel such placebo reluctance; in 2006, the American Medical Association cautioned that "[p]hysicians may use [a] placebo for diagnosis or treatment only if the patient is informed of and agrees to its use." Fostering an educational climate in which students can explore this taboo topic, both scientifically and clinically, is essential to advancing placebo science knowledge and subsequent discussions on the ethical and responsible use of placebos in modern medicine.

Physician surveys reveal significant confusion and inconsistency regarding the definitions of placebos and placebo effects as well as the therapeutic potential of placebo therapies in clinical practice. Distinctions between pure and impure placebos, for instance, are often vague or misunderstood. The relevant literature only recently began to clearly distinguish between these two types of placebos; understandably, without proper education in this field, physicians are left in the dark. Internationally, physicians use impure placebos much more frequently than pure placebos (Fässler et al. 2010; Harris and Raz 2012), yet many who report using impure placebos—even in the absence of proven or expected efficacy—deny prescribing placebos at all. In our Canadian study, whereas 19% of physicians reported using placebos, over 75% reported prescribing at least one unwarranted treatment (e.g., vitamins or antibiotics without evidence or expectation of benefit) (Raz et al. 2011). Our survey also revealed that 12% of psychiatrists and 27% of non-psychiatrists believed that placebos had neither psychological nor physiological benefits for neurological disorders. Considering that Parkinson's disease is a much-discussed model system of placebo effects, this is surprising. In addition, many types of pain, including chronic pain and migraines, are both neurological and highly studied in terms of placebo (De Craen et al. 2000; Wager et al. 2007). Medical education, therefore, should aim to clarify such vague conceptualizations and fill in these knowledge gaps—especially considering findings that physicians use impure placebos in the clinic.

6.6.2 Students: a Canadian case study

Few, if any, published studies address either the inclusion of placebo in medical school curricula or the opinions of students on the subject. Our laboratory recently investigated placebo attitudes, knowledge, and beliefs among students at a leading Canadian medical school. We hypothesized that the dearth of placebo science in medical education would result in a lack of appreciation for psychosomatic medicine. We used an online survey to obtain 125 anonymous responses from medical students. The survey explored themes such as student knowledge of current placebo science research findings, their positions on the use of placebos as part of routine care, and their belief in the placebo effect. Despite studies reporting that parameters such as pill number, color, brand, and cost strongly influence therapeutic outcome, respondents consistently underestimated the impact of these factors. Approximately 40% of respondents reported that they would prescribe a placebo in clinical practice; no respondents reported that placebos had no clinical benefit. Complementing reports regarding placebo use among practicing physicians, our findings suggest that medical students are amenable to the benefits of placebos and their non-drug effects, yet unfamiliar with related scientific findings. While students had clearly developed opinions about placebos and the placebo effect, our study demonstrates the need for primary and continuing education regarding placebo science.

Although anecdotal, an additional observation may provide insight into student attitudes toward the biological underpinnings and therapeutic potential of placebos. As part of our ongoing research and educational program on placebos, we replicated demonstrations of Blackwell's pioneering placebo study on medical students (Blackwell et al. 1972). In these demonstrations, medical students receive either red or blue placebo pills, with the impression that they are receiving either stimulants or sedatives. However, demonstrators never explicitly assign color to activity (e.g., red pills with stimulants). We collect subjective psychological measures such as alertness, tension, drowsiness, and sluggishness before and twenty minutes after the ingestion of the pills. After analyzing the data, we return to the class to report and discuss the results. To date, we have conducted the demonstration with diverse student populations. Regardless of educational background, students who receive red pills are consistently more stimulated and less sedated than those who receive blue ones, and vice versa. Interestingly, upon seeing the results, the student population most suspicious of and resistant to the validity of the experiment are reliably fourth-year medical students. First-year medical students, in contrast, accept the results and implications far more readily, suggesting that skepticism towards placebo effects may develop over the course of medical training.

6.7 How can we integrate placebo science into medical education?

Traditionally, in Canada and the United States, professional medical programs for mind–body practices and CAM offer certification or diplomas independently of medical schools. As a result, such perspectives and expertise are separated and nearly excluded from conventional medical education. However, medical schools in North America are beginning to add courses in integrative and mind–body medicine to their curricula. Taking it a step further, the Arizona Center for Integrative Medicine at the University of Arizona College of Medicine developed a leading educational program in integrative medicine. In 1997, the Center created the first residency program in integrative medicine in the United States. With nearly 1000 Fellows having graduated in integrative medicine by 2012, the Center currently offers one of the largest Fellowships in the world. Similar programs across North America, however, are few and far between. Moreover, although some North American medical school programs currently include aspects of mind–body regulation (e.g., classes devoted to CAM), few specifically offer courses on placebo science.

Introducing placebo science into an already overextended curriculum poses many challenges. However, a carefully tailored syllabus on this topic, integrated with the current educational system, offers many benefits. Currently, medical students usually form their opinions about placebos indirectly, by gleaning information from modules dedicated to clinical research, medical ethics, historical accounts, physicianship (e.g., bedside manners, physician–patient rapport) and physician mentors. The four-year curriculum at McGill University (Montreal, Canada), for example, comprises a physicianship module centered on the concept of the doctor as both a healer and professional (Boudreau et al. 2007). This module, which emphasizes observation, attentive listening, and clinical reasoning, stresses the importance of the physician–patient relationship. Beyond this interaction, however, knowledge of additional psychosocial factors in medicine could include mini-lectures, structured discussions, or small-group demonstrations (e.g., ethical variations of Blackwell's 1972 study, as discussed in the section "The current state of placebo science knowledge"). One of us (AR) was the first to offer a structured elective on placebo science to fourth-year medical students at McGill University in 2009. Since its introduction and for every consecutive year to date, many students have rated this course as one of the most meaningful and informative in their entire medical education. In addition to being highly popular, the placebo course has garnered much media attention and inquiries from both colleagues and students worldwide.

As an alternative to introducing placebo science in a formal classroom setting, medical schools could provide future physicians with recent, major publications in this burgeoning field. Such a method would allow students to be well-versed in a subject that imbues so many aspects of medicine. Publications could be easily transmitted through medical school journals, websites, e-mails, or newsletters. As the ethical debate on the use of deceptive placebos continues, recent articles could keep physicians up to date on policies and stances regarding this delicate issue. Another example of a topical article in the field would be Kirsch's "The placebo effect revisited: lessons learned to date" which summarizes six main lessons that can be learned from over a half century of scientific research on the placebo effect (Kirsch 2013). With such articles that succinctly summarize much of the extensive research in placebo science, future physicians would undoubtedly be able to extract the relevance to their own fields. For example, Kirsch suggests that physicians spend more time with their patients and take more care forming a therapeutic alliance, which would in turn enhance the placebo effect of treatment. Future physicians, no matter what their specialty, could employ such suggested methods.

Beyond class lectures and group discussions, therefore, modern multimedia provides many platforms by which to disseminate relevant information on placebos—something that medical schools could use to their advantage. Beyond medical education, hospitals and universities could share relevant articles with many members of the healthcare community, including currently practicing physicians.

The learning objectives of placebo science education, however disseminated, should include:

1 understanding of the neurological, immune, and endocrine correlates of placebo effects;

2 appreciating the potential of expectations, suggestions, context, symbolic thinking, framing, cultural biases, and related psychosocial factors in health and illness;

3 recognizing and interpreting the role of placebos and their effects in various clinical settings;

4 navigating the tenuous ethical issues surrounding the use of placebos in the clinic.

Reference materials would cover relevant concepts and paradigms central to placebo research, the proposed underlying mechanisms of placebo effects and responses, and the widespread significance of placebos in basic and clinical science.

6.8 **Closing remarks**

Presently, scientific evidence reveals that placebo factors contribute to the effectiveness of any treatment, in both conventional and complementary disciplines. Whether recognizing the therapeutic potential of placebo-like interventions or the limitations of conventional medicine, capitalizing on opportunities to promote placebo effects can improve patient outcomes in a clinical setting. In order to capitalize on such effects, future physicians must be equipped with relevant knowledge. This knowledge would provide physicians with increased awareness regarding many tools at their immediate disposal. Thus, incorporating placebo science topics into medical education would aid in developing and implementing treatments aimed at harnessing placebo effects in an ethical manner.

Acknowledgments

The authors would like to thank the members of the Raz Lab for their support and editorial insights. In particular, "thank you" to Constance Yuen for her thorough research assistance and to Dr. Cory Harris for his thoughtful comments and suggestions on several earlier drafts. We would also like to extend our thanks to Drs. Donald Boudreau and Abraham Fuks, for sharing their expertise.

Note

1 Many disparate definitions of conventional or alternative medicine appear in the literature. In this chapter, we define conventional medicine as the primary curriculum taught in established medical schools; in other words, what is licensed and regulated as medicine by governing authorities. Complementary medicine, on the other hand, is defined by exclusion: it is not conventional medicine. Once proven "effective" by evidence-based standards, a treatment is no longer regarded as complementary and/or alternative medicine (CAM) (Singh and Ernst 2008).

References

American Medical Association (2006). *American Medical Association code of medical ethics, opinion 8.083: placebo use in clinical practice.* http://www.ama-assn.org/ama/pub/physician-resources/medical-ethics/code-medical-ethics/opinion8083.shtml.

Amin, Z. and Eng, K. H. (2003). *Basics in medical education.* Toh Tuck Link, Singapore: World Scientific Publishing Co. Pte. Ltd.

Bausell, R. B. (2007). *Snake oil science: the truth about alternative and complementary medicine.* New York: Oxford University Press.

Beecher, H. K. (1955). The powerful placebo. *Journal of the American Medical Association,* **159**, 1602–1606.

Benedetti, F., Amanzio, M., Rosato, R. and Blanchard, C. (2011). Nonopioid placebo analgesia is mediated by CB1 cannabinoid receptors. *Nature Medicine,* **17**, 1228–1230.

Benedetti, F., Mayberg, H. S., Wager, T. D., Stohler, C. S. and Zubieta, J.-K. (2005). Neurobiological mechanisms of the placebo effect. *The Journal of Neuroscience,* **25**, 10390–10402.

Benedetti, F., Pollo, A., Lopiano, L., et al. (2003). Conscious expectation and unconscious conditioning in analgesic, motor, and hormonal placebo/nocebo responses. *The Journal of Neuroscience,* **23**, 4315–4323.

Bensoussan, A., Talley, N. J., Hing, M., et al. (1998). Treatment of irritable bowel syndrome with Chinese herbal medicine: A randomized controlled trial. *Journal of the American Medical Association,* **280**, 1585–1589.

Blackwell, B., Bloomfield, S., and Buncher, C. R. (1972). Demonstration to medical students of placebo responses and non-drug factors. *The Lancet,* **299**, 1279–1282.

Boudreau, J. D., Cassell, E. J., and Fuks, A. (2007). A healing curriculum. *Medical Education,* **41**, 1193–1201.

Brody, H. (2009). Medicine's continuing quest for an excuse to avoid relationships with patients. *American Journal of Bioethics,* **9**, 13–15.

Buckman, R. and Sabbagh, K. (1993). *Magic or medicine? An investigation of healing and healers.* Amherst, New York: Prometheus Books.

Chaput De Saintonge, D. M. and Herxheimer, A. (1994). Harnessing placebo effects in health care. *Lancet,* **344**, 995–998.

Colloca, L. and Finniss, D. (2012). Nocebo effects, patient–clinician communication, and therapeutic outcomes. *The Journal of the American Medical Association,* **307**, 567–568.

Colloca, L. and Miller, F. G. (2011). The nocebo effect and its relevance for clinical practice. *Psychosomatic Medicine,* **73**, 598–603.

Daniels, A. M. and Sallie, R. (1981). Headache, lumbar puncture, and expectation. *The Lancet*, **317**, 1003.

De Craen, A. J. M., Moerman, D. E., Heisterkamp, S. H., et al. (1999). Placebo effect in the treatment of duodenal ulcer. *British Journal of Clinical Pharmacology*, **48**, 853–860.

De Craen, A. J. M., Tijssen, J. G. P., De Gans, J., and Kleijnen, J. (2000). Placebo effect in the acute treatment of migraine: subcutaneous placebos are better than oral placebos. *Journal of Neurology*, **247**, 183–188.

Engel, G. (1977). The need for a new medical model: a challenge for biomedicine. *Science*, **196**, 129–136.

Engel, G. L. (1997). From biomedical to biopsychosocial: being scientific in the human domain. *Psychosomatics*, **38**, 521–528.

Ernst, E. (2001). Towards a scientific understanding of placebo effects. In: *Understanding the placebo effect in complementary medicine: theory, practice and research* (ed. D. Peters). London: Churchill Livingstone.

Fässler, M., Meissner, K., Schneider, A., and Linde, K. (2010). Frequency and circumstances of placebo use in clinical practice—a systematic review of empirical studies. *BMC Medicine*, **8**, 15.

Flexner, A. (1910). *Medical education in the United States and Canada: a report to the Carnegie Foundation for the Advancement of Teaching [Carnegie Foundation Bulletin No. 4]*. New York, NY: Carnegie Foundation for the Advancement of Teaching.

Harrington, A. (1997). *The placebo effect: an interdisciplinary exploration*. Cambridge, MA: Harvard University Press.

Harris, C. S. and Raz, A. (2012). Deliberate use of placebos in clinical practice: what we really know. *Journal of Medical Ethics*, **38**, 406–407.

Hodges, B. D., Albert, M., Arweiler, D., et al. (2011). The future of medical education: a Canadian environmental scan. *Medical Education*, **45**, 95–106.

Jarcho, J., Chang, L., Berman, S., et al. (2008). Neural and psychological predictors of treatment response in irritable bowel syndrome patients with a 5 HT3 receptor antagonist: a pilot study. *Alimentary Pharmacology and Therapeutics*, **28**, 344–352.

Jonas, W. B. (2011). Reframing placebo in research and practice. *Philosophical Transactions of the Royal Society B: Biological Sciences*, **366**, 1896–1904.

Kaptchuk, T. J., Friedlander, E., Kelley, J. M., et al. (2010). Placebos without deception: a randomized controlled trial in irritable bowel syndrome. *PLoS One*, **5**, e15591.

Kelley, J. M., Kaptchuk, T. J., Cusin, C., Lipkin, S., and Fava, M. (2012). Open-label placebo for major depressive disorder: a pilot randomized controlled trial. *Psychotherapy and Psychosomatics*, **81**, 312–314.

Kermen, R., Hickner, J., Brody, H., and Hasham, I. (2010). Family physicians believe the placebo effect is therapeutic but often use real drugs as placebos. *Family Medicine*, **42**, 636–642.

Kirsch, I. (2003). Hidden administration as ethical alternatives to the balanced placebo design. *Prevention and Treatment*, **6**, 1–5.

Kirsch, I. (2013). The placebo effect revisited: lessons learned to date. *Complementary Therapies in Medicine*, **21**, 102–104.

Kolber, A. (2009). How placebo deception can infringe autonomy. *American Journal of Bioethics*, **9**, 25–26.

Levine, J. D., Gordon, N. C., and Fields, H. L. (1978). The mechanism of placebo analgesia. *Lancet*, **2**, 654–657.

McGuire, W. J. (1969). Suspiciousness of experimenter's intent. In: *Artifact in behavioral research* (eds. R. Rosenthal and R. L. Rosnow). New York, NY: Academic Press.

Meissner, K., Höfner, L., Fässler, M., and Linde, K. (2011). Widespread use of pure and impure placebo interventions by GPs in Germany. *Family Practice*, **29**, 79–85.

Moerman, D. E. (2002). *Meaning, medicine, and the "placebo effect."* Cambridge, UK/ New York: Cambridge University Press.

Phillips, E. D. (1987). *Aspects of Greek medicine*. Philadelphia, Pennsylvania: The Charles Press Publishers.

Pittler, M. H. and Ernst, E. (1998). Peppermint oil for irritable bowel syndrome: a critical review and metaanalysis. *American Journal of Gastroenterology*, **93**, 1131–1135.

Poynard, T., Naveau, S., Mory, B., and Chaput, J. C. (1994). Meta-analysis of smooth muscle relaxants in the treatment of irritable bowel syndrome. *Alimentary Pharmacology and Therapeutics*, **8**, 499–510.

Raz, A., Campbell, N., Guindi, D., et al. (2011). Placebos in clinical practice: comparing attitudes, beliefs, and patterns of use between academic psychiatrists and non-psychiatrists. *Canadian Journal of Psychiatry*, **56**, 198–208.

Scott, D. J., Stohler, C. S., Egnatuk, C. M., et al. (2007). Individual differences in reward responding explain placebo-induced expectations and effects. *Neuron*, **55**, 325–336.

Shah, K. R. and Goold, S. D. (2009). The primacy of autonomy, honesty, and disclosure: Council on Ethical and Judicial Affairs' placebo opinions. *American Journal of Bioethics*, **9**, 15–17.

Shapiro, A. K. and Shapiro, E. (1997). *The powerful placebo: from ancient priest to modern physician*. Baltimore: Johns Hopkins University Press.

Sherman, R. and Hickner, J. (2008). Academic physicians use placebos in clinical practice and believe in the mind–body connection. *Journal of General Internal Medicine*, **23**, 7–10.

Singh, S. and Ernst, E. (2008). *Trick or treatment? alternative medicine on trial*. London: Bantam Press.

Varelmann, D., Pancaro, C., Cappiello, E. C., and Camann, W. R. (2010). Nocebo-induced hyperalgesia during local anesthetic injection. *Anesthesia and Analgesia*, **110**, 868–870.

Wager, T. D., Scott, D. J., and Zubieta, J.-K. (2007). Placebo effects on human mu-opioid activity during pain. *Proceedings of the National Academy of Sciences*, **104**, 11056–11061.

Weatherall, D. J. (2006). Science in the undergraduate curriculum during the 20th century. *Medical Education*, **40**, 195–201.

Part 3

The cultural lens

PART 3

The cultural lens

Chapter 7

Looking at placebos through a cultural lens and finding meaning

Daniel E. Moerman

7.1 Introduction

In this chapter, I will examine a powerful healing effect through a cultural lens.

The human healing process is complicated and involves a number of different dimensions that are sometimes interacting, sometimes apparently orthogonal. The most important component is probably the action of the immune system, operating independently. Also involved are the natural histories of many self-limiting illnesses (e.g., colds, flu, sprains, simple broken bones); a certain amount of conditioning or learning, as we face an illness for the second or third time; regression to the mean (that is, things sometimes just return to "normal"); and biases of patients or investigators who are trying to please one another and, perhaps, themselves. Medication can play a role, as can *meaning*. The latter term describes the cognitive and emotional response to objects of thought that are especially lively in times of crisis, such as an illness of a spouse, or child, or one's self.

7.1.1 Issues of meaning

None of these are particularly controversial, save perhaps the last. This is usually understood (or as I would prefer, misunderstood) as the "placebo effect." This important element in the human healing project occasions periodic scorn, with reports denying either that these forces exist at all, or, if they do, claiming they are trivial and short-lasting. I am sure most readers are familiar with the mini-industry of papers by Drs. Hróbjartsson and Gøtzsche which, if nothing else, have drawn attention to some of the very worst papers ever written within the history of medicine (Hróbjartsson and Gøtzsche 2001).

There is a long history of such articles, global attempts to explain away one of the most important and interesting forces in human life as simple delusion. Why such skepticism persists while powerful evidence continues to accumulate for the biological consequences of the fact of medical care, its meaning (rather than its content), is a striking question about a cultural phenomenon. I believe that the answer to that question has at least two parts. First, while reductionism is utterly essential for a scientific approach to human biology, the fact is that some matters are more easily "reduced" than others; some phenomena, like the construction of meaning, are emergent properties of human mental, emotional, religious, and historical processes. These phenomena engage the interactions of people, communities, history, and culture in ways that are as richly interesting as they are challenging. Many of these processes are utterly invisible to us at the same time as we embody them; in a sense, I embody meaning in the same way that I embody my liver—unless something very bad is happening, I am ordinarily completely unaware of both. By confusing these things with related, yet vastly simpler, communication systems (e.g., bird song, chimpanzee signing), we trivialize the most astonishing aspects of our being that are so enormous and powerful that we often do not recognize them for what they are. We can find and explore within such meaning by means of an array of cultural processes: rituals, dance, music, literature. Most of it we do not understand, and do not need to: none but the most skillful and educated linguist can plot out the ins and outs of ordinary language, and even linguists have their limits. Yet we can all talk (well, we can try). For a primer on meaning, see Michael Polanyi's book *Meaning* (Polanyi and Prosch 1975).

Second, physicians often find matters of linguistic interpretation onerous, as it seems to increase their burdensome liability for patient outcomes. "My gosh," they say, "now I'm responsible for my 'bedside manner.'" It appears easiest to ignore the issue. However, to do so is, in my view, to miss a point of striking human and medical importance. This extraordinary will to disbelieve is an interesting and complicated question in itself, but not one we can resolve today.

7.1.2 Meaning is everywhere

Hróbjartsson and Gøtzsche's research aside, studies in both the laboratory and clinic have shown that people receiving inert treatments display significant benefit. Of this literature, few paradigms are as elegant and persuasive as those by Fabrizio Benedetti. In a classic study of experimentally induced pain, an open injection of saline—described, in about six to eight words, as a helpful pain reliever—is given to the members of one group. The outcome is compared to another group, which receives the same injection but "hidden," with no words. The use or non-use of words is the only difference between the groups. Yet the open saline treatment group shows a persistent decline in pain reports, while the hidden infusion group shows a continued rise in pain (Benedetti 1996). Let me qualify this: does this show us that placebos have effects? No, *because both groups received placebos.* The difference between the two groups was the inclusion, or not, of words, or more specifically, of a *meaningful utterance.*[1]

It is more challenging to get such clear evidence of this in a clinical setting, since—largely for ethical reasons—it is difficult to deny sick or injured patients treatment, whether it be placebo or otherwise. There are, however, a few such studies, including one looking at third molar extraction. Gracely's results from a three-arm trial with subjects following removal of third molars shows that pain in a placebo treatment group declined while in a comparable but untreated group, pain continued to increase for several hours after surgery. Both visual analog scale and verbal descriptor scale pain reports dropped substantially after inert treatment, as compared to no treatment (Gracely et al. 1979).

One of the biggest difficulties in all this follows from the confusion of what is happening during placebo treatment. Imagine that patients in some mythical trial are given inert tablets called placebos. A week later, they are different than at baseline; this difference is the "placebo effect." Of course, it is not. Placebos are inert; they do not do anything. One reason why people may be different is regression to the mean, which is not caused by placebos but by study selection criteria (select 1000 people with hypertension, leave them alone for three months, and many of them will now have "normal" blood pressure as things set themselves right). Placebos do not cause changes due to natural history, and they do not cause conditioning (for this to occur, you have to train the subject with an active drug, one which has an unconditioned response). If placebos do not do anything, then it seems possible that what we call "placebo effects" might occur without placebos.

In an important study, 835 women who reported that they regularly treated headaches with over-the-counter analgesics were randomly placed in four groups: one group received an unlabeled placebo; one received a placebo marked with a widely advertised brand name, known as "one of the most popular . . . analgesics in the United Kingdom widely available for many years and supported by extensive advertising"; one received unbranded aspirin; and one received branded aspirin. They noted the amount of headache pain relief an hour after taking the pills (Branthwaite and Cooper 1981). The results showed that, first, aspirin was more effective than placebo. However, the brand name aspirin was more effective than the generic aspirin, and the brand name placebo was more effective than the generic placebo. In particular, 55% of headaches reported by branded placebo users improved after an hour (rated 2, 3, or 4 on the scale), while only 45% of 410 headaches were reported to be that much better by unbranded placebo users ($X^2 = 6.76$, $p < 0.01$). Aspirin relieves headaches, but so does the knowledge that the pills you are taking are good ones, which many patients have learned via television. The difference here is to be attributed not to the placebo (which is, after all, inert) but to the brand name (which clearly is not): it enhances the effect of both placebo and aspirin.

Similarly, Benedetti reported on a clinical experiment where surgery patients were treated with four different drugs appropriate to their conditions; however, half the patients received their drugs openly, with an injection by a clinician, while half received equivalent doses of the same drugs by hidden infusion through an intravenous line (Benedetti et al. 2003). Patients receiving the medication openly, who were told they were about to receive it, reported more pain relief than those who received equivalent amounts of drugs secretly. Pain researcher Don Price, in an accompanying editorial, described this study as "assessing placebo effects without placebo groups" (Price 2001). As much as I respect Don Price, this is an unfortunate use of language. There were no placebos here. So obviously, there were not any "placebo effects." What differentiated the separate groups in this study were *human interaction* and *words*.

Price did, however, note that although the increase in pain relief in the study was probably not, by itself, clinically significant, "both pain research scientists and the pharmaceutical industry go to the ends of the earth to make improvements of this magnitude [to existing drugs]. Adding one or two sentences to each pain treatment might help to produce them." Placebos are inert, but language is not!

Note that most of the examples I have given deal with pain, clearly the system most fully mapped for meaningful responses. However, there are other systems that can also respond to language and meaning. Benedetti has replicated his open/hidden drug experiment in three other areas: diazepam in anxiety states, stimulation of the subthalmic nucleus in patients with Parkinson's disease, and administration of beta-blocker (propranalol) and muscarinic antagonists (atropine) in healthy volunteers. In all these cases, when the treatment was given openly, it was more effective than when given secretly (Benedetti et al. 2003; Colloca et al. 2004).

7.2 **The meaning response**

Given that there are no placebos in most of these experiments, it seems unwise to call the responses "placebo effects." The aspirin study shows that the brand name can enhance the effect of an inert drug *and* of an active drug, indicating that at least one dimension of benefit is the effect of what medications *mean*. I define the meaning response as "the psychological or physiological effects of meaning in the treatment of illness." Much of what is called the placebo effect— that is, meaning responses elicited with inert medications—is a special case of the meaning response, as is much of what is called the "nocebo effect."

I am interested particularly in the responses that people have to what things mean or to what they know, to what others often call their expectations or expectancies. I do not use these terms since they seem to me, as an anthropologist, insensitive to culture; I anticipate, before the fact, that people in different parts of the world with varying cultural backgrounds will know the world differently, and might construct different meanings of apparently similar objects or experiences. I would suggest that, more often than not, expectancies are the outcome of a complex play of meanings. The two approaches are not fundamentally different, but have a distinct emphasis.

It is also important to note that the influence of meaning on health and mortality can occur well outside the ordinary bounds of the clinic.

Dr. P. D. Phillips and colleagues have shown that, in the presence of a broad range of diseases in Chinese Americans in California, those who are understood by Chinese traditions of astrology to be particularly susceptible to these conditions—by virtue of the year of their birth—die significantly earlier than those with the same conditions born in other years. Here are two examples that Phillips described (Phillips et al. 2001):

Earth years: Chinese born in "earth years" (years ending with 8 or 9)—and consequently deemed by Chinese medical theory to be especially susceptible to diseases involving lumps, nodules, or tumors—*and* who have lymphatic cancer, die, on average, 4 years sooner than Chinese with lymphatic cancer born in other years.

Lung diseases: Those with lung diseases born in "metal years" (years ending in 0 or 1)—in Chinese theory, "the lung is the organ of metal"—die, on average, 5 years younger (roughly 7% of length of life!) than those born in other years.

There were no such differences found in a similar examination of the mortality of thousands of non-Chinese Californians (Phillips et al. 1993). These are very compelling examples of "meaning responses."

In another study, Phillips showed that Chinese Americans and Japanese Americans were more likely to die on the fourth day of the month than any other because four is an unlucky number; if thirteen is an unlucky number for Californians in general, it is not unlucky enough to increase the mortality rate (Phillips et al. 2001). It is worth noting that these meanings—of metal and the lung, or of earth and lumps, or of unlucky fours—are not notions concocted by individual patients or therapists; they are icons of a sort which permeate the language and culture of, in this case, immigrant Chinese and/or their American-born children, to some degree or other. Phillips shows, in one case, that the effects of these beliefs are influenced by the degree of commitment to Asian culture. These relationships have nothing to do with having Asian genes, but with having Asian ways of living, thinking, behaving, and being. At least some of the time, biological processes can be "activated," or perhaps "suppressed," by that system of meanings we call culture.

Although these effects occur widely in human life, they are often most clearly and visibly displayed in the clinic. People bring to their engagements with physicians many things; patients are not blank slates. However, one of the most powerful influences on patients is their doctor. Dozens of studies have demonstrated this; here, I will summarize one example.

Physician attitudes can be conveyed to patients in extremely subtle and delicate ways. Rick Gracely has described a phased experiment in which dental patients were told they would receive a placebo, which might reduce the pain of third molar extraction, or might do nothing; naloxone, which might increase their pain, or do nothing; the synthetic narcotic analgesic, fentanyl, which might reduce their pain, or do nothing; or no treatment at all. Subjects were all recruited from the same patient stream, with consistent selection criteria by the same staff. In the first phase of the study, clinicians (but not patients) were told fentanyl was not yet a possibility because of administrative problems with the study protocol, yielding the placebo-naloxone (PN) group. It is worth noting that fentanyl is well-known in medical circles as a very powerful drug, a hundred times more potent than morphine.

In the second phase, clinicians were told that now patients might indeed receive fentanyl, yielding the PNF group. Placebo-treated patients reported no relief during the first phase of the study; moreover, after an hour, their pain reports increased significantly. In the second phase of the study, placebo-treated patients experienced significant pain reduction from their inert treatments. The only apparent difference between the two groups was that the clinicians knew that no one in the first group would get fentanyl, while the patients in the second group might (in fact, they all received only placebo). It is not at all clear how physicians elicited these effects from their patients in a double-blind trial, but they did (Gracely et al. 1985). The clinicians were clearly more impressed by fentanyl than were the patients.

The significance of clinician belief, enthusiasm, or commitment seems to be a fairly broadly applicable principle that can be seen in a number of different contexts.

7.2.1 Old treatments become less effective as new ones come along

It is a commonplace belief in medicine that drugs must be used quickly before they lose their effectiveness. This quip has been attributed to William Olser, among others. Here are some data from a meta-analysis of treatment of ulcer disease (Moerman 2000). Figure 7.1 shows the healing rates of drug groups in endoscopically controlled trials of two anti-secretory drugs, plotted by year of publication of the study. At least in the pre-internet world of the 1970s and 1980s, it was doctors, not patients, who knew what the "hot" new drug was, and, apparently, old drugs become less effective as new ones come along.

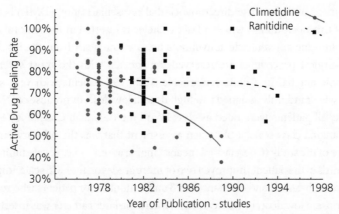

Fig. 7.1 Effectiveness studies (by date of publication) for Cimetidine and Ranitidine, introduced to research in 1977 and 1980, respectively.

7.2.2 **Meaning responses occur throughout medicine, in surgery as well as in internal medicine**

I do not have space to recall here the curious history of the bilateral internal mammary artery ligation, which gained popularity in the later 1950s (Kitchell et al. 1958). Suffice it to say, in two rare double-blind trials of a surgical procedure, combined here, people seriously ill with angina and coronary artery disease did as well (maybe a little better) with the sham procedure as with the "real" one. The sham surgery patients received local anesthesia, and two small incisions on the chest, which were then closed (Cobb et al. 1959; Dimond et al. 1960). Seventy-five to eight-five percent of patients experienced substantial subjective and objective improvement, leading to an increase in exercise tolerance and dramatically reducing nitroglycerine consumption. These figures are well within the range of improvement for the best contemporary treatments that exist a generation later.

A recent study showed the effects of inactive versus active pacemakers in obstructive hypertrophic cardiomyopathy. Three months after installation of pacemakers, randomly activated or not, all patients were better than at baseline. Sham and active pacemaker patients were better on most dimensions of the study: palpitations, dizziness, shortness of breath, chest pain, self-perceived health, and so on. While pacemakers worked better when they were turned on, they were not much better. Patients with active pacemakers showed signs of seemingly lowered cognitive functioning, which was improved in patients fitted with inactive pacers (Linde et al. 1999).

Additionally, a recent study in heart surgery, particularly involving laser transmyocardial revascularization (TMR), has shown evidence of significant meaning responses as well. Biosense direct myocardial revascularization (DMR) is a variation of this operation in which a laser catheter is inserted in the femoral artery, guided into the left ventricle, and shoots holes in the heart from the inside out. These surgical procedures are reserved for patients with the most severe and retractable angina. In a quite remarkable study, 299 patients with very serious angina were randomly assigned to a high dose, a low dose, or no dose of DMR. At baseline, all patients were rated as class IV on the Canadian Cardiology Society (CCS) angina class scale, a physician assessment that was the primary outcome measure of the study (CCS class IV means "angina at rest"—i.e., severe limitation). Two-thirds of the patients improved two or more grades on the CCS scale. Improvement was substantial and constant after 3 and 6 months, for patients who received a high dose, a low dose, or no treatment (where the laser catheter was inserted but not fired). Disease perception was dramatically improved, as were a broad range of other secondary outcome measures (Leon et al. 2000; Leon et al. 2005).[2]

Alan Johnson made, in my opinion, a prescient observation in 1994: "Electrical machines have great appeal to patients [and doctors] and recently anything with the word 'laser' attached to it has caught the imagination" (Johnson 1994, p. 1141). He left out the word "doctors," but I do not! I urge you to take a look at the websites of the companies that make and market these laser instruments, a primary source of patient education for this surgery. Watch very compelling meaning being created out of virtual laser beams with advanced computer programs.

What we know, what we think, what we are led to believe, or what we understand, whether we know it or not, can have a significant effect in the context of medical care. Let me add an important caveat; while it is always prudent to imagine that every medical intervention includes some portion of the meaning response, it is not always the case. A study of a statin (Rosuvastatin) and its effect on cholesterol showed a very classic dose–response rate: eight groups of patients were given increasing doses of the drug, from 0 mg to 80 mg per day. The group given 0 mg had no response (Olsson et al. 2001). This is unusual, and very interesting: it suggests that the liver operates in a way somehow insulated from cognitive influence, which seems odd but not impossible. This also shows that we are dealing with a complex form of physiology here, not magic. If it is not magic, what is it?

I would argue that it is here that we confront one of the biggest and most interesting challenges in this whole arena; and I would suggest that they are very big, very important, and very interesting challenges—Nobel Prize challenges. One of the classic ways that people have dismissed these matters in the past has been by saying, "Well, it's all in your head." It turns out they are right, but not in the dismissive way they intended.

Parkinson's disease has long been known by clinicians to be susceptible to influence by inert treatments. Imaging studies by a group from British Columbia, Canada, have shown a neurological basis for this common clinical observation. Using positron emission tomography (PET) scanning, the authors showed a substantial increase in occupancy of D2 receptors with dopamine in the striatum after an injection of saline solution to a patient with Parkinson's disease, when presented as his standard medication. These effects are similar in magnitude to the effect of amphetamine administration in healthy populations. The authors note that an area of the nucleus accumbens is also susceptible to placebo effect in Parkinson's disease (de La Fuente-Fernandez et al. 2001).

In a somewhat more complex study, regional glucose metabolism in PET scans following administration of fluoxetine (sold as Prozac in the United States) appears to overlap the metabolic pattern of placebo in depressed patients (Leuchter et al. 2002). Although the clinical response of drug and placebo patients was very similar in this study, the drug response showed somewhat more generalized brain activity than the placebo response. In another study, the authors concluded that "[a]ctive fluoxetine treatment was associated with additional and unique changes in the brainstem, striatum and hippocampus" (Mayberg et al. 2002). This may help to account for why it is that while placebo treatment of depression is often very nearly as effective as treatment with selective serotonin reuptake inhibitors (SSRIs), there is often substantially less evidence of unwanted side-effects with a placebo (Kirsch et al. 2002).

7.3 **Variability in meaning response**

Given that the meaning response is "all in your head" and that it involves language, it seems reasonable to imagine that cultural factors—different ways of knowing the world through language and meaning—will shape different responses to the same "placebos" around the world. There is a great deal of variability in the response to meaning in medicine, which I wish to briefly examine now.

If there is a single shibboleth of the effect of meaning or of placebos, it is that "placebo effects occur about a third of the time." I cannot address the history of this idea here, but I can assure you that it is wrong (see de Craen et al. 1999a). My study of the healing rates of 117 control groups in trials of anti-secretory medications for peptic ulcer disease showed patient improvements ranging from 0.0% to 100% (Moerman 2000). As seen here, meaning responses can be extremely variable. I am convinced that the study of this variability can be a key to developing a fundamental understanding of how meaning interacts with human biology.

7.3.1 **Color**

Color makes a difference: changing the color of a pill can change its effects in a variety of ways. With regard to one particular aspect, a dozen or more studies have shown that red pills tend to act as uppers/stimulants, while blue ones tend to act as downers/sedatives. Moreover, although they probably do not realize they are doing it, drug manufacturers tend to follow suit, coloring their drugs to match these cultural expectations. De Craen has shown that this is more generally true. He and his colleagues did a study of forty-nine medicines that affect the nervous system, available for sale in Holland. They found that stimulant medications tend to be marketed in red, orange, or yellow tablets, while depressants or tranquilizers tend to marketed in blue, green, or purple ones (de Craen et al. 1996).

There are some interesting exceptions to this pattern. In a series of experiments in Italy, it was shown that blue sleeping tablets, or blue placebos presented as sleeping tablets, worked better than did tablets of other colors, but only for Italian women; blue tablets tended to have a stimulating effect on men (Cattaneo et al. 1970; Lucchelli et al. 1978)! Checking with an Italian American anthropologist colleague, we arrived at this speculation. Many Italian women have a special relationship with the Virgin Mary. In Roman Catholic tradition, she is the protector of women. In religious art, the Virgin Mary is almost always shown in blue. This iconography of the blue Virgin extends well beyond Italy, but the relationship to women seems to be particularly strong in Italy, although it may be so elsewhere as well. What about men? "Azzuri" is both the name and color of the Italian national football team. Blue, for many Italian men, is not a color of solace but of excitement and stimulation, of joy and madness, of exhilaration and, too often, of catastrophe—while the Italian team won the World Cup in 2006, they lost in the first round in 2010. It is hardly the color of sleep!

Symbols are often polysemic; a single color, the same blue, can be associated with stimulation and excitement, and also associated with solace and protection. It seems a plausible way to think about the experimental results. Anecdotally, it may be worth mentioning that Italian football fans holler "Forza Azzurri" to cheer on their team. Let me note that I have a certain sympathy for this proposition, since a good translation of "Forza Azzuri" is "Go Blue," the chant of the University of Michigan Wolverines who wear maize and blue colors as they routinely play (another sort of) football in Michigan Stadium in front of 110,000 screaming fans. Not a soporific sight, even for a jaded fan like me. It is also true that the French national football team, the World Cup Champions in 1998, are known as "Les Bleus." I am aware of no evidence to show that this has any effect on sleeping tablets in that country, or in Michigan, for that matter.

7.3.2 **Form**

As color can make a difference in the meaning of medicine, so can form. For example, Ton de Craen has shown that injected placebo is more effective than oral placebo in the treatment of migraine headache (de Craen et al. 2000). When the drug sumatriptan (known in the United States as Imitrex, and as Imgran elsewhere) was first introduced, it was only available in the form of an injection; today, it is still available that way, but also as tablets and nasal spray. De Craen did a meta-analysis of thirty-five trials. In placebo-treated patients, among those treated with an oral pill, 26% of patients reported that their headache was better (defined as more mild or gone) after two hours. Of those treated with a placebo injection, 32% of patients were better. This difference is small (6.7%) but it is statistically significant ($X^2 = 9.4$, p = 0.002).

7.3.3 **Number**

Similarly, the number of pills can make a difference. In a very subtle meta-analysis, Ton de Craen showed that in some eighty studies of anti-secretory medications for peptic ulcer, there was a significant difference in the healing rates for those who took two placebos per day (36%) compared to those who took four per day (44%): a difference of 8%, where $X^2 = 21.7$, p < 0.0000 (de Craen et al. 1999b).

7.3.4 **National cultural differences**

There are also other cultural factors that are associated with some variation, in addition to color. Recall the study of inert injection versus inert tablet for migraine, where it was shown that injections worked better than pills. In studies carried out in the United States, the same pattern appeared: 22% oral versus 34% subcutaneous placebo relief rate. In studies done in Europe, however, the difference disappeared: 27% oral versus 25% subcutaneous placebo relief rate (de Craen et al. 2000; Moerman 2002, pp. 78–79). Injections work better than pills, but only in the United States. There are cultural differences shaping the placebo effect.

In my work with peptic ulcers, the mean healing rate for placebos (again, 4-week duration, endoscopically controlled) in six German studies is 59%; the rate in three Brazilian studies is 7%. For ulcer patients taking placebo, the NNTb (the number needed to treat for a benefit[3]) among German patients is two. There is no obvious reason why this should be the case; to contextualize these differences would have required a challenging and complex research study (for which I never received funding, despite years of effort).

Perhaps Brazilians and Germans have fundamentally different kinds of ulcers—although there is no evidence for this at all. Sticking geographically closer to home, and comparing the six German studies to five studies from Germany's northern neighbors in Denmark and the Netherlands, the German healing rate for placebo treatment is 59% compared to the Danish/Dutch rate of 22%. For ulcer patients taking placebo, the NNTb among Germans (not Danish or Dutch) is three.

Note that the situation is not a simple one. These differences seem to vary by illness: the control group healing rates in treating hypertension are substantially lower in Germany than in other Western nations (Moerman 2000). These are not generic cultural or "racial" phenomena, but seem to be specific cultural ones as different conceptualizations, or understandings, or constructions of illness in different cultures seem to have a real impact on health and healing.

7.3.5 Historical variation

These kinds of differences can be seen not only between different cultures but also through as attitudes and understandings change. Walsh and colleagues reviewed seventy-five published trials of various antidepressants (tricyclics and SSRIs) compared with placebo. The effectiveness of drug treatment for depression trended up substantially between 1981 and 2000, so that the proportion of patients responding to tricyclics and to SSRIs had increased from about 40% to about 55%. Over the same period, the proportion of patients responding to placebos increased from about 20% to about 35%. The proportion responding was strongly correlated with the year of publication of the study for both drug and placebo treatment. The authors conclude that "Some factor or factors associated with the level of placebo response must therefore have changed significantly during this period. Unfortunately, we were not able to identify these factors" (Walsh et al. 2002, p.1844).

However, the matter does not seem too complicated to me. Over the past generation, there has been a clear shift in consciousness among doctors, patients, friends, and, generally, everyone, to the effect that depression can be treated with drugs. This was simply not the case (or at least not broadly shared) 20 or 25 years ago. As recently as 1970, for example, Goodman and Gilman's *Pharmacological basis of therapeutics*, one of the standard reference sources, was clearly more enthusiastic about electroconvulsive therapy (ECT) than it was about treatment with imipramine or amitriptyline, which were said never to be more effective than ECT (Goodman and Gilman 1970).

Today, while we practically never hear of ECT[4], we all "know" that drugs are effective for depression; we read it in the newspapers and in the scientific journals; we see it on television dramas; and, in the United States at least, we see it in drug company advertisements everywhere, both in professional media and on television commercials, blogs, and, of course, in our spam e-mail, plus on Twitter and Facebook.

Antidepressant drugs are available in the drugstore and, in the form of St. John's Wort, at the drug section of your local supermarket.[5] As we change our views about the effectiveness of drugs, their effectiveness changes, as do their placebo mimics in trials. Meanings change, and so do meaning responses.

Although I have yet to find any indication of it in the medical literature, there are press reports (Silberman 2009) which suggest that, recently, many large drug companies have become very concerned after losing millions of dollars in drug development once their investigational drugs failed to outperform placebos in Phase II trials. There are indications that they have formed a secret committee to compare all their own trial results to determine what is happening and why the effect of "dummy" drugs is increasing.

7.4 **Placebo dilemmas—meaning strikes back**

In the fall of 2009, the *New England Journal of Medicine* published two remarkable articles in the same issue describing two randomized controlled trials, one from the Mayo Clinic (Kallmes et al. 2009) and one from a group of investigators in Melbourne, Australia (Buchbinder et al. 2009). The trials looked at a surgical procedure called vertebroplasty of painful osteoporotic vertebral fractures. Older persons, especially women, often have osteoporosis. This condition leads to a weakening of the vertebrae which sometimes simply break. With vertebroplasty, the broken vertebrae are repaired with an injection of polymethylmethacrylate (PMMA), a medicinal glue. There are an estimated 750,000 persons in the United States with such fractures; there are as many as nine vertebroplasty procedures per 1000 persons in the United States annually, and the annual direct care for these fractures was estimated to range from $12 to $18 billion in 2002 (Weinstein 2009). This is, then, a substantial industry.

In the Australian study, seventy-one patients finished the trial. The verum group had the standard procedure, while the control group underwent a sham procedure where no needle was inserted into the bone. In the Mayo Clinic trial, 131 patients completed the trial. Both groups received anesthesia in the fractured vertebra, but the control group did not receive the subsequent injection of PMMA. In both studies, PMMA was opened and released in the operating chamber, since it has a distinctive odor (although it would probably not be all that distinctive to patients).

In the Mayo Clinic study, at one month after surgery, "there was no significant difference between the vertebroplasty group and the control group . . . [and] both groups had immediate improvement in disability and pain scores after the intervention" (Kallmes et al. 2009, p. 569). In the Australian study, "there were significant reductions in overall pain in both study groups at each follow-up assessment. At 3 months, the mean reductions" in overall pain score were the same for both groups. "Similar improvements were seen in both groups with respect to pain at night and at rest, physical functioning, quality of life and perceived improvement" (Buchbinder et al. 2009, p. 557). In both studies, nearly all the patients got better, with active or sham surgery. It is important to note the dilemma here: ordinarily, if the treatment is not better than the control, it is abandoned as a treatment. However here, both the treatment and the control made significant improvements in the lives of elderly patients (treatment: 74.2 years old; control: 78.9 years old), mostly women.

Complicating matters are two recent studies of acupuncture for low back pain, one conducted in Germany (the GERAC trial), and one at several sites on the American west coast. In the GERAC trial, 1162 patients participated in a three-arm trial: traditional Chinese acupuncture in one group, sham acupuncture (superficial needling at non-acupuncture points) in the second group, and conventional care (drugs, physical therapy, and exercise following the standard German guidelines) in the third. Outcome was measured in terms of response to one of two standard pain questionnaires. The results at 6 months showed that 48% of the verum acupuncture group was better; 44% of the sham acupuncture group was better; and 27% of the standard care group was better. "Low back pain improved after acupuncture treatment for at least six months. Effectiveness of acupuncture, either verum or sham, was almost twice that of conventional therapy" (Haake et al. 2007, p. 1892).

The American trial enrolled 638 adults who were randomly assigned to four groups: individualized acupuncture, standardized acupuncture, simulated acupuncture (using a toothpick in a guide tube), and standard care (at the patient's and their physicians' choice, usually a combination of drugs and physical therapy). Primary outcome was based on telephone interviews centered around the Roland-Morris disability questionnaire; there were a range of secondary outcome measures. The patients in the acupuncture groups all gained 4.4 to 4.5 points on the disability scale compared with 2.1 points for the usual care group, 8 weeks after treatment. These changes generally were still evident, in the same pattern, after 52 weeks. "In conclusion, acupuncture-like treatments significantly improved function in persons with chronic low back pain" (Cherkin et al. 2009, p. 865).

These remarkable studies demonstrate just how effective "inert" therapy can be. In particular, the bone surgery in each group was complex and dramatic; there is not room here to describe the elaborate fluoroscope suites where such work is done. There are elaborate and technologically rich diagnostic procedures involved that narrow down a complex, aching, debilitating pain to a simple, visible line on an X-ray, repairable with a little drop of super glue.

Likewise, acupuncture has led a charmed life in America since James Reston's Chinese appendectomy in 1971. Millions of Americans have had acupuncture treatments, though perhaps only a half dozen of them understand anything about qi (in Chinese, 氣; the character represents steam rising from cooking rice). We now know that acupuncture is better for treating low back pain (a major nemesis of conventional medicine) than is ordinary medical care, but it is not substantially better than sham treatment. (Note that it is not better than sham acupuncture; we do not know if it is better than sham conventional therapy.)

How to reconcile these studies with our everyday understanding of medical causality is challenging. However, they do force us to consider the role—throughout all of medicine—of the power of medicine's ritual, narrative, and performance, which, more and more often, seem to trump its "evidence-based" remedies.

7.5 **The mind/body problem**

I am regularly asked, "How does this work?" or "How does the mind influence the body to *do* these things?" I routinely say, "I don't know." I am an anthropologist, not a physiologist, neurologist, psychologist, or any other kind of scientist. Indeed, if you look carefully, you will notice that, until this paragraph, I have not once used the word "mind" in this chapter, and only once the word "body" (while referring to my embodied liver). Personally, I found the mind/body problem to be so devastatingly difficult when I first stumbled on it thirty years ago that I decided simply to ignore it, as I have so far done in this chapter. I remember discussing this issue with a bright young student once, perhaps in the early 1970s. She had no doubt about it, asserting confidently that, "The mind just tells the body what to do." I pondered that response, which used the metaphor of "speaking" to account for the matter. I replied something like this: "That implies that the body has some sort of ears to hear what the mind is saying, and that it can decode language; but for that, it would probably have to have . . . a mind." I recalled for her a joking variation on a Native American cosmological myth, which stated that the earth sat on the back of a giant turtle. When asked what the turtle stood on, the informant replied "another turtle," and, when pressed as to what *that* turtle stood on, he simply noted that "it's just turtles all the way down."

This story pleases me greatly, but does not help a lot. On the other hand, I think that it is plausible to imagine that the "connection" between mind and body is some sort of operation similar or analogous to "induction," as occurs, for example, in an electromagnet, where an insulated copper wire is coiled around an iron bar. The two parts, the copper and the iron, are separated from one another by inert plastic. If we send an electric current through the copper wire, it will create a "field," which will generate a magnetic force in the iron (not the copper). The field will occur without the iron, but it will be much stronger with it. The field is the result of the interaction of the electricity in the wire, amplified by the magnetized iron. One thing changes the other without ever touching it. Also, the magnetism can "do things," that is, it can attract other iron objects and so act, for example, as a switch, or a solenoid, like the one in an automobile starter motor.

Another analogy is with the "transducer cells" in the hypothalamus which, by mechanisms far beyond my pay grade, translate, in effect, information from the rest of the brain to the endocrine system, and vice versa. Generally, people think of the brain as an "electrical" organ, and the endocrine system as a "chemical" one (clearly an oversimplification), but there is something to it. The hypothalamus is clearly both. (Well, "clearly" may be an exaggeration.)

I think that mind and body, such as they are, interact by means of some sort of metaphorical "fields" or inductions or transductions. Other metaphors come to mind: the mind might "seduce" the body into doing one thing or another (at some different level than we ordinarily think of seduction). I try to avoid "trigger" metaphors, but who knows, some powerful stimulus may explode through the brain, like the powder in a cartridge, having either very widespread consequences or perhaps very focused, projectile-like effects (as you leap out of the way of an oncoming train).

My hunch is that mind and body influence one another in many different ways. However, the image of an electrical current creating a magnetic field is the one I prefer. I also like the image of language tickling my ears, which send messages, seducing my anterior cingulate cortex into producing endorphins. I sort of hope my brain works that way, at least some of the time. I have no idea how "hope" works.

7.6 **Conclusions**

What we know, understand, think, and feel; what we are told and believe; our cultural background; the relationships we have with our clinicians—our doctors, residents, interns, nurses, aids, orderlies, and probably receptionists and parking lot attendants—can very directly affect our response to medicines, inert or otherwise. These matters are, these days, largely left to chance, or to ideology, or to market forces, but are rarely subject to robust science (although that is less true today, thankfully, than it was a decade ago). The clinical implications of these matters are clearly rich and virtually unexamined.

Acknowledgments

This chapter was originally published as: Daniel E. Moerman, Examining a powerful healing effect through a cultural lens, and finding meaning, *The Journal of Mind–Body Regulation*, 1 (2), pp. 63–72, © The Authors, 2011.

Several versions of this chapter have preceded it, including talks in Bologna in 2008, and Auckland in 2004. My friend and colleague Lola Romanucci-Ross suggested to me the hypothesis about gender differences in the reaction to blue pills in Italy. Friend and colleague—and native speaker of Italian—Emanuela Appetiti contributed to this interpretation, and assisted with the translation of the highly idiomatic phrase "Forza Azurri." The presentation of the paper and discussion about it at the workshop in Montreal, "Using social science to elucidate placebos," were particularly helpful. Workshop participant Elia Abi-Jaoude clarified my understanding of the NNT (see footnote 3). Among others, Abraham Fuks, Ian Gold, Irving Kirsch, Steve Silberman, Laurence Kirmayer, Bennett Foddy, Vratislav Hadrava, and Cory Harris were particularly cogent and helpful commentators; several of them urged me to address the interaction of "mind and body" as I have attempted to do toward the end of this chapter. For Anne Harrington.

Notes

1 Note that this experiment was a replication, on a whole new level of complexity, of the pioneering study done a generation earlier by Levine, Gordon, and Fields (1978).

2 It may be worth noting that this research, done in the 1990s, was first reported at the American College of Cardiology meetings in Florida in 2000. The paper itself was not published for nearly 6 years; reading it shows, at least to this retired editor, a clear case of a paper dramatically damaged by peer review. The original abstract, published online in 2000, is no longer available online.

3 The NNT, or number needed to treat, is a clinically relevant statistic describing the value of a drug or treatment. If in a trial with 100 in each of two groups, and all of the drug group got better while none of the control group did, then the NNT to get one person better is 1. If (more realistically) 50 of the drug group and 25 of the control group improved, the NNT would be 100 divided by the absolute risk reduction ($100/(50–25) = 100/25 = 4$), or simply, the inverse of the absolute risk reduction expressed as a proportion ($1/(0.5–0.25) = 1/0.25 = 4$); that is, you would need to treat four people to get one person better.

4 It is also true that, whatever public opinion might be about ECT after *One flew over the cuckoo's nest*, it remains a valuable treatment of choice for many with the most severe and debilitating depression (Kelly and Zisselman 2000).

5 In a complex randomized controlled trial, Hypericum was shown to be as effective as sertraline (Zoloft); both were as effective as the placebo control. All three treatments led to quite satisfactory outcomes for about a third of patients treated (HDTSG 2002).

References

Benedetti, F. (1996). The opposite effects of the opiate antagonist naloxone and the chole-cystokinin antagonist proglumide on placebo analgesia. *Pain*, **64**(3), 535–543.

Benedetti, F., Maggi, G., Lopiano, L., Rainero, I., Vighetti, S., and Pollo, A. (2003). Open versus hidden medical treatments: the patient's knowledge about a therapy affects the therapy outcome. *Prevention and Treatment*, **6**(1), June 2003. http://dx.doi.org/10.1037/1522-3736.6.1.61a.

Branthwaite, A. and Cooper, P. (1981). Analgesic effects of branding in treatment of headaches. *British Medical Journal (Clinical Research Ed)*, **282**(6276), 1576–1578.

Buchbinder, R., Osborne, R. H., Ebeling, P. R., et al. (2009). A randomized trial of vertebroplasty for painful osteoporotic vertebral fractures. [Multicenter study randomized controlled trial research support, non-U.S. government.] *New England Journal of Medicine*, **361**(6), 557–568. DOI: 10.1056/NEJMoa0900429

Cattaneo, A. D., Lucchilli, P. E., and Filippucci, G. (1970). Sedative effects of placebo treatment. *European Journal of Clinical Pharmacology*, **3**, 43–45.

Cherkin, D. C., Sherman, K. J., Avins, A. L., et al. (2009). A randomized trial comparing acupuncture, simulated acupuncture, and usual care for chronic low back pain. *Archives of Internal Medicine*, **169**(9), 858–866.

Cobb, L., Thomas, G. I., Dillard, D. H., Merendino, K. A., and Bruce, R. A. (1959). An evaluation of internal-mammary artery ligation by a double blind technic. *New England Journal of Medicine*, **260**(22), 1115–1118.

Colloca, L., Lopiano, L., Lanotte, M., and Benedetti, F. (2004). Overt versus covert treatment for pain, anxiety, and Parkinson's disease. *Lancet Neurology*, **3**(11), 679–684.

de Craen, A. J., Kaptchuk, T., Tijssen, J. G., and Kleijnen, J. (1999a). Placebos and placebo effects in medicine: historical overview. *Journal of the Royal Society of Medicine*, **92**(10), 511–515.

de Craen, A. J., Moerman, D. E., Heisterkamp, S. H., Tytgat, G. N., Tijssen, J. G., and Kleijnen, J. (1999b). Placebo effect in the treatment of duodenal ulcer. [In process citation.] *British Journal of Clinical Pharmacology*, **48**(6), 853–860.

de Craen, A. J., Roos, P. J., Leonard de Vries, A., and Kleijnen, J. (1996). Effect of colour of drugs: systematic review of perceived effect of drugs and of their effectiveness. *British Medical Journal*, **313**(7072), 1624–1626.

de Craen, A. J., Tijssen, J. G., de Gans, J., and Kleijnen, J. (2000). Placebo effect in the acute treatment of migraine: subcutaneous placebos are better than oral placebos. *Journal of Neurology*, **247**(3), 183–188.

de La Fuente-Fernandez, R., Ruth, T. J., Sossi, V., Schulzer, M., Calne, D. B., and Stoessl, A. J. (2001). Expectation and dopamine release: mechanism of the placebo effect in Parkinson's disease. *Science*, **293**(5532), 1164–1166.

Dimond, E. G., Kittle, C. F., and Crockett, J. E. (1960). Comparison of internal mammary ligation and sham operation for angina pectoris. *American Journal of Cardiology*, **5**, 483–486.

Goodman, L. S. and Gilman, A. (1970). *The pharmacological basis of therapeutics* (4th edn.). New York: The Macmillan Company.

Gracely, R. H., Deeter, W. R., Wolskee, P. J., et al. (1979). The effect of naloxone on multidimensional scales of postsurgical pain in nonsedated patients. *Society for Neuroscience Abstracts*, **5**, 609.

Gracely, R. H., Dubner, R., Deeter, W. R., and Wolskee, P. J. (1985). Clinicians' expectations influence placebo analgesia. [Letter.] *Lancet*, **1**(8419), 43.

Haake, M., Muller, H. H., Schade-Brittinger, C., et al. (2007). German acupuncture trials (GERAC) for chronic low back pain: randomized, multicenter, blinded, parallel-group trial with 3 groups. *Archives of Internal Medicine*, **167**(17), 1892–1898. DOI: 167/17/1892 [pii]

Hróbjartsson, A. and Gøtzsche, P. C. (2001). Is the placebo powerless? An analysis of clinical trials comparing placebo with no treatment. *New England Journal of Medicine*, **344**(21), 1594–1602.

Hypericum Depression Trial Study Group (HDTSG) (2002). Effect of Hypericum perforatum (St John's wort) in major depressive disorder: a randomized controlled trial. *Journal of the American Medical Association*, **287**(14), 1807–1814.

Johnson, A. G. (1994). Surgery as a placebo. *Lancet*, **344**(8930), 1140–1142.

Kallmes, D. F., Comstock, B. A., Heagerty, P. J., et al. (2009). A randomized trial of vertebroplasty for osteoporotic spinal fractures. *New England Journal of Medicine*, **361**(6), 569–579.

Kelly, K. G. and Zisselman, M. (2000). Update on electroconvulsive therapy (ECT) in older adults. *Journal of the American Geriatrics Society*, **48**(5), 560–566.

Kirsch, I., Moore, T. J., Scorboria, A., and Nicholls, S. S. (2002). The emperor's new drugs: an analysis of antidepressant medication data Submitted to the U.S. Food and Drug Administration. *Prevention and Treatment*, **5**, article 23.

Kitchell, J. R., Glover, R. P., and Kyle, R. H. (1958). Bilateral internal mammary artery ligation for angina pectoris: preliminary clinical considerations. *American Journal of Cardiology*, **1**, 46–50.

Leon, M. B., Baim, D. S., Moses, J. W., Laham, R. J., and Knopf, W. (2000). A randomized blinded clinical trial comparing percutaneous laser myocardial revascularization (using Biosense LV Mapping) vs. placebo in patients with refractory coronary ischemia. Paper presented at American Heart Association, November, 2000.

Leon, M. B., Kornowski, R., Downey, W. E., et al. (2005). A blinded, randomized, placebo-controlled trial of percutaneous laser myocardial revascularization to improve angina symptoms in patients with severe coronary disease. *Journal of the American College of Cardiology*, **46**(10), 1812–1819.

Leuchter, A. F., Cook, I. A., Witte, E. A., Morgan, M., and Abrams, M. (2002). Changes in brain function of depressed subjects during treatment with placebo. *American Journal of Psychiatry*, **159**(1), 122–129.

Levine, J. D., Gordon, N. C., and Fields, H. L. (1978). The mechanism of placebo analgesia. *Lancet*, **2**(8091), 654–657.

Linde, C., Gadler, F., Kappenberger, L., and Ryden, L. (1999). Placebo effect of pacemaker implantation in obstructive hypertrophic cardiomyopathy. PIC study group. Pacing in cardiomyopathy. *American Journal of Cardiology*, **83**(6), 903–907.

Lucchelli, P. E., Cattaneo, A. D., and Zattoni, J. (1978). Effect of capsule colour and order of administration of hypnotic treatments. *European Journal of Clinical Pharmacology*, **13**(2), 153–155.

Mayberg, H. S., Silva, J. A., Brannan, S. K., et al. (2002). The functional neuroanatomy of the placebo effect. *American Journal of Psychiatry*, **159**(5), 728–737.

Moerman, D. E. (2000). Cultural variations in the placebo effect: ulcers, anxiety, and blood pressure. *Medical Anthropology Quarterly*, **14**(1), 1–22.

Moerman, D. E. (2002). *Meaning, medicine and the "placebo effect."* Cambridge, UK: Cambridge University Press.

Olsson, A. G., Pears, J., McKellar, J., Mizan, J., and Raza, A. (2001). Effect of rosuvastatin on low-density lipoprotein cholesterol in patients with hypercholesterolemia. *American Journal of Cardiology*, **88**(5), 504–508.

Phillips, D. P., Liu, G. C., Kwok, K., Jarvinen, J. R., Zhang, W., and Abramson, I. S. (2001). The hound of the Baskervilles effect: natural experiment on the influence of psychological stress on timing of death. *British Medical Journal*, **323**(7327), 1443–1446.

Phillips, D. P., Ruth, T. E., and Wagner, L. M. (1993). Psychology and survival. *Lancet*, **342**(8880), 1142–1145.

Polanyi, M. and Prosch, H. (1975). *Meaning*. Chicago, IL: The University of Chicago Press.

Price, D. D. (2001). Assessing placebo effects without placebo groups: an untapped possibility? *Pain*, **90**(3), 201–203.

Silberman, S. (2009). Placebos are getting more effective. Drugmakers are desperate to know why. *Wired*, **17**(9), 1–8. http://www.southdevonacupuncture.net/pdf/Placebos-Are-Getting-More-Effective-July2011.pdf

Walsh, B. T., Seidman, S. N., Sysko, R., and Gould, M. (2002). Placebo response in studies of major depression: variable, substantial, and growing. *Journal of the American Medical Association*, **287**(14), 1840–1847.

Weinstein, J. N. (2009). Balancing science and informed choice in decisions about vertebroplasty. *New England Journal of Medicine*, **361**(6), 619–621. DOI: 361/6/619 [pii] 10.1056/NEJMe0905889

Chapter 8

Unpacking the placebo response: insights from ethnographic studies of healing

Laurence J. Kirmayer

8.1 Introduction

Placebo responding stands at the heart of the symbolic efficacy of all forms of medicine (Brody 2010). Although most research on placebos has focused on psychological and psychophysiological processes, studying the social contexts of healing can illuminate the interpersonal and wider social determinants of placebo response. As this chapter will argue, understanding the effectiveness of placebos or any healing intervention requires knowledge of the person's social world, contexts, and commitments.

The focus on depression in many of the contributions to this volume is especially interesting and important for several reasons. Contemporary psychiatry tends to view depression as a biological condition, hence treatments that alter brain functioning are viewed as plausible. However, it is clear that feedback loops between cognition and emotion and between behavior and social response contribute to exacerbating and maintaining depression and, in some theories, may be primary causes. Understanding the nature of these loops points to many sites where expectations or other placebo-related phenomena can occur. Meta-analyses showing that medication has only a small advantage over placebos for mild to moderate depression can also be interpreted as evidence for the power of placebos (or for naturalistic processes of recovery). The blurred and sometimes contentious boundaries between depression and common experiences of sadness, grief, and demoralization encourage the search for interventions that bolster ordinary processes of resilience and healing. Finally, the recognition of depression as a major contributor to the global burden of disease, with calls for better screening and treatment, raises concerns about the wholesale promotion of psychopharmaceuticals for everyday problems in living or social structural problems that demand political attention. All of these issues make it critical to consider the extent to which the use of medications, psychotherapy, or any therapeutic intervention for depression, including the doctor–patient relationship itself, can be understood in terms of placebo mechanisms. This understanding can provide guidance on how best to deploy interventions for maximum effectiveness both in clinical care and public health.

The sections that follow first consider some epistemological and methodological issues central to placebo theory and research, and then briefly review work on the great variety of mechanisms that underlie placebo responding. The section on healing as a placebo, summarizes some insights that have come from anthropological efforts to develop a general theory of symbolic or ritual healing. Turning this analogy around, the next section considers the clinical and experimental use of placebos as a type of symbolic healing ritual. The final section outlines some implications for ethical and pragmatic issues in clinical practice of understanding placebo responding as embodied processes that are socially situated and culturally mediated. In particular, I argue that the attempts to justify the deceptive use of placebos ignore crucial facts about the science of placebos and the social context of the clinical encounter.

8.2 Clinical and experimental epistemics of placebos

Speaking of an intervention as a placebo draws attention to the externally administered agent, often a pill or some other visible form of treatment. This encourages the observer to attribute any healing efficacy to the intervention itself. Because the placebo treatment is, by definition, inert, this poses a puzzle. If the placebo really has no (biological) effect, those who claim to benefit must be dissimulating or simply gullible, talking themselves into something that is not really happening. More accurately, since the placebo has no immediate biological activity that could elicit its therapeutic outcomes, if it has some physiological effect, this must be through some longer causal chain of psychophysiological processes that translate symbolic meaning into physiological response.

Clinical trials often involve comparing an active treatment to an inactive (placebo) control. Of course, this experimental paradigm does not measure the placebo effect per se, because any improvement over time in the group receiving the placebo may reflect a myriad of other factors associated with the course of the condition being treated, including unmeasured effects of the environment or host responses. To identify the placebo effect itself, we must compare a group given a placebo (a biologically inactive treatment) to a group not receiving any treatment at all (Ernst and Resch 1995; Hrobjartsson et al. 2011). Indeed, we can begin to disentangle components of placebo responding by varying this comparison: for example, giving one group an inert pill accompanied by a strong positive message ("This will make your headache go away") and another group the same pill with less emphatic message ("This pill *may* make your headache go away") or the same message but a differently colored pill.[1] We can also measure the strength of individuals' expectations of improvement before and after the placebo administration and see whether this correlates with positive outcome. Alternatively, in the "open–hidden" drug treatment paradigm devised by Benedetti (2009), the response of subjects who are aware they are receiving an active treatment is compared to that of subjects who are unaware they are receiving the same treatment. Any difference between groups can then be attributed to psychologically mediated responses associated with knowing that one is receiving a treatment.[2]

These types of experiment can help identify the parameters that influence placebo effects and point to the underlying processes that may mediate placebo responses including cognitive expectations, emotional arousal, and the impact of relationships (Finniss et al. 2010). A growing body of work of this type has produced some surprising results that challenge conventional medical understandings of placebos. In particular, the "hidden drug versus open drug paradigm" makes it clear that a large part of the observed efficacy of many drug treatments comes from their symbolic effects (Benedetti 2008). Being given a medication surreptitiously does not have the same degree of benefit as knowing one is taking it. Placebo effects then are part of every medical treatment and may account for a substantial part of the observed benefit of drugs, surgery, and other medical interventions. Calling a treatment a "placebo," while often meant as a dismissal, actually points to the endogenous healing capacities of human beings, which deserve intensive study and systematic incorporation into every aspect of medical care (Harrington 2006).

8.3 **Varieties of placebo responding**

Although references to the placebo effect imply a unitary phenomenon, there are as many types of placebo responding as there are forms of learning and adaptation that can give rise to physiological anticipation or psychological expectation. We can organize these varieties of placebo responding in terms of specific physiological systems (autonomic, endocrine, immune, motor, pain, etc.), expected effects (e.g., analgesia, anxiety reduction, mood elevation, impact on specific disease processes), or contexts (type of medical system, healthcare setting, religious ritual, etc.) (Benedetti 2008; Benedetti et al. 2011; Linde et al. 2011; Meissner 2011; Pollo et al. 2011; Price et al. 2008). Alternatively, drawing from hierarchical systems theory, we can think of placebo effects in terms of the level of regulatory process and the corresponding mediating mechanisms that are influenced by learning, cognition, or social interaction (Figure 8.1; see Kirmayer 2004).

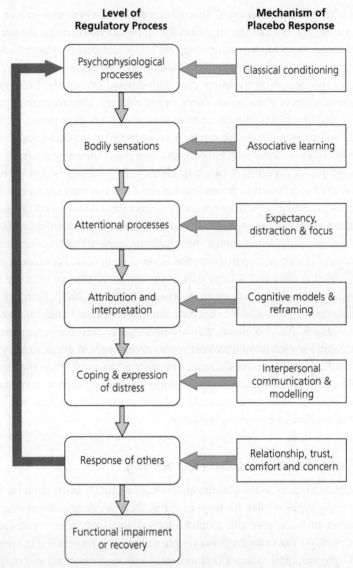

Fig. 8.1 Levels of regulation and varieties of placebo response. Regulatory processes involved in placebo responding may be mediated and modified by learning mechanisms that operate at multiple levels.

Adapted from Kirmayer L. J. Unpacking the placebo response: Insights from ethnographic studies of healing. *Journal of Mind-Body Regulation*. 1(3), pp 112–124, The Author © 2011.

Table 8.1 Potential pathways for placebo influence on depression

Level	Mechanism	Pathways
Neural systems involved in depression	Classical conditioning	Conditioned responses link stimulus of the placebo to alterations in neural pathways regulating mood and reinforcement
Emotional experience	Evocation of emotion	Anticipation of improvement associated with feelings of pleasure or happiness
	Anxiety reduction	Decreased worry and fear of negative course of illness diminishes sadness and anxiety
Cognitive processes	Attention	Increased attention to positive social cues leads to improved mood
	Attribution	Expectation of improvement leads to increased morale, hope, and optimism
Coping behaviors	Behavioral activation	Anticipation of improvement leads to less social withdrawal and increased engagement in rewarding activities
Social interaction	Social reinforcement	Change in expectations of others leads to more positive response

Some of the potential ways in which placebos could affect depression are listed in Table 8.1. Depression spans a continuum from common fluctuations in mood that are self-righting to more severe and enduring mood states characterized by disruption of physiological regulation (e.g., autonomic symptoms including slowed gut motility, increased muscle tension), lack of pleasure in ordinarily enjoyable activities (*anhedonia*), and resistance to the activating effects of positive events or social reinforcers. Current theories of depression emphasize alterations of mood regulatory systems in the brain, but processes involving cognitive appraisal, attribution of action, and social withdrawal likely also play a role, as do interpersonal responses. These different levels of process may interact to form vicious circles that exacerbate and maintain negative mood. The beneficial effects of any treatment of depression, including placebos, may then involve action at any place along the vicious circles that maintain depression and that prevent normal processes of mood regulation, self-righting, restitution, and recovery. These processes vary substantially across cultures (Kirmayer and Jarvis 2005).

8.3.1 **Psychological mediation**

At the level of psychological mediation, placebo effects have been explained in three broad ways as a result of (i) enhancing positive emotions and optimism, (ii) reducing anxiety and other negative emotions that cause distress, and (iii) shaping attentional and interpretive or attributional processes that give meaning to experience (Geers et al. 2005). Clearly, these mediators can interact in many ways. Positive and negative emotions may compete for attention and mutually suppress each other. Attention and interpretation are influenced by emotional state but also can give rise to positive or negative emotions, setting up feedback loops. All of these potential mediators may be influenced by other cognitive, affective, and motivational processes.

Although we think of expectations as conscious processes, there are various kinds of expectation or anticipatory responding that involve non-conscious mechanisms based on learning processes mediated by specific neural systems. Simply handling a pain medication can increase the person's subsequent ability to tolerate pain (Rutchik and Slepian 2013). This may occur through unconscious associations or classically conditioned responses.

Much of what we know about the physiology of placebos comes from work on placebo analgesia. Placebo analgesia involves the activation of endogenous opioid pain control systems in the brainstem (Levine et al. 1978). Indeed, much of the individual variability in response to both opiate and non-opiate analgesics may be determined by individual differences in the response of endogenous opiate pain-modulation systems (Amanzio et al. 2001). Placebo responding to analgesics also involves additional top–down influences from the frontal cortex acting on the rostral anterior cingulate cortex, along pathways that do not involve endogenous opioid neurotransmission (Petrovic et al. 2010). Placebo analgesia involves activation of an internal regulatory system that normally functions to control pain. These systems have multiple effects so that, for example, placebo effects on enhancing memory may also be mediated by endorphins (Stern et al. 2011). Similar systems exist for regulating inflammatory processes and various autonomic, endocrine, and immune functions and these may provide the basis for a variety of other specific placebo responses (Ader 1997; Meissner 2011; Murray and Stoessel 2013; Pollo et al. 2011).

Placebo responses may also be mediated by classical or Pavlovian conditioning (Stewart-Williams and Podd 2004; Wickramasekera 1980). Classical conditioning is based on adaptive responses (e.g., salivating in anticipation of eating to aid in the digestion of food) that can be linked to new contextual stimuli. Physiological responses that are linked to stimuli by classical conditioning tend to have a compensatory physiological function that reflects specific regulatory systems (Siegel 2002). For example, a sensory cue that has been linked to the presentation of food triggers the release of insulin in anticipation of eating. Other classically conditioned responses are based on linking symbolic stimuli to specific responses of regulatory systems.

Classical conditioning has been shown for a wide range of physiological responses involving motor, autonomic, endocrine, and immune systems, each of which may mediate specific types of placebo response (Ader 1997). These mechanisms could build associations between particular environmental cues and physiological responses that have clinical significance. The strength and direction of these responses will depend in part on each individual's learning history, which in turn will reflect culturally patterned frameworks of meaning, as well as shared and idiosyncratic experiences. Classically conditioned effects constitute forms of non-conscious expectations or predispositions to respond that are part of each individual's enculturation and personal biography. Similarly, other forms of operant and sensory associative learning can link salient stimuli to bodily responses (Hinton et al. 2008). These embodied processes of learning can contribute to placebo responding even in the absence of awareness (Frenkel 2008). Of course, cognitive and classically conditioned learning processes usually coexist and interact and, in some situations, cognitive expectations may trump classically conditioned effects (Kirsch 2004).

Attentional mechanisms also may play a central role in placebo responses. Focusing attention on discomfort can intensify symptoms and, conversely, distraction, or absorption in other sensations, imagery, or activity can markedly reduce symptoms like pain, nausea, and other forms of discomfort (Pennebaker 1982). This attentional capacity may underlie some of the phenomena associated with clinical hypnosis (Raz 2007; Raz and Buhle 2006). Suggestions and expectations, whether direct or implicit, can guide attention. Focus of attention and expectations interact in symptom experience (Cioffi 1991; Geers et al. 2006, 2011). Simply knowing that one has begun an effective treatment may lead to shifts in attention in which the person looks for cues of improvement. In the case of depression, low mood and low self-esteem may lead people to pay more attention to negative social cues (e.g., a frown on another person's face). Paying closer attention to positive social cues can improve mood and bolster self-esteem (Dandeneau et al. 2007; Wadlinger and Isaacowitz 2011).

Expectations generally involve cognitive models or frameworks and affective attitudes or stances. These models can be encoded as stories, propositions, metaphors, or images that may be explicit (conscious) or implicit (non-conscious). Both implicit and explicit cognitive models can direct thinking in ways that amplify or diminish symptomatology and distress. Indeed, cognition can influence symptoms through the ways in which sensations are focused on, interpreted, labeled, and attributed (Kirmayer and Sartorius 2007). These processes represent levels or sites where the symbolic effects of placebos may exert effects. Because attributional processes are central to symptom experience, any suggestion, instruction, or contextual cue that shifts attention, attributions, and coping responses will, in turn, change symptom experience. These shifts can occur through reattribution, engaging with new images or metaphors, or re-narrating distress in a new story-frame.

8.3.2 Social mediation

Social interaction is a powerful vehicle for conveying treatment expectations. Modeling and observational learning can result in placebo effects that are stronger than those elicited by direct verbal suggestion (Colloca and Benedetti 2009). The doctor–patient relationship involves all of these cognitive, emotional influences, but therapeutic relationships can have additional effects through neurobiological mechanisms that are fundamental to human sociality (Benedetti 2010). For example, experiences of trust can stimulate brain oxytocin release, which increases feelings of comfort and trust, with potentially far-reaching effects on well-being, interpersonal relationships, and long-term health outcomes. This feedback loop from quality of relationships to physiology and back (depicted in Figure 8.1) is just one of many such potential loops which may involve larger social processes. Of course, relationships of trust are embedded in larger social structures. For some marginalized individuals or groups, mistrust in healthcare institutions and professionals may reduce help seeking and undermine the effectiveness of interventions, thus aggravating the health disparities associated with social inequities.

The sociopsychological processes involved in placebo responding are not specific to placebos; they apply to every type of treatment. The individual's psychological and interpersonal responses to a medical intervention are embedded in larger sociocultural systems that give meaning to experience. Changes in the social meaning of specific treatments can, therefore, reshape expectations, vastly increasing hope or undermining confidence in a good outcome. There may be complex social patterns of anticipation that depend on interactions with others, social context, and cultural systems of meaning which are embedded in social practices. Based on such cultural and personal meanings, people may invest in a treatment because it is consonant with their values and motivations and respond positively because of the emotional meaning of the treatment (Hyland and Whalley 2008).

Thompson and colleagues (2009) suggest that placebo responses can reflect embodied learning and contextual responding that are independent of consciousness awareness. The symbolic, affective, and esthetic responses to treatments cannot be reduced to expectations; they are part of cultural performance and participation (Myers 2010). This means that responses to placebos or other treatment interventions need not be based on cognitive models or representations carried by the individual but may be part of a performance that involves distributed knowledge and that, therefore, can only be enacted through concerted social action. These enactments depend on interactions with others who are essential to create the context and shape the response. In this sense, placebo responses may be understood as social phenomena that depend on embodied experience, socially distributed or embedded knowledge, and situated practice. The positive expectations and responses of others are important components of placebo-responding real-life contexts.

8.4 **Healing ritual as a placebo**

There is a vast anthropological literature on healing rituals in diverse cultures. Much of this has focused on the esthetics of performance and explored the parallels between healing practices and larger cultural myths, values, and social structures (Csordas and Lewton 1998). The actual effectiveness of healing has been examined less often, but authors have attributed the potential efficacy of ritual to non-specific effects of meaning, expectation, and belief that may be related to placebo effects (Frank 1961; Moerman 2002).

Ethnographic studies of healing emphasize the multiple sources and complex dynamics of belief and expectation, the interpersonal processes of renegotiating illness and healing experiences, and the embedding of healing practices in larger cultural ontologies and ideologies of the person (Kirmayer 2004; Kleinman 1980; Waldram 2008). These ontologies recognize different types of agency or influence as sources of healing efficacy. For example, in different systems of medicine, spirits, humors, "energies," chemicals, or human relationships may be invoked as a powerful mediator of effective healing. These notions of agency are part of larger cultural differences in notions of the person that shape the diagnostic systems, goals, and methods of healing (Kirmayer 2007).

There are many reasons why people may believe in the potential efficacy of a treatment and have positive expectations. These sources of hope and conviction include the causal logic of the treatment, which may be grounded in a specific ontology or simply part of an extended metaphor that is popular, appealing, or compelling; the extent of individuals' investment in the larger healing system, which may be part of religious or other cultural identities, values, and commitments; the degree to which they reject conventional biomedicine and, therefore, are open to alternative systems of medicine that challenge the hegemony of biomedicine; and, especially, compelling experiences of their own or of others that seem to demonstrate impact and positive outcomes (Kirmayer 2006). These expectations or believed-in efficacy then give rise to a variety of responses that can contribute to positive outcomes.

8.4.1 **Theories of ritual healing**

The classic account of expectancy effects in healing is found in the work of social psychiatrist Jerome Frank (1961). Frank identified four components common to all systems of healing that were part of a "shared assumptive world" between sufferer and healer: theories of affliction with particular ontologies;

defined roles for healers which confer healing power, authority, and legitimacy; a designated place and time for healing (often imbued with sacred qualities); and the symbolic action of the healing ritual which aims to transform the status of the sick person. Frank saw positive expectations (based on a "shared assumptive world" and the evocative power of healer, context, and treatment) as reducing "demoralization"—a common dimension of many forms of affliction (Young 1988). Demoralization is a broader category than depression in psychiatry, but there is much overlap between the constructs. The hallmark of demoralization is a subjective feeling of incompetence, and anything that mobilizes and engages the person in effective action can help to remoralize them (de Figueiredo and Gostoli 2013).

In later versions of his theory, Frank considered a diversity of healing processes relevant to specific conditions (Frank and Frank 1991). He also came to see the relevance of studies of rhetoric which examine how communication can persuade and transform experience (Frank 1995). The study of rhetoric takes on new significance in societies with high levels of cultural diversity where Frank's notion of a shared assumptive world is challenged. In contemporary societies, people often participate in systems of healing with little shared experience or understanding of the specific tradition. The appeal of these heterodox traditions must be explained by the persuasive power of rhetoric and the imaginative appeal of novel models and metaphors for illness and healing (Kaptchuk and Eisenberg 1998; Kirmayer 2006, 2014).

In an influential paper on the effectiveness of symbolic healing, the anthropologist Claude Lévi-Strauss (1967) considered how a shamanic ritual could evoke physiological changes. For Lévi-Strauss, the formal analogy or parallels between the structure of the healing ritual and the patient's experience accounted for the healing transformation. In effect, the patient's experience of bodily affliction was mapped, by analogy, onto a mythic landscape. This mapping might occur through divination or other forms of diagnosis before or during the healing ritual, which sometimes takes the form of a search for the nature of the affliction. Traversing this mythic landscape in image, narrative, or metaphor, through ritual incantations, the healer or his spirit guide then moves from a place representing affliction to one that corresponds to health. This metaphoric movement somehow causes corresponding changes in attention, cognition, and experience that result in healing.

The appeal of Lévi-Strauss's account lies in its formal structure, but this also is its limitation. The process of healing seems under-theorized and the mechanisms involved remain unclear (Kirmayer 1993). In the actual example of Kuna shamans used by Lévi-Strauss, the patient may not understand the healer's incantations, hence the impact of the ritual must be through non-linguistic aspects of the healing performance (Sherzer, 1983). Nevertheless, the notion that healing involves a transformative process mediated by the evocation of and participation in a mythic or "virtual world" remains a useful way to understand the rich symbolism and formal structure of healing practices (Kapferer 2005).

Anthropologist James Dow (1986) addressed the question of the dynamics of healing, building on the work of Lévi-Strauss, with the suggestion that the transformative effects occur by attaching experience to emotionally meaningful symbols. It is the moving quality of emotion itself that ultimately does the psychophysiological or psychological work. Rituals then exert their effects by influencing emotional experience. This fits with observations that healing rituals often are structured like dramatic performances that elicit emotional catharsis (Scheff 1979). It is also consistent with studies showing that some aspects of placebo responding may be mediated by changes in emotional state (Flaten et al. 2011).

8.4.2. The metaphoric mediation of healing

In my own work, I have extended these models to consider how the metaphors used in healing practices map experience onto images or mythic narratives with different sensory, affective, and cognitive qualities (Kirmayer 1993, 2003, 2004, 2008). There is now a wealth of research showing how metaphors emerge from bodily experience and how employing a metaphor can, in turn, change bodily sensations, cognition, and action (Barsalou 2008; Gibbs 2006). Metaphors mediate bodily experience and overarching mythic narratives that are viewed as compelling or sacred truths. The metaphoric elaboration of experience can occur through listening and imaginative representation or through ritual enactment.

In a healing ritual, the sufferer's experience is mapped analogically onto a metaphoric representational space. This representation is extended and transformed according to the metaphoric logic and imagery of the ritual. The transformed metaphoric representation is embodied and enacted by the afflicted person. In practice, this process of transformation occurs through an ongoing cycle of embodiment and enactment both during the healing ritual and in subsequent re-experiencing, recollection, and narration of the ritual or its expected consequences.

Esthetics play an important role in healing rituals, making the performance attractive, compelling, absorbing, or entrancing.[3] Esthetic elements of the ritual portray the predicament of the suffering person and dramatize the transition from darkness and affliction to goodness, positivity, health, and harmony (Kapferer and Papigny 2005). The form, structure, and sensory qualities of healing can convey specific metaphoric qualities (e.g., vigor, strength, power) (Kirmayer 1993, 2008). These metaphors influence processes of attention, cognition, and behavior that evoke the anticipated mode of experiencing and amplify its intensity.

Healing rituals have received so much attention from anthropologists not only because of their claims for efficacy but also because of their dramatic and esthetic qualities. The arcane, numinous, arresting, and authoritative aspects of ritual performance are serve to mobilize symbolic power which has material, social, emotional, and cognitive dimensions. The power of ritual is often felt within the body in ways that convey a sense of immediacy and conviction that something significant is happening. The power that healing rituals mobilize is often understood as not simply social or physiological but as drawing from spiritual or transcendental realms.

All of this theoretical work on ritual is somewhat idealized and must be set against the observation that, in everyday experience, healing rituals often do not work—at least not as advertised. For example, a study of healing by Chinese shamans (*dang-ki*) in Singapore found that many of the people resorting to this form of ritual healing did not have strong beliefs or expectations in the treatment; they sought out the healer with some tentative hope or open-minded interest to see if it might work (Lee et al. 2010). People sought evidence during and after the healing that something significant had happened, noticing changes in bodily sensations or other signs. In many cases, the healing did not work quite as expected. While some people then gave up on the healer, many maintained their hope and commitment by identifying another change in symptoms or life events that they interpreted as a positive sign of healing efficacy. In this way, they could preserve and strengthen a belief in the healing efficacy. The pragmatic, tentative, subjunctivizing ("what if it works?") stance, the active search for evidence of effectiveness, and the shifting criteria for a positive outcome seen in this ethnographic study are probably not unique to this particular cultural context but are features of help seeking in many contemporary settings and healing systems, including biomedicine.

8.5 **Placebos as ritual healing**

Examining the parallels between ritual healing and placebo administration can advance our understanding of the mechanisms of placebo response. Noting that most of the clinical contexts where placebos are used can be viewed as rituals, Brody proposed a "meaning model" of placebo responding, suggesting that a positive therapeutic response occurs when the patient:

i feels listened to and attended to by the caregiver;

ii receives an explanation of the illness that is consistent with his or her own worldview;

iii feels care and compassion from the helper or healer; and

iv experiences an increased sense of mastery or control over the illness (Brody 2010, p. 161).

Like Frank before him, Brody assumes that shared, culturally grounded notions of illness and healing govern the relationship with the healer. Through enacting and affirming shared ontologies, "the performance of a healing ritual becomes a bodily enactment of reconnection with the community" (Brody 2010, p. 162).

Consistent with contemporary Western notions of psychotherapy, Brody emphasizes the positive effects of supportive, caring, and compassionate emotional relationships. In fact, many forms of traditional healing do not involve much listening, communication, or explicit support to the patient. These modes of healing must mobilize other social processes to facilitate healing. Much ritual healing is aimed not at the suffering individual but at their social and spiritual context. It aims to put right the sociomoral world of the afflicted person, as well as that of his or her family and community (Turner 1977). This may be deemed successful even if the patient continues to be symptomatic.

Brody summarizes his view of placebo as the outcome of medical ritual in this way:

> A simple way of expressing what we know about the placebo response is that the human brain seems to be hard-wired to get better in illness, and that certain sorts of mental stimuli seem capable of turning on this hard-wired system to produce symptom relief. The elements that make up ritual seem to be especially effective in turning on the wiring circuits. (2010, p. 163)

Though deliberately phrased in informal language that makes no claim for scientific precision, it is instructive to consider the implications of Brody's choices of metaphor because similar locutions are common in both mass media and the medical literature. My aim in unpacking Brody's account is not to take him more literally than he intends, but to show how the metaphors in this passage convey certain common assumptions about mind, brain, and personhood that influence the way that both professionals and patients think about placebos. Exposing these assumptions can help us appreciate the sense in which all forms of healing, including placebo use, constitute forms of ritual action.

First, Brody emphasizes an endogenous "hard-wired" healing system or mechanism. Although he uses the singular ("*the* hard-wired system"), clearly there are multiple regulatory systems involved and, in most treatment contexts, multiple systems will be activated and interact to give rise to any observed effects. More significantly, he brackets off the developmental and learning history of these systems by calling them "hard-wired." In describing the effect of these systems, Brody uses grammar that implies it is the brain that gets better.

This metonymic use of the brain for the person is increasingly common in popular and scientific discourse (Vidal 2009). Of course, placebo effects do involve alterations in brain chemistry and function (Benedetti 2011). Generally speaking though, it is not the brain that is afflicted and that gets better in healing but the *person*. This distinction is important because the person is much more than a brain and its regulatory systems. The person includes cognitive processes that are embodied, socially embedded, and enacted, and hence, not reducible to the brain (Kirmayer and Gold 2011). Moreover, it is not simply illness that is modified by ritual healing but *sickness*—that is, the sufferer's social identity as a person with an affliction (Young 1992). This is why healing may be judged successful even when symptoms and disability continue. As well, the stimuli or cues that activate the endogenous healing systems are not strictly "mental" (in the sense of being located in our psychological processes) but also social, and their power and evocativeness derive from larger cultural systems of meaning.

Ritual healing then is not simply a matter of turning on endogenous self-regulatory or healing systems, but an ongoing process of modulation of experience that involves interpersonal interactions that can reinforce or undermine the therapeutic effect. In terms of placebo as ritual healing, this means that the impact of any intervention extends beyond the clinical interaction or the moment of treatment administration to include socially mediated processes of reflection, narration, re-interpretation, and re-evaluation that precede and follow the treatment.

Closer attention to particular systems of healing reveals other commonalities but also distinctive features that may point to unique mechanisms and sources of efficacy. In a recent paper, Kaptchuk (2011) examines the parallels between the healing rituals of Navajo healing, acupuncture, and biomedical treatments. Although these systems of healing differ profoundly in theory and practice, all three involve rituals that invoke positive expectations and engagement, affective experiential warranting of the power and authority of the healer or the treatment, and cognitive perceptual transformations of illness experience. Kaptchuk suggests that healing rituals engender a receptive mode of participation that makes the participant more open to therapeutic suggestion.

The nature of the rituals involved in biomedicine influences the specific processes involved in clinical engagement, warranting of medical power and authority, and therapeutic transformations of experience. Indeed, all three of these functions may be fused in a single medical act or intervention. Naming a disease and prescribing a treatment are interventions that only doctors can perform as a function of their particular social power, status, and authority. This social power, in turn, imbues the acts of diagnosis and treatment with symbolic transformative power. Simply diagnosing or labeling a symptom or illness sets up a whole set of expectations, possibilities, and ways to think about and interpret experience. The consequences depend not only on the patient's own expectations but also on how others respond to the diagnostic label.

The acts of prescribing and taking a pill usually occur in the context of a relationship between patient and physician, and the meaning of that relationship and of the medication itself are embedded in larger cultural systems of meaning and practice (Miller and Kaptchuk 2008). These practices involve social institutions, rules, and norms that give biomedical treatments *performative efficacy*. These same institutions inform self-care (e.g., taking non-prescription medication) that occurs outside the context of a patient–physician relationship and lend that action its cultural meaning and symbolic power.

Rituals are *performative* in the sense of bringing into being specific social states of affairs and, as a by-product, new configurations of the person. Performative speech acts are statements that create the social reality they name as when, for example, a justice of the peace pronounces a man and woman "husband and wife" (Austin 1975; Searle 1995). These rituals work because we all agree that the verbal act—performed by the appropriate authority—transforms the person's social status. Similarly, physicians are assigned a specific type of social authority to make clinical diagnoses and prescribe medications or other types of medical treatment. Prescribing a treatment, whether active or placebo, conveys the message "you are being treated and will get better." However, the transformative effects of a placebo occur not only because the doctor says "this will help" or declares the patient healed but because the patient undergoes cognitive, emotional, and experiential changes in response to contextual cues. The biomedical intervention is usually not a declarative statement (like a faith healer emphatically saying "Now you are healed!") but an implicit suggestion built into an intervention, and reinforced by statements framed as possibilities ("This should make you feel better") or even questions ("Are you starting to feel better yet?"). These forms of suggestion have their own distinct pragmatic linguistic and psychological dynamics.

Ultimately, healing rituals, including the techno-scientific practices of biomedicine, are not abstract performative acts but emotionally engaging social events in which both healer and patient are active. As such, healing involves processes of thinking, feeling, and imagining one's way into new modes of experiencing. A more complete account of the effects of symbolic healing will therefore require theories of the psychophysiology of imagination and enactment, the social psychology of rhetorical persuasion, and the politics and economy of medical practices (Kirmayer 2006, 2014).

8.6 **Implications for clinical epistemology, ethics, and practice**

The perspective on placebos as ritual performance sketched in this chapter has implications for the ways in which placebos are used in current biomedical research and diagnostic situations, as well as for arguments recently advanced for the increased use of placebos in clinical care.

In clinical settings, placebos are sometimes used to support diagnostic claims about the nature of a patient's symptoms or condition (Fässler et al. 2010). A positive response to a placebo is interpreted as evidence that a patient's symptoms and distress are exaggerated, fabricated, or psychogenic in origin. It is, perhaps, not unreasonable to think that in forms of pathology, where beliefs and expectations play a central role (e.g., the vicious circles of a panic attack or hypochondriasis), an intervention that directly targets beliefs and expectations would have great efficacy. Hence, to the extent that giving a placebo creates expectancy effects, we might expect greater responses in such conditions compared to illnesses where cognitive processes appear to play a less central role. For example, those who respond to placebo analgesia are sometimes taken to have had symptoms of psychogenic rather than organic pain—notwithstanding the fact that the distinction between psychogenic and organic has been challenged by pain researchers who find that precisely the same central pathways are involved in pain of diverse origins (Gatchel et al. 2007; Melzack and Katz 2006) and even from words or other social stimuli like interpersonal rejection (Eisenberger and Lieberman 2004; Richter et al. 2010).

The reasoning behind this diagnostic use of placebos is fallacious for several reasons. As discussed earlier (see the section "Varieties of placebo responding"), placebo analgesia is mediated by the same endogenous pain control systems that may be activated in coping with pain of any origin. Moreover, the processes involved in placebo responding occur with biologically active treatments and account for much of their efficacy. The mechanisms of symptom control can be influenced by placebos regardless of the original cause of symptoms or illness. Similar arguments hold for distinguishing "real depression" from milder dysphoria. Hence, the placebo response cannot be used diagnostically to show that an individual's clinical condition is primarily due to psychological or social mechanisms.

The placebo response also cannot be viewed as a neutral baseline in clinical trials against which to measure the effectiveness of interventions because, like any "active" agent or treatment, it is also responsive to many contextual factors involved in clinical trials. As a result, the mechanisms of placebo response overlap and interact with the unique mechanisms of efficacy of the intervention. At the same time, the clinical experimental context of the randomized clinical trial is a fraught situation that engenders complex expectancies of its own. People may hope they are receiving active treatment but must contend with the possibility they are not (Kaptchuk et al. 2009). They thus may experience some mitigation of the benefit that might be achieved if they were confident they were receiving the best possible treatment. In contemporary biomedical research and clinical settings, where risk and benefits are presented probabilistically, people must judge the likelihood that will get benefit. Individuals may respond differently to these complex communications. In a randomized trial, some participants may have diminished expectations due to the possibility of receiving an ineffective treatment; others may convince themselves that they are receiving active treatment (Rutherford and Roose 2013).

The recognition that placebos "really work" might encourage their deliberate use in medical care. However, giving a biologically inactive treatment while claiming it is active constitutes a type of deception. Recently, Foddy (2009) and others (e.g., Gold and Lichtenberg 2014) have argued for the deceptive use of placebos when they would have a stronger beneficial effect than other available treatments. These authors are able to advance this argument because they adopt a minimalist view of the practice of medicine in which the physician is a technician applying a one-off treatment. However, medicine involves building therapeutic relationships with the clinician and with the healthcare system as a whole. It is these trusting relationships and institutions that the patient will count on for help in the future.

Arguments for the benefits of the deceptive use of placebos in medical care tend to be based on a narrow, instrumental view of the doctor–patient relationship as well as limited understanding of the nature of placebo responding. The clinical encounter involves dimensions of empathic recognition, relationship building, trust, education, and advocacy that may contribute to the efficacy of any treatment intervention, including placebos (Benedetti 2011). To explore these dimensions of care, Kaptchuk and colleagues developed a paradigm for decomposing elements of the placebo response, comparing, for example, sham acupuncture with and without various ritual components of treatment (e.g., a warm and attentive interaction with the practitioner) (Kaptchuk et al. 2008; Kelley et al. 2009). Each element added something to the effectiveness of a treatment, with a warm and supportive patient–practitioner relationship probably accounting for the largest single component. This observation has important implications for the potential use of placebos in clinical care. If the clinician–patient relationship is actually the most powerful component of a placebo response, protecting and preserving the relationship is crucial, and bad faith may ultimately destroy the positive effect. Of course, it is possible to have a lot of faith in a warm and personable or authoritative and rhetorically powerful charlatan and, indeed, go to one's grave secure in the illusion one is being well cared for. However, the widespread deceptive use of placebos would alter the nature of the doctor–patient relationship and of medical institutions more broadly.

Lying, subterfuge, and misrepresentation are corrosive to trust in individuals and institutions. Discovering that the doctor "lied" will damage future collaboration (both with this doctor and with others, by association). Indeed, if it was widely known that doctors give placebos deceptively, then the effectiveness of every existing treatment might be reduced since people could always suspect they were receiving an "ineffective" treatment. If patients knew that it was always a possibility that they were being given placebos, this might erode the efficacy of treatments in general (but see Martin and Katz 2010), as well as undermining confidence in the trustworthiness of doctors and in the reliability of the institution of medicine as a whole. In the end, any analysis of the effects of deception that remains at the level of the individual is inadequate because medicine is also a social institution: healthcare contributes to the fabric of civil society. Knowing that doctors in general may lie would damage trust in individual physicians, in the whole institution of medicine, and, potentially, also in broader social institutions that underwrite medical care.

The arguments in favor of the deceptive use of placebos may be moot, however, because, in fact, placebos demonstrably *do not* depend on deception (Kaptchuk et al. 2010). Moreover, there are ways to openly prescribe placebos and strengthen their effects without engaging in deception. For example, referring to the "power of the mind" is both a plausible and culturally consonant non-deceptive explanation of a placebo effect that is, in fact, reinforced in certain cultural and religious contexts.

In summary, the meaning and context effects that underlie placebo responding are important components in any effective medical treatment. Giving people positive expectations, realistic hope, and optimism is crucial both for strengthening the healing relationship and ensuring treatment efficacy. Prescribing the best effective treatment will also maximize placebo effects, strengthen expectations, and increase the potential for positive responding in the future. However, there is no ethical or pragmatic justification for the use of subterfuge or deceit in the delivery of placebos because the much the same beneficial effects can be achieved by truthful communication that also strengthens and maintains a working alliance and confidence in the healthcare system.

8.7 **Conclusion: embodiment, enactment, and the rhetorics of healing**

The idea of placebos is a biomedical construction because it is only in the disenchanted world of biomedicine that the therapeutic effectiveness of words, symbols, and rituals are viewed as suspect. When only direct chemical or physical effects are recognized as causal agents, then the power of symbolic interventions requires special explanations. However, placebo effects are ubiquitous and intrinsic to all healing practices. Placebo research has clearly shown that symbolic stimuli and positive expectations set in motion specific physiological processes that mediate a wide range of therapeutic responses. These mechanisms vary according to the type of symbolic stimulus or context and the resultant expectations. For example, under specific circumstances, symbolic interventions may activate endogenous opioid pain control systems to produce analgesia, dopaminergic reward systems to produce elevated mood, and immunological responses to reinforce host resistance to infection.

The term "placebo" names a social situation not a substance. Placebo responding reflects the ways that people think, act, feel, and respond physiologically to an intervention they believe and expect will be of help. Defined in this way, placebo responses clearly are based on individuals' psychological processes of belief, expectation, trust, and conviction. However, these processes are complex and only partially dependent on individuals' cognitive models or explanations of illness and healing. Health beliefs and treatment expectations may follow from bodily experiences, actions, and commitments that are socially embedded and enacted. Indeed, these same processes of embodiment and enactment may give rise to placebo responses in the absence of explicit beliefs and conscious expectations (Kirmayer 2003).

A view of biomedical treatment as ritual healing leads us toward a model that bridges the psychological view of placebo responding as based on endogenous healing mechanisms and the social view that focuses on the ways in which placebo responses are mediated by cultural models of affliction and healing. These two views can be integrated through theories metaphor and communicative action that link embodied experience and social discourse. The mechanisms of ritual healing involve both *sociopsychological* (persuasive, rhetorical) and *psychophysiological* processes of imaginative enactment. Unpacking the mechanisms that subserve these processes can provide the basis for an integrative theory of symbolic healing that includes the many varieties of placebo response alongside the social, psychological, and biological processes that accompany every biomedical intervention.

Acknowledgments

An earlier version of this chapter appears as: Laurence J. Kirmayer, Unpacking the placebo response: insights from ethnographic studies of healing, *The Journal of Mind–Body Regulation*, 1 (3), pp. 112–124, © The Authors, 2011.

I thank Amir Raz and Cory Harris for the workshop and creative exchanges that informed this essay.

Notes

1 Expectations may follow not just from verbal instructions but from every aspect of the placebo. For example, the color, size, and shape of pills can influence the placebo response and there may be some cultural regularities in the metaphoric connotations of specific stimuli. Surprisingly, this fact sometimes often seems to be ignored not only by clinicians but also by pharmaceutical companies (Khan et al. 2010).

2 Of course, the difference between "open" and "hidden" administration is not clear-cut because, for both ethical and pragmatic reasons, people usually know they are in a situation where this may happen. Similarly, participants in placebo trials know there is some probability that they may receive active treatment (Rutherford and Roose 2013). They also may be able to detect whether they are receiving active medication based on sensory cues. While this can be controlled for by debriefing and post-hoc statistical analysis, it reflects an important set of issues related to the ways that cultural systems—in this case, the instrumental rationality of modernity—influence individuals' attention to the body and interpretation of sensations, symptoms, and clinical interventions.

3 The etymology of the word "empathy," from the German *einfühlung*, stems from this experience of aesthetic absorption.

References

Ader, R. (1997). The role of conditioning in pharmacotherapy. In: *The placebo effect: an interdisciplinary exploration* (ed. A. Harrington). Cambridge, MA: Harvard University Press, pp. 138–165.

Amanzio, M., Pollo, A., Maggi, G., and Benedetti, F. (2001). Response variability to analgesics: a role for non-specific activation of endogenous opioids. *Pain*, **90**, 205–215.

Austin, J. L. (1975). *How to do things with words*. Cambridge, MA: Harvard University Press.

Barsalou, L. W. (2008). Grounded cognition. *Annual Review of Psychology*, **59**, 617–645.

Benedetti, F. (2008). Mechanisms of placebo and placebo-related effects across diseases and treatments. *Annual Review of Pharmacology and Toxicology*, **48**, 33–60.

Benedetti, F. (2009). *Placebo effects: understanding the mechanisms in health and disease*. Oxford: Oxford University Press.

Benedetti, F. (2010). *The patient's brain: the neuroscience behind the doctor–patient relationship*. New York, NY: Oxford University Press.

Benedetti, F., Carlino, E., and Pollo, A. (2011). How placebos change the patient's brain. *Neuropsychopharmacology*, **36**(1), 339–354.

Brody, H. (2010). Ritual, medicine and the placebo response. In: *The problem of ritual efficacy* (eds. W. S. Sax, J. Quack, and J. Weinhold). Oxford: Oxford University Press, pp. 151–167.

Cioffi, D. (1991). Beyond attentional strategies: cognitive-perceptual model of somatic interpretation. *Psychological Bulletin*, **109**(1), 25–41.

Colloca, L. and Benedetti, F. (2009). Placebo analgesia induced by social observational learning. *Pain*, **144**(1–2), 28–34.

Csordas, T. J. and Lewton, E. (1998). Practice, performance, and experience in ritual healing. *Transcultural Psychiatry*, **35**(4), 435–512.

Dandeneau, S. D., Baldwin, M. W., Baccus, J. R., Sakellaropoulo, M., and Pruessner, J. C. (2007). Cutting stress off at the pass: reducing vigilance and responsiveness to social threat by manipulating attention. *Journal of Personality and Social Psychology*, **93**(4), 651–666. DOI: 10.1037/0022-3514.93.4.651

de Figueiredo, J. M. and Gostoli, S. (2013). Culture and demoralization in psychotherapy. *Advances in Psychosomatic Medicine*, **33**, 75–87.

Dow, J. (1986). Universal aspects of symbolic healing: a theoretical synthesis. *American Anthropologist*, **88**, 56–69.

Eisenberger, N. I. and Lieberman, M. D. (2004). Why rejection hurts: a common neural alarm system for physical and social pain. *Trends in Cognitive Sciences*, **8**(7), 294–300.

Ernst, E. and Resch, K. L. (1995). Concept of true and perceived placebo effects. *British Medical Journal*, **311**(7004), 551–553.

Fässler, M., Meissner, K., Schneider, A., and Linde, K. (2010). Frequency and circumstances of placebo use in clinical practice: a systematic review of empirical studies. *BMC Medicine*, **8**, 15.

Finniss, D. G., Kaptchuk, T. J., Miller, F., and Benedetti, F. (2010). Biological, clinical, and ethical advances of placebo effects. *Lancet*, **375**(9715), 686–695.

Flaten, M. A., Aslaksen, P. M., Lyby, P. S., and Bjorkedal, E. (2011). The relation of emotions to placebo responses. *Philosophical Transactions of the Royal Society of London: Series B, Biological Sciences*, **366**(1572), 1818–1827.

Foddy, B. (2009). A duty to deceive: placebos in clinical practice. *American Journal of Bioethics*, **9**(12), 4–12.

Frank, J. D. (1961). *Persuasion and healing: a comparative study of psychotherapy*. Baltimore: Johns Hopkins Press.

Frank, J. D. (1995). Psychotherapy as rhetoric: some implications. *Clinical Psychology-Science and Practice*, **2**(1), 90–93.

Frank, J. D. and Frank, J. B. (1991). *Persuasion and healing: a comparative study of psychotherapy*. Baltimore: Johns Hopkins University Press.

Frenkel, O. (2008). A phenomenology of the "placebo effect": taking meaning from the mind to the body. *Journal of Medicine and Philosophy*, **33**(1), 58–79.

Gatchel, R. J., Peng, Y. B., Peters, M. L., Fuchs, P. N., and Turk, D. C. (2007). The biopsychosocial approach to chronic pain: scientific advances and future directions. *Psychological Bulletin*, **133**(4), 581–624.

Geers, A. L., Helfer, S. G., Weiland, P. E., and Kosbab, K. (2006). Expectations and placebo response: a laboratory investigation into the role of somatic focus. *Journal of Behavioral Medicine*, **29**(2), 171–178.

Geers, A. L., Weiland, P. E., Kosbab, K., Landry, S. J., and Helfer, S. G. (2005). Goal activation, expectations, and the placebo effect. *Journal of Personality and Social Psychology*, 89(2), 143–159.

Geers, A. L., Wellman, J. A., Fowler, S. L., Rasinski, H. M., and Helfer, S. G. (2011). Placebo expectations and the detection of somatic information. *Journal of Behavioral Medicine*, 34(3), 208–217.

Gibbs, R. W. (2006). *Embodiment and cognitive science.* New York: Cambridge University Press.

Gold, A. and Lichtenberg, P. (2014). The moral case for the clinical placebo. *Journal of Medical Ethics.* DOI: 10.1136/medethics-2012-101314, 40, 219–224.

Harrington, A. (2006). The many meanings of the placebo effect: where they came from, why they matter. *BioSocieties*, 1, 181–193.

Hinton, D. E., Howes, D., and Kirmayer, L. J. (2008). Toward a medical anthropology of sensations: definitions and research agenda. *Transcultural Psychiatry*, 45(2), 142–162.

Hrobjartsson, A., Kaptchuk, T. J., and Miller, F. G. (2011). Placebo effect studies are susceptible to response bias and to other types of biases. *Journal of Clinical Epidemiology*, 64(11), 1223–1229.

Hyland, M. E. and Whalley, B. (2008). Motivational concordance: an important mechanism in self-help therapeutic rituals involving inert (placebo) substances. *Journal of Psychosomatic Research*, 65(5), 405–413.

Kapferer, B. (2005). Ritual dynamics and virtual practice: beyond representation and meaning. In: *Ritual in its own right* (eds. D. Handelman and G. Lindquist). New York: Berghahn Books, pp. 35–54.

Kapferer, B. and Papigny, G. (2005). *Tovil: exorcism & healing rites.* Negombo: Viator Publications.

Kaptchuk, T. J. (2011). Placebo studies and ritual theory: a comparative analysis of Navajo, acupuncture and biomedical healing. *Philosophical Transactions of the Royal Society of London: Series B, Biological Sciences*, 366(1572), 1849–1858.

Kaptchuk, T. J. and Eisenberg, D. M. (1998). The persuasive appeal of alternative medicine. *Annals of Internal Medicine*, 129, 1061–1065.

Kaptchuk, T. J., Friedlander, E., Kelley, J. M., et al. (2010). Placebos without deception: a randomized controlled trial in irritable bowel syndrome. *PLoS One*, 5(12), e15591.

Kaptchuk, T. J., Kelley, J. M., Conboy, L. A., et al. (2008). Components of placebo effect: randomised controlled trial in patients with irritable bowel syndrome. *British Medical Journal*, 336(7651), 999–1003.

Kaptchuk, T. J., Shaw, J., Kerr, C. E., et al. (2009). "Maybe I made up the whole thing": placebos and patients' experiences in a randomized controlled trial. *Culture, Medicine and Psychiatry*, 33(3), 382–411.

Kelley, J. M., Lembo, A. J., Ablon, J. S., Villanueva, J. J., Conboy, L. A., Levy, R., et al. (2009). Patient and practitioner influences on the placebo effect in irritable bowel syndrome. *Psychosomatic Medicine*, 71(7), 789–797.

Khan, A., Bomminayuni, E. P., Bhat, A., Faucett, J., and Brown, W. A. (2010). Are the colors and shapes of current psychotropics designed to maximize the placebo response? *Psychopharmacology*, 211(1), 113–122.

Kirmayer, L. J. (1993). Healing and the invention of metaphor: the effectiveness of symbols revisited. *Culture, Medicine and Psychiatry*, **17**(2), 161–195.

Kirmayer, L. J. (2003). Reflections on embodiment. In: *Social and cultural lives of immune systems* (ed. J. Wilce). New York: Routledge, pp. 282–302.

Kirmayer, L. J. (2004). The cultural diversity of healing: meaning, metaphor and mechanism. *British Medical Bulletin*, **69**(1), 33–48.

Kirmayer, L. J. (2006). Toward a medicine of the imagination. *New Literary History*, **37**(3), 583–605.

Kirmayer, L. J. (2007). Psychotherapy and the cultural concept of the person. *Transcultural Psychiatry*, **44**(2), 232–257.

Kirmayer, L. J. (2008). Culture and the metaphoric mediation of pain. *Transcultural Psychiatry*, **45**(2), 318–338.

Kirmayer, L. J. (2014). Medicines of the imagination: cultural phenomenology, medical pluralism and the persistence of mind–body dualism. In: *Asymmetrical conversations: contestations, circumventions and the blurring of therapeutic boundaries* (eds. H. Naraindas, J. Quack, and W. S. Sax). London: Berghahn, pp. 26–55.

Kirmayer, L. J. and Gold, I. (2011). Re-socializing psychiatry: critical neuroscience and the limits of reductionism. In: *Critical neuroscience: a handbook of the social and cultural contexts of neuroscience* (eds. S. Choudhury and J. Slaby). Oxford: Blackwell.

Kirmayer, L. J. and Jarvis, G. E. (2005). Depression across cultures. In: *Textbook of mood disorders* (eds. D. Stein, A. Schatzberg, and D. Kupfer). Washington: American Psychiatric Press, pp. 611–629.

Kirmayer, L. J. and Sartorius, N. (2007). Cultural models and somatic syndromes. *Psychosomatic Medicine*, **69**(9), 832–840.

Kirsch, I. (2004). Conditioning, expectancy, and the placebo effect: comment on Stewart-Williams and Podd (2004). *Psychological Bulletin*, **130**(2), 341–343, discussion 344–345.

Kleinman, A. M. (1980). *Patients and healers in the context of culture*. Berkeley: University of California Press.

Lee, B. O., Kirmayer, L. J., and Groleau, D. (2010). Therapeutic processes and perceived helpfulness of dang-ki (Chinese shamanism) from the symbolic healing perspective. *Culture, Medicine and Psychiatry*, **34**(1), 56–105.

Lévi-Strauss, C. (1967). The effectiveness of symbols. In: Structural Anthropology. New York: Basic Books.

Levine, J. D., Gordon, N. C., and Fields, H. L. (1978). The mechanism of placebo analgesia. *Lancet*, **23**, 654–657.

Linde, K., Fässler, M., and Meissner, K. (2011). Placebo interventions, placebo effects and clinical practice. *Philosophical Transactions of the Royal Society of London: Series B, Biological Sciences*, **366**(1572), 1905–1912.

Martin, A. L. and Katz, J. (2010). Inclusion of authorized deception in the informed consent process does not affect the magnitude of the placebo effect for experimentally induced pain. *Pain*, **149**(2), 208–215.

Meissner, K. (2011). The placebo effect and the autonomic nervous system: evidence for an intimate relationship. *Philosophical Transactions of the Royal Society of London: Series B, Biological Sciences*, **366**(1572), 1808–1817.

Melzack, R. and Katz, J. (2006). Pain in the 21st century: the neuromatrix and beyond. In: *Psychological knowledge in court* (eds. G. D. Young, A. W. Kane, and K. Nicholson). New York: Springer, pp. 129–148.

Miller, F. G. and Kaptchuk, T. J. (2008). The power of context: reconceptualizing the placebo effect. *Journal of the Royal Society of Medicine*, **101**(5), 222–225.

Moerman, D. E. (2002). *Meaning, medicine, and the "placebo effect."* New York: Cambridge University Press.

Murray, D. and Stoessel, A. J. (2013). Mechanisms and therapeutic implications of the placebo effect in neurological and psychiatric conditions. *Pharmacology and Therapeutics*, **140**(3), 306–318.

Myers, W. B. (2010). The placebo as performance: speaking across domains of healing. *Qualitative Health Research*, **20**(9), 1295–1303.

Pennebaker, J. W. (1982). *The psychology of physical symptoms.* New York: Springer.

Petrovic, P., Kalso, E., Petersson, K. M., Andersson, J., Fransson, P., and Ingvar, M. (2010). A prefrontal non-opioid mechanism in placebo analgesia. *Pain*, **150**(1), 59–65.

Pollo, A., Carlino, E., and Benedetti, F. (2011). Placebo mechanisms across different conditions: from the clinical setting to physical performance. *Philosophical Transactions of the Royal Society of London: Series B, Biological Sciences*, **366**(1572), 1790–1798.

Price, D. D., Finniss, D. G., and Benedetti, F. (2008). A comprehensive review of the placebo effect: recent advances and current thought. *Annual Review of Psychology*, **59**, 565–590.

Raz, A. (2007). Hypnobo: perspectives on hypnosis and placebo. *The American Journal of Clinical Hypnosis*, **50**(1), 29–36.

Raz, A. and Buhle, J. (2006). Typologies of attentional networks. *Nature Reviews Neuroscience*, **7**(5), 367–379.

Richter, M., Eck, J., Straube, T., Miltner, W. H., and Weiss, T. (2010). Do words hurt? Brain activation during the processing of pain-related words. *Pain*, **148**(2), 198–205.

Rutchick, A. M. and Slepian, M. L. (2013). Handling ibuprofen increases pain tolerance and decreases perceived pain intensity in a cold pressor test. *PLoS One*, **8**, e56175. DOI: 10.1371/journal.pone.0056175

Rutherford, B. R. and Roose, S. P. (2013). A model of placebo response in antidepressant clinical trials. *American Journal of Psychiatry*, **170**(7), 723–733. DOI: 10.1176/appi.ajp.2012.12040474

Scheff, T. J. (1979). *Catharsis in healing, ritual, and drama.* Berkeley, CA: University of California Press.

Searle, J. R. (1995). *The construction of social reality.* New York: Free Press.

Sherzer, J. (1983). *Kuna Ways of Speaking: An Ethnographic Perspective.* Austin: University of Texas Press.

Siegel, S. (2002). Explanatory mechanisms for placebo effects—Pavlovian conditioning. In: (Eds.), *The science of the placebo: toward an interdisciplinary research agenda* (eds. H. A. Guess, A. Kleinman, J. W. Kusek, and L. W. Engle). London: BMJ Books, pp. 133–157.

Stern, J., Candia, V., Porchet, R. I., et al. (2011). Placebo-mediated, naloxone-sensitive suggestibility of short-term memory performance. *Neurobiology of Learning and Memory*, **95**(3), 326–334.

Stewart-Williams, S. and Podd, J. (2004). The placebo effect: dissolving the expectancy versus conditioning debate. *Psychological Bulletin*, **130**(2), 324–340.

Thompson, J. J., Ritenbaugh, C., and Nichter, M. (2009). Reconsidering the placebo response from a broad anthropological perspective. *Culture, Medicine and Psychiatry*, **33**(1), 112–152.

Turner, V. W. (1977). *The ritual process: structure and anti-structure*. Ithaca, NY: Cornell University Press.

Vidal, F. (2009). Brainhood, anthropological figure of modernity. *History of the Human Sciences*, **22**(1), 5–36.

Wadlinger, H. A. and Isaacowitz, D. M. (2011). Fixing our focus: training attention to regulate emotion. *Personality and Social Psychology Review*, **15**(1), 75–102.

Waldram, J. B. (ed.). (2008). *Aboriginal healing in Canada: studies in therapeutic meaning and practice*. Ottawa: Aboriginal Healing Foundation.

Wickramasekera, I. (1980). A conditioned response model of the placebo effect: predictions from the model. *Biofeedback and Self-Regulation*, **5**(1), 5–18.

Young, A. (1992). The anthropologies of illness and sickness. *Annual Review of Anthropology*, **11**, 257–285.

Young, A. (1988). Unpacking the demoralization thesis. *Medical Anthropology Quarterly*, **2**(1), 3–16.

Chapter 9

Pills in a pretty box: social sources of the placebo effect

Stewart Justman

9.1 **The influence of others**

Imagine consuming tonic water in the belief that it is vodka and tonic. As suggested by many authors in this volume, you might well experience some of the ordinary—that is, expected—effects of vodka. Now, however, enliven this scenario and imagine yourself at a gathering with a dozen others also drinking tonic water in the belief that it contains alcohol. Once again, you seem to sense the effects of alcohol coming on, but in this case they are the product not of your expectation alone but one held implicitly by everyone present. A degree of intoxication follows. With your belief in the beverage mirrored by the beliefs of others, the situation itself acts as a kind of intoxicant. If the tonic water can be considered a placebo, its action in this instance is fueled by the setting in which it operates. Rarely in the literature, however, is the social dimension of the placebo effect noted.

The literature does document that not only the content but even the size and color of pills contribute to their experienced effects. Yet colors have a social component—witness the finding that "people taking red or pink placebo pills tend to feel stimulated, and those taking blue pills tend to feel more sedated, regardless of active ingredients" (Barrett et al. 2006, p. 184), a result replicated many times (see Chapter 6 for a similar example). One doubts these reported experiences trace back in each and every case to the pill-taker's history with red and blue pills respectively. As Moerman explains in Chapter 7, these colors take on certain associations derived from the world around us: red with fire, passion, energy ("red hot"); blue with coolness, languor, melancholy ("the blues"). Moreover, the original experiment with pink and blue placebos was complicated with social factors that seem to have passed unnoticed in the literature. Though blue is no more strongly associated with sedation than red with passion, the "blue" reaction was much stronger, possibly because responses were measured after the medical students who served as the study subjects sat through an hour-long lecture (Blackwell et al. 1972). Not only can a lecture act as a sedative in itself, but the drowsiness of some audience members can readily pass to others. As in the case of a social gathering with misconstrued tonic water, the placebo effect operates here in a social medium—in the first instance a lecture theater, but secondarily a world we all inhabit in which even colors have connotations.

Though the meaning of a color may be a curiosity, the social contribution to placebo effects in medicine is far more. Unless we were under the belief that a medication has helped others like ourselves, we would be less likely to expect good things of it, which is why placebo effects are "smaller when patients are told their treatment might be a placebo, as is routinely done in clinical trials, and . . . larger when people are told that their treatment has been shown to be powerful" (Kirsch 2010, p. 110). It is also why doctors used to, and perhaps still, say things like, "I'm going to have you get some B-12 injections. They have helped many other patients, but I cannot explain to you why they work and I cannot promise you they will work. I can simply say that many patients tell me they feel better and stronger after such a course of therapy" (Spiro 1986, p. 1), thereby arousing an expectation that the patient will enjoy the same benefits enjoyed by others. (On the prescription of B-vitamins for placebo purposes in Denmark, see Hróbjartsson and Norup 2003.) However, while few at this point would deny that the rites and props of medicine are significant in their own right and have considerable placebo potential, it would be a mistake to assume that a social force can be monopolized and administered by doctors. Advertisements choreographing the message that this or that medication or quasi-medication has "helped many other patients" are now ubiquitous in the United States—a point that has a bearing, surely, on this volume's frequently discussed question of antidepressants.

In discussions of antidepressants it is sometimes overlooked that one who takes them does so in tandem with untold millions of others, as if swept up in a common wave. Indeed, within three years of the Food and Drug Administration (FDA) approving direct-to-consumer advertising in 1997, antidepressants were the best-selling class of drugs in the United States (Horwitz and Wakefield 2007). Clearly, advertising has had something to do with the triumph of these wonder-drugs whose actual performance compares so unimpressively with placebo in clinical trials. Aside from their specific content, though, the mere fact of the ads was significant, announcing as it did that the time had come for depression to step out of the shadows and into the light of public notice, medical legitimacy, and hope.

The basic message of antidepressant advertising may be, therefore, that it is no longer necessary to be depressed about being depressed, as Irving Kirsch puts it in Chapter 2; the downward spiral can be broken. Precisely in addressing itself to a mass audience, advertising for antidepressants also reminds the depressed, in the strongest way, that they are not alone; and as a medical commentator on the placebo effect reminds us, misery loves company (Spiro 1997). If the knowledge that others benefit from the treatment we are taking is known to boost the placebo effect, this principle can hardly be confined to the doctor's office or the clinical trial. The folklore surrounding antidepressants since the advent of Prozac; the scientific ring of the theory of chemical imbalance; the power of the corporations behind the pills; the morale-building effect generated by the "social movement" that the cause of depression has become (Horwitz and Wakefield 2007, p. 26); the resonant message that it is no longer necessary to suffer in silence; the assurance that multitudes of others seem to find antidepressants beneficial—all such factors contribute their share to a placebo effect that cannot be reduced to the expectation of a patient in a social vacuum like those engineered in many studies where placebos serve either as controls or the target of research.

Antidepressants themselves are the product of a constellation of conditions, notable among them the introduction of diagnostic criteria in the 1980 edition of the *Diagnostic and statistical manual* at once "medical" enough to drive pharmaceutical research and justify insurance coverage, yet loose enough to allow for the massive expansion of the population diagnosed with depression (Horwitz and Wakefield 2007). With the incidence of depression fueled not only by depression per se but by "normal sadness," and with the opportunistic marketing of antidepressants that were offspring of circumstance in their own right, little wonder that depression shows itself responsive to a socially mediated placebo effect.

9.2 **The placebo effect: early investigations**

As it happens, the original research on the placebo effect (though it did not yet have that name) was in connection with a movement sensational enough to alter the bodily sensations of many who came within its orbit. The movement was Mesmerism. The fascination of France in the latter years of the pre-revolutionary era, Mesmerism was the brainchild of a medical doctor convinced that a physical but ethereal fluid called animal magnetism suffused the universe and that ailments were caused by blockages of this power in the human body, which could be cleared by his ministrations. Students of the placebo effect remind us of the ritualized or theatrical nature of the medical encounter. Mesmer was a theatrical virtuoso. Employing costume (lilac robes), sound effects (the tones of a glass harmonica, whose ethereality spoke for that of the universe), and impressive props such as magnetic tubs, he staged healing sessions that were charged occasions in themselves, so much so that attendees were thrown into cathartic "crises." "As a master of manipulation, Mesmer surely recognized the social value of treatment in groups—both the reinforcing effect of numerous crises and the simple value of conviviality in spreading any vogue as a joint social event and medical cure" (Gould 1992, pp. 185–86).

That Mesmer's subjects were in touch with each other—physically in his sessions and figuratively through the written and oral reports surrounding the Mesmer movement—is of the essence. Intensity flowed from person to person. It was the energy animating the movement, the heightened, almost sexual interest it provoked, that accounts for the sensations felt by those under its influence—sensations they attributed to a theorized magnetism that does not exist. "Men, women, children, everyone is involved, everyone mesmerizes," observed a commentator at the time (Darnton 1968, p. 40), much as if everyone were mesmerized by everyone else. As the atmosphere of my non-alcoholic get-together acts as an intoxicant in its own right, so the phenomenon of Mesmerism was itself highly magnetic. Indeed, the universal power that Mesmerism claimed to tap—one flowing through us whether we know it or not—resembles nothing so much as the power of example, which as the incomparable literary critic Dr. Johnson observed in 1750, "is so great as to . . . produce effects almost without the intervention of the will" (Johnson 1750, Rambler no. 4). Johnson's estimate of the power of human models over the imagination reads almost like a description of hypnotism, an eventual outgrowth of Mesmerism.

By an irony of history, the glass harmonica that provided the aural atmosphere for the maestro's performances was invented by the man who presided over the refutation of Mesmerism. In 1784, the King of France commissioned a distinguished panel, chaired by Benjamin Franklin, to investigate the suspect phenomenon—suspect less because of its claim to scientific legitimacy, perhaps, than because of the suggestive physical drama it licensed, the utopianism of its rhetoric, and the not-so-secret societies it spawned. Working in his gardens outside Paris, Franklin and his fellow experimenters, including Lavoisier, tested whether subjects could actually tell the difference between water magnetized à la Mesmer and ordinary water, or could tell, indeed, whether they themselves had been magnetized while blindfolded. They could not. Franklin and his fellows concluded that animal magnetism had no physical existence. As reported to the Academy of Sciences in September of that year, the investigators

> discovered we could influence [blindfolded subjects] ourselves so that their answers were the same, whether they had been magnetized or not. This means we were dealing now with the power of the imagination . . . We succeeded in manipulating the

> imagination. Without being touched or signaled, the subjects who thought themselves
> magnetized felt pain, felt heat, a very great heat. In some cases, we provoked convul-
> sions and what is known as crises. The subjects' imagination could be brought to the
> point of the loss of speech. It allowed us to produce all the so-called effects of magnet-
> ism, even the calming down of convulsions. (Lopez 1993, p. 329)

The experiments in Franklin's garden were as elegant as they were conclusive. However, precisely because they were conducted elegantly, they could not capture the social energy charging the phenomenon of Mesmerism—the general fascination and impassioned chatter surrounding the movement, the reports of crises and convulsions that fed into the very behavior witnessed by the experimenters. Neither a tree nor water could be magnetized, but Mesmer's followers could still be magnetized to one another. The refutation of Mesmerism was precedent-setting not only in the sense that it inspired similar experiments in England and indeed laid the groundwork for modern clinical research, but in that its studied exclusion of the forces behind the Mesmer movement anticipates the neglect of social forces in placebo literature to this day.

A few years after Mesmerism went into eclipse with the onset of the Revolution, another medical craze broke out—this time in the United States, and secondarily in England—in which bodily ailments were treated by channeling a theorized elemental fluid, in this case labeled "animal electricity." As a result of haphazard trials, apparent successes, and diligent salesmanship, the idea caught on that certain patented metal rods, known as tractors (for their power to draw things from the body), were capable of curing everything from ordinary aches and pains to epilepsy if simply passed over the subject. Invented by the physician Elisha Perkins, the tractors were championed after his death by his son Benjamin, who indignantly denied that their operation bore any similarity to Mesmerism, which he regarded as pure charlatanism. However, while the Perkins tractor was wrapped in republican simplicity and Mesmerism in exotic charisma, these were clearly kindred phenomena. Not only was Perkins' rod, like Mesmer's, wielded like a wand, but both evoked the imagery of the lightning rod, and both were said to be in touch with a physical force too profound and subtle for ordinary perception. More fundamentally, and in contrast to a medical treatment said to be specific, both therapies addressed themselves to humanity in general and to ailments of all kinds. Both presumed that a single force is at work in all bodies, somehow responsible for well-being or illness, and both activated this presumption of universality by inviting those in search of healing to experience the same thing that many others had already experienced.

In the case of the Perkins tractor, the invitation to feel what others feel was all but explicit. Where Mesmerism drew followers as though socially magnetic,

Benjamin Perkins attracted interest in the tractor by citing the reports of respected persons one after another, all documenting the sort of benefits to be had by anyone who might use it. When it was Perkins' turn to be exposed as a sham, the principal investigator—John Haygarth of Bath (1740–1827), a physician of skeptical mind trained at Edinburgh under a friend of Hume—turned the social mechanism of the Perkins movement against itself with a deftness worthy of Franklin. Before treating a number of patients with wooden tractors made to look indistinguishable from the genuine, patented article, Haygarth and his confederates made sure to tell study subjects of the cures wrought by the Perkins tractor in many other cases. Most subjects promptly reported the sort of sensations that animal electricity might be supposed to produce, even though the only electricity at work was the social electricity of the Perkins movement (Justman 2011).

9.3 **Contemporary applications**

Replicating Haygarth's experiment, a colleague told a patient in the nearby Bristol Infirmary "that I had an instrument in my pocket which had been very serviceable to many in his state," (Haygarth 1800, p. 7), an equivocation no doubt accompanied with a secret laugh. Surprisingly, some placebo researchers now contend in all seriousness that statements of this kind—for example, "The agent you have just been given is known to significantly reduce pain in some patients" (Vase et al. 2003, p. 19)—are not really deceptive and that the use of placebos is therefore potentially compatible with ethical medical practice. In a groundbreaking placebo experiment where both disguise and equivocation were explicitly abandoned, subjects were still told emphatically that others had benefited from the sugar-pill-like treatment they received (Kaptchuk et al. 2010). Presumably, however, those others, who after all were not participants in an open-placebo experiment, found the treatment beneficial because they believed it was not a sugar pill. It would be interesting to compare the responses of subjects told that their inert treatment has proven beneficial to others and subjects told only that their treatment is inert but may benefit them.

It is not only in its use of artful language that Haygarth's exposé of a now-forgotten medical craze continues to resonate.

Among the powerful disclosures of Irving Kirsch's *The emperor's new drugs* (2010), perhaps none was more so than his discovery that in most trials of antidepressants filed with the FDA, the drug failed to outperform placebo. Because American law does not compel the publication of these failures and a manufacturer is required to show only that a drug outstrips placebo in two trials, the negative trials are simply buried. In Haygarth's time, the practice of disregarding failures in estimates of efficacy seems to have been common— common enough, anyway, for him and his associates to censure it (Tröhler 2000). In granting that the Perkins tractor was successful in some cases (though not by virtue of its composition), Haygarth does not concede its merit but completes his indictment of it, showing that these successes imply the concealment of failure. "The cases which have been published [by Perkins] are selected from many which were unsuccessful, and passed over in silence" (Haygarth 1800, p. 5).

On other grounds, too, the antidepressant phenomenon of our day recalls an exploded medical fashion. As Irving Kirsch demonstrates in this volume (Chapter 2), antidepressants have such competing, indeed contradictory, modes of chemical action that it is impossible that they actually work as advertised. To a true believer, however, how a drug works does not matter, only that it works (and precisely as placebos, antidepressants do work). The same was said about the Perkins tractor by its promoter—exactly how it worked was a mystery best left to the Author of the Universe, but that it worked was an undeniable fact.

> We frequently hear men, whose wisdom is perhaps confined to their significant looks and manner of expression, observe, on a relation of any newly discovered phenomena, that "These things *cannot* be: I know of no principle, or possible operation in nature, by which such effects can be produced." As if the great Creator of the Universe had made no laws relating to the economy of nature, which had not been communicated to them, and familiarized to their understandings. I shall take the liberty to observe, as a well known fact, that mere hypothetical reasoning, unaccompanied by experiment, never accurately investigated the properties of any medicine, or predetermined its effects upon the human body. (Perkins 1798, p. 34)

In some cases the Perkins tractor worked, but it could not outperform placebo because, as Haygarth classically demonstrated, it *was* a placebo. What then was its power source? It was none other than the reports, testimonials, whispers of wonder, salesmanship, and social energy that propelled it from New England to England, where Perkins had sales agents and the son of Benjamin Franklin became an officer of the Perkins Institute. (Indeed, the Perkins phenomenon spread as far as Denmark.)

The enthusiasm for antidepressants that has swept the United States, with fully 10% of the population now taking these drugs, recalls the Perkins enthusiasm, in that both are marketing triumphs and both tap what I call social energy: the energy that the Perkins user felt as electricity and the depressed as morale. Within a few years after its exposure by Haygarth, the Perkins phenomenon faded away. The fate of antidepressants remains to be seen.

9.4 **Placebos in fiction**

If the placebo effect has social sources, such that we are more likely to expect benefit when we believe others have experienced it as well, by far the richest descriptions of the social realm available to us belong to the literature of the imagination. A corrective for the abstract cases and schematic descriptions all too common in medical papers, literature also offers examples of socially powered placebos or their inverse (nocebo effects). Perhaps literature's most explicit portrayal of medicine as a social proceeding is the description in Tolstoy's *War and peace* of Natasha's illness and recovery following her disastrous escapade with a man she did not know to be married. Upon learning the truth, she attempts suicide, albeit ambiguously, by swallowing "a little" arsenic; then a condition Tolstoy names "grief" sets in, marked by such symptoms as loss of appetite, loss of sleep, and low spirits, each of which appears among the *DSM* criteria for depression. How then is Natasha's depression treated?

> Doctors came to see her singly and in consultation, talked much in French, German, and Latin, blamed one another, and prescribed a great variety of medicines for all the diseases known to them, but the simple idea never occurred to any of them that they could not know the disease Natasha was suffering from, as no disease suffered by a live man can be known.

Less philosophically, the doctors cannot know what Natasha is suffering from because, like her parents, they do not know the story behind it; they do not even know she attempted suicide. However, even though their show of medical knowledge is a charade, the doctors are not absolutely useless.

> Their usefulness did not depend on making the patient swallow substances for the most part harmful . . . but they were useful, necessary, and indispensable because they satisfied a mental need of the invalid and of those who loved her—and that is why there are, and always will be, pseudo-healers, wise women, homeopaths, and allopaths. They satisfied that eternal human need for hope of relief, for sympathy, and that something should be done, which is felt by those who are suffering . . . The doctors were of use to Natasha . . . assuring her that [her illness] would soon pass if only the coachman went to the chemist's in the Arbat and got a powder and some pills in a pretty box for a ruble and seventy kopecks, and if she took those powders in boiled water at intervals of precisely two hours, neither more nor less. (Tolstoy 1991, pp. 700–701)

The doctors set social wheels in motion—there are orders to follow, errands to run, concoctions to prepare—and it is this make-work, not the specific composition of the antidepressant powders and pills, that does some good, albeit more for the household than the patient.

Medicine per se does not contribute to Natasha's eventual return toward health. Of that Tolstoy says, with a kind of caustic simplicity, "youth prevailed. Natasha's grief began to be overlaid by the impressions of daily life, it ceased to press so painfully on her heart, it gradually faded into the past, and she began to recover physically" (p. 702). (Nothing could be farther from the instantaneous healing of Mesmerism and its cousin, the Perkins movement, than that word "gradually.") Though serious, Natasha's depression is not an uncaused sadness that preys from within but a transient condition born of the circumstantial misfortunes of human life. It remits, more or less, when it is ready to remit. The specifics of her treatment are nothing but placebo—the term means *I shall please,* and she is said to find the attention lavished on her "pleasant"—and the placebo effect does not hasten recovery. In essence, the ritual of regular dosing simply gives Natasha some comfort while her condition subsides in its own time, not as a result of medical ministrations. The case reminds us why, in clinical trials, reported improvement in a placebo group does not necessarily arise from the placebo per se (Krøgsboll et al. 2009).

In Tolstoy's denial of the very possibility of medical knowledge, and corresponding reduction of medical practice to dumb show and imposture, philosophy fuses with satire. It is possible to represent medicine as a social art without subjecting it to such contempt. To my mind, the most suggestive portrayal of a drug's social action occurs in *The odyssey*, in connection with one of the earliest references in Western literature to the origin of medicine. In Book Four, Telemachus, in company with Nestor's son Peisistratus, journeys to the palace of Menelaus and Helen in Sparta, where he is recognized as the son of Odysseus and honored accordingly. Given the importance of trust (see Chapter 5), this is especially significant in that Telemachus confessed to the disguised Athena in Book One that he did not know who his father was, which is tantamount to distrusting the story of his identity. From Helen and Menelaus he learns in the most indubitable way that such disbelief is unfounded.

If Natasha's household is her hospital, Telemachus and Peisistratus receive all the rites of hospitality. Although Menelaus grieves the loss of so many warriors for his sake; Peisistratus, the loss of a brother; and Telemachus, the disappearance of his father, they proceed to dine in due course. To crown the dining ritual, Helen mixes into the wine a mysterious preparation said to originate from the motherland of medicine, Egypt.

> Into the bowl that their wine was drawn from she threw a drug that dispelled all grief and anger and banished remembrance of every trouble. Once it was mingled in the wine-bowl, any man who drank it down would never on that same day let a tear fall down his cheeks, no, not if his father and mother died, or if his brother or his own son were slain with the sword before his eyes. Such were the cunning powerful drugs this daughter of Zeus had in her possession; they had been a gift from a woman of Egypt, Polydamna, wife of Thon. In Egypt, more than in other lands, the bounteous earth yields a wealth of drugs, healthful and baneful side by side; and every man there is a physician. (Homer 1980, p. 40)

As in Tolstoy, a certain medical compound is ceremonially administered, although in this case without being enveloped in authorial derision. What makes the mystery drug all the more intriguing is that this is the last time it is mentioned, quite as if it had dissolved not only into the wine—and note that Helen is seen to add the drug, in accordance with what the placebo literature calls the *open condition*—but into the occasion itself. If the drug is stamped with the extraordinary, so is the moment, albeit in a different sense. Never before have these four stood in one another's presence, nor perhaps will they ever again after this one encounter. With the drug being administered in a radiant palace by the daughter of Zeus, with the bond between the recognized sons of two noble fathers creating a reinforcing effect, with the setting in every respect powerfully heightened, the action of the drug (sometimes rendered as "heartsease") seems supported by the context in which it is given and received. Not after the mixing of the drug but even before the dining ritual, Menelaus says, "Come then, let us put aside weeping" (p. 40). Perhaps the power of Helen's compound is no more and no less than that of the occasion itself.

The central activity of the occasion is storytelling. If indeed "all sorrows can be borne if you put them into a story or tell a story about them," as Hannah Arendt has written, attributing the saying to Isak Dinesen (Arendt 1957, p.175), then the anodyne effect of Helen's drug in fact resembles that of narrative—resembles it so suggestively as to make the two almost one. The action of the drug is virtually that of storytelling. While we do not discover whether it can really make a man indifferent to the murder of a brother, we have already learned that storytelling can reconcile a man to such a loss, or at least begin to. The murder of Menelaus' brother Agamemnon is probably the most frequently told story in *The odyssey*; and while Menelaus laments his death, he does not (as he tells us) grieve it so much as the disappearance of Odysseus, whose fate, precisely because he *has* disappeared from view, cannot be commemorated in story. Story itself is consolation, is heart's ease.

9.5 **Ambiguous potential**

The manner in which medical care is given and received is now recognized as a strong source of the placebo effect.

> Healing resulting from the clinical encounter consists of a causal connection between clinician–patient interaction (or a particular component of the interaction) and improvement in the condition of the patient. That aspect of healing that is produced, activated or enhanced by the context of the clinical encounter, as distinct from the specific efficacy of treatment interventions, is contextual healing. (Miller and Kaptchuk 2008, p. 224)

However, many doctors are simply too hurried, remote, or indifferent to culti-vate the placebo potential of the clinical encounter; nor are patients themselves necessarily invested. In the notable case of antidepressants, patients commonly short-circuit the clinical encounter by employing doctors "as mere conduits to get fabled products rather than as counselors capable of using the doctor-patient relationship itself therapeutically" (Shorter 1997, p. 314). Few would contend that the placebo effect of antidepressants is accounted for by the man-ner in which they are described and prescribed by the doctor. The mythology, advertising, and social buzz surrounding these reputed wonder-drugs surely have something to do with expectations of efficacy.

If, as I claim, the placebo effect has social sources, this is also to say that its potential is as various as that of the forms of social life in which we participate. The doctor's office, Benjamin Franklin's gardens, Natasha's household, and Menelaus' palace are different settings to be sure, but all are circumscribed and highly ordered; in more open spaces the placebo effect has more room to unfold its mixed possibilities, as with the ads seen on American television not only for antidepressants but for miscellaneous placebo-like remedies and boosters including vitamins, supplements, and probiotics. Even psychotherapy, nor-mally a confidential proceeding (with a strong placebo component), has spilled over into the public realm in the form of self-help books and therapeutic cant. While one fashionable mode of psychotherapy—eye movement desensitization and reprocessing—has been convincingly likened to Mesmerism (McNally 1999), the books and workshops it has generated also look back to Mesmerism as a therapy surrounded by print and enacted in gatherings.

Medicine too has spilled over into public spaces, and in some questionable ways. Even though prostate cancer, for example, is recognized in the medical literature to be greatly over-diagnosed and there is a nascent consensus that mass screening for the disease may well yield a net harm, campaigns prompting men to get screened are conducted daily. The screening movement is driven not only by clinical advice but message-bearing postage stamps and license plates, early-detection folklore, public service announcements, emotive headlines, blue ribbons, workplace programs, and—not least—the knowledge that friends and associates get screened (Justman 2010). Leading as it does to unnecessary treatment on a large scale with accompanying adverse effects, mass screening for prostate cancer resembles a nocebo event, as when numbers of people fall ill of exposure to noxious fumes that elude investigation (Jones et al. 2000), except that in this case, investigation uncovers evidence of disease that would other-wise in all likelihood lie dormant. Coincidentally or not, the 1990s—the decade that saw the institutionalization of mass screening for prostate cancer and an ensuing spectacular increase in disease incidence—also witnessed any number of pseudo-epidemics, from chronic fatigue syndrome to recovered memories (Showalter 1997). Many treated for screening-detected prostate cancer firmly believe they had their life saved, but if that were generally true, the disease's mortality rate would be considerably higher than the actual rate of 3.5% (Brawley and Kramer 2005).

To estimate the tidal effect of social trends in our common life, we need only consider the interest at this moment in the issue of placebos and their enigmatic potential. However, the most potent social influences on health are at once more durable than trends and less conspicuous than the sort of messages that compete for public attention. Two decades ago, a paper in *Science* demonstrated that the less socially integrated enjoy poorer health and are significantly more likely to die: a striking confirmation of the medical import of purely social influences (House et al. 1988). In an also striking confirmation of the Tolstoyan principle that facts of patent importance somehow escape our notice (Morson 2007), the *Science* finding has not left much of a mark in the medical literature. We neglect the medical import of our connections, or indeed frayed connections, because we take them for granted; they are simply the element in which we live.

Antidepressants seem to be the Tolstoyan pills of today, with advertising and popular lore as the pretty box. The rising incidence of depression—or of discontents and anxieties interpreted as depression—is driven by mass marketing and the use of simplistic diagnostic criteria, but also, arguably, by the instability of the social bonds that sustain well-being. So contends Edward Shorter in a social history of the doctor–patient relationship published just before the advent of Prozac:

> One may describe the postmodern couple as being in a state of almost permanent instability . . . These changes have certain consequences for health, not so much creating more illness as making people more *sensitive* to the symptoms they already have . . . For a generation accustomed to translating human conditions into medical terms, unhappiness becomes "depression," a treatable disorder. (Shorter 1985, p. 218)

However, just as not everything that calls itself depression is depression, so not everything deemed a treatment is really a treatment.

With the growing recognition that the placebo effect is potentially an element of any medical proceeding, attention is now turning to ways of translating the power of the placebo from the realm of experiment into clinical practice. Arguably, though, the best way for doctors to cultivate the power of the placebo is simply through the attentive care of the patient—that is, through the mindful performance of the rituals of medicine to which we all respond strongly as social beings. The placebo effect should not be thought of as a medical short-cut or a secret resource to be drawn from the doctor's bag as a colleague of John Haygarth took from his pocket a facsimile of the Perkins tractor. Mindful practice also calls on doctors to take note of the medical or quasi-medical trends sweeping their society—trends that may or may not be worthy of their endorsement. If the placebo effect can enhance good medical practice, it can also free-ride on treatments and medications of little or no medical merit. Its potential is in fact as ambiguous as the potential of our social responsiveness itself.[1]

Note

1 For further reading, please see Justman, S. *To feel what others feel: social sources of the placebo effect* (San Francisco: University of California Medical Humanities Press, 2012).

References

Arendt, H. (1957). *The human condition.* Chicago: University of Chicago Press.

Barrett, B., Muller, D., Rakel, D., Rabago, D., Marchand, L., and Scheder, J. (2006). Placebo, meaning, and health. *Perspectives in Biology and Medicine,* **49,** 178–198.

Blackwell, B., Bloomfield, S., and Buncher, C. R. (1972). Demonstration to medical students of placebo responses and non-drug factors. *The Lancet,* **299,** 1279–1282.

Brawley, O. and Kramer, B. (2005). Cancer screening in theory and practice. *Journal of Clinical Oncology,* **23,** 293–300.

Darnton, R. (1968). *Mesmerism and the end of the Enlightenment in France.* Cambridge, MA: Harvard University Press.

Gould, S. (1992). *Bully for brontosaurus: reflections in natural history.* New York: Norton.

Haygarth, J. (1800). *Of the imagination as a cause and as a cure of disorders of the body.* Bath: Cruttwell.

Homer (1980 edn.). *The odyssey* (trans. W. Shewring). Oxford: Oxford University Press.

Horwitz, A. and Wakefield, J. (2007). *The loss of sadness: how psychiatry transformed normal sadness into depressive disorder.* Oxford: Oxford University Press.

House, J., Landis, K., and Umberson, D. (1988). Social relationships and health. *Science,* **241,** 540–545.

Hróbjarttson, A. and Norup, M. (2003). The use of placebo interventions in medical practice—a national questionnaire survey of Danish physicians. *Evaluation and the Health Professions,* **26,** 153–165.

Johnson, S. (1750). *Rambler* No. 4.

Jones, T., Craig, A., Hoy, D., et al. (2000). Mass psychogenic illness attributed to toxic exposure at a high school. *New England Journal of Medicine,* **342,** 96–100.

Justman, S. (2010). How did the PSA system arise? *Journal of the Royal Society of Medicine,* **103,** 309–312.

Justman, S. (2011). To feel what others feel: two episodes from 18th-century medicine. *Medical Humanities,* **37,** 34–37.

Kaptchuk, T., Friedlander, E., Kelley, J., et al. (2010). Placebos without deception: a randomized controlled trial in irritable bowel syndrome. *PLoS ONE,* **5**(12), e15591. DOI: 10.1371/journal.pone.0015591.

Kirsch, I. (2010). *The emperor's new drugs: exploding the antidepressant myth*. New York: Basic Books.

Krøgsboll, L., Hróbjartsson, A., and Gøtzsche, P. (2009). Spontaneous improvement in randomised clinical trials: meta-analysis of three-armed trials comparing no treatment, placebo and active treatment. *BMC Medical Research* Methodology, **9**, 1–10. DOI: 10.1.1186/1471-2288-9-1.

Lopez, C.-A. (1993). Franklin and Mesmer: an exchange. *Yale Journal of Biology and Medicine*, **66**, 325–331.

McNally, R. (1999). EMDR and Mesmerism: a comparative historical analysis. *Journal of Anxiety Disorders*, **13**, 225–236.

Miller, F. and Kaptchuk, T. (2008). The power of context: reconceptualizing the placebo effect. *Journal of the Royal Society of Medicine*, **101**, 222–225.

Morson, G. S. (2007). *"Anna Karenina" in our time: seeing more wisely*. New Haven: Yale University Press.

Perkins, B. D. (1798). *The influence of metallic tractors on the human body*. London: J. Johnson.

Shorter, E. (1985). *Doctors and their patients: a social history*. New Brunswick, NJ: Transaction.

Shorter, E. (1997). *A history of psychiatry: from the era of the asylum to the age of Prozac*. New York: Wiley.

Showalter, E. (1997). *Hystories: hysterical epidemics and modern media*. New York: Columbia University Press.

Spiro, H. (1986). *Doctors, patients, and placebos*. New Haven: Yale University Press.

Spiro, H. (1997). Clinical reflections on the placebo phenomenon. In: *The placebo effect: an interdisciplinary exploration* (ed. A. Harrington). Cambridge, MA: Harvard University Press.

Tolstoy, L. (1991 edn.). *War and peace* (trans. L. Maude and A. Maude). New York: Oxford University Press.

Tröhler, U. (2000). *"To improve the evidence of medicine": the 18th century British origins of a critical approach*. Edinburgh: Royal College of Physicians.

Vase, L., Robinson, M., Verne, G. N., and Price, D. (2003). The contributions of suggestion, desire, and expectation to placebo effects in irritable bowel syndrome patients: an empirical investigation. *Pain*, **105**, 17–25.

Chapter 10

Healing words: the placebo effect and journalism at the mind–body boundary

Steve Silberman

10.1 Introducing "the placebo problem"

One morning last fall, I woke up to find an unexpected torrent of email in my in-box. Friends and strangers were asking me if I had seen the previous night's broadcast of *The Colbert Report*. For those who do not know, *The Colbert Report* is a popular show on cable television in America starring Stephen Colbert, a comedian who plays the role of a slick, relentlessly self-possessed conservative commentator. Colbert had based one of the segments of the previous night's broadcast on an article of mine, entitled "The placebo problem", that had just been published in *Wired* magazine. In his wry and engaging way, Colbert played with the notion that pharmaceutical companies are suddenly facing the challenge of sugar pills that have become miraculously powerful in clinical trials—indeed, proving more effective than the drugs that these companies are trying to test. Colbert suggested that taking sugar pills might be a better idea.

This was a satirical version of the real problem that I had written about, which has been an open secret in big pharma for a decade or more, but had not been talked about much in the mainstream press. An astonishing range of the pharmaceutical industry's biggest-selling products, accounting for billions of dollars in sales each year worldwide—including antidepressants, anti-anxiety medications, pain relievers, blood pressure pills, even antihistamines—are having an increasingly hard time demonstrating their efficacy in trials, because the health of volunteers in placebo control groups improves as much, or more than, the health of volunteers in the groups receiving the real drugs. While researching the article, I was told by a senior drug developer for Merck and Lilly that even drugs that had been approved by the Food and Drug Administration (FDA) a couple of decades ago, such as Prozac, might not be approved now because their therapeutic effects would be swamped by placebo effects in clinical trials.

As scientists have written about, at length, in books like Irving Kirsch's *The emperor's new drugs,* this is a highly complex issue involving a web of social, cultural, medical, and statistical factors, ranging from where clinical trials are conducted (that is, increasingly among the desperately poor in countries like China and India, rather than among students and housewives on college campuses in North America) to the medical establishment's ever-broadening definitions of disease and particularly of mood disorders (diagnoses that often seem to have as much to do with drug companies seeking to extend their patent protection on blockbuster products as with serving the needs of patients). It is important to understand some of the social dynamics behind the placebo effect, which is becoming an increasingly popular item of cultural fascination, with more and more articles and news broadcasts devoted each month to the subject.

One of the luckiest things that can happen to a journalist is when multiple stars align to encourage the creation of a large readership that is eager to absorb the substance and implications of a subject that he or she is writing about. I would like to talk about some of the reasons why even television comedians and young internet surfers, who would normally be barely interested in the intricacies of clinical trials, might have been intrigued enough to read my article, as well as some of the challenges I faced when writing it—some of which had to do with the complexity of the subject itself, and some to do with the realities of science journalism. I also want to say straight out that I attribute the somewhat surprising level of response to the article not to my own journalistic abilities, but to a great unmet need in our culture to acknowledge the role that factors beyond the contents of a pill play in healing. I believe that while many people first become beguiled by the placebo effect because it seems like some interesting kind of fraud or trick, the subject is inherently haunting and provocative because it hints at the deeper truth that what we think and how we interact with other people—particularly those in positions of medical authority—has a profound, demonstrable, physical, measurable effect on our well-being.

As several people pointed out in the course of my research, the term "placebo effect" is really a misnomer, because by their very definition, placebos have no effect at all—unless they are so-called active placebos, designed to trigger side-effects like a dry mouth or feelings of dizziness, and thus deepen the deception necessary to incite the body's natural healing response. As Daniel Moerman has articulated so wonderfully, a more accurate term would be "the meaning effect," because it depends on the meaning that we invest in the fake pills, the people who give them to us, the settings in which we take them, and how we conceptualize health and disease.

It is also important to remember that while the social factors contributing to this meaning effect are varied and subtle, we all experienced the placebo effect at the age of three or so, when, in the wake of some playtime mishap, our mother told us that she would kiss the "boo boo" and make it better. As every parent and child knows, a mother's kind words or a ride on a father's shoulders can be marvelously effective medicine—and the need for that kind of attention from someone we trust is something we never outgrow, even when the problems that ail us become enormously complex and daunting.

Behind the cartoon notion of mysteriously powerful sugar pills is a desperate hunger for people to feel that they are, in some way, in control of their health, within certain limits. In that sense, though my article focused on the problems for drug companies that placebo effects create in clinical trials, I think its real appeal was a subtext hinting at the indivisible unity of mind and matter, thought and physiology, the individual and the social group, biology and belief.

We live in an increasingly polarized world, in which right wingers and left wingers, liberals and conservatives, scientists and lay people, New Agers and skeptics, bloggers and mainstream media pundits, people of faith and people of skepticism, those in the medical establishment and those who challenge the assumptions of the medical establishment, seem to have less and less common ground, and more and more of what the American author Jack Kerouac (whose parents were Québecois) called "new reasons for spitefulness." We are getting better at distrusting one another, yelling at one another, and preaching to the choir, and worse at understanding one another and exploring issues with people who have different opinions or come from different backgrounds. Meanwhile, the placebo effect flickers on the horizon of body and mind, insisting on the salubrious power of transcending the categories that enslave us.

10.2 The *woo,* power and paradox of placebos

One of the reasons that my article was able to draw people into the cultural conversation about placebos who might not otherwise be interested in suspiciously soft-sounding topics like "mind–body healing" is that the editor-in-chief of *Wired* magazine, Chris Anderson, is profoundly allergic to what he might call "woo." Sounding appropriately like a word drawn from the lexicon of Chinese herbal medicine or some other ancient healing art, *woo* has become the catchphrase du jour among hipsters for anything that reeks of junk science, quackery, hippie mysticism, religious fundamentalism, or other forms of irrational belief. I was painfully aware that even using the phrase "mind–body" (with a hyphen) would immediately set off Chris Anderson's *woo* alarms, and that unless my evocative subject was approached from a strictly hard-nosed, business-oriented, quantifiable perspective, I would be asking for trouble.

My strategy was to craft the article as a kind of journalistic Trojan horse. From the outside, it would look like a no-nonsense story about big pharma and its multiple billions of dollars lost annually in research and development because of this unexpectedly unruly variable in clinical trials. On the inside, however, the story would engage concepts that are harder to quantify, such as the therapeutic value of bedside manner. In short, I was trying to write a story that might catch the interest even of someone who might never read an article about meditation, hypnosis, or psychedelics. My Trojan horse strategy seems to have succeeded in getting people like Ezra Klein at the *Washington Post* to link to the article, but it also meant that I was unable to include certain intriguing anecdotes that I came across in my research, while others were eliminated by editors who were all well aware of the editor-in-chief's visceral distrust of anything that cannot be plotted on a spreadsheet or rendered as a cheeky infographic.

I would like to mention a couple of those lost pieces of the story here, partly because they will never see the light of day anywhere else, and partly since I feel that they are indeed a piece of the big picture that we are attempting to clarify and describe in this volume. One story was told to me by Harvard's Ted Kaptchuk, whom some of you may know personally. Certainly almost anyone who has studied the placebo effect in an academic setting has come across his work. I first heard his name many years ago as the author of a book called *The web that has no weaver*, one of the primary texts that made readers in the West aware of acupuncture and Chinese herbal medicine. In fact, I believe that Kaptchuk was the first Westerner to earn a graduate degree in Chinese medicine in China. I remember seeing copies of this book on many a bookshelf in Santa Cruz, California, alongside copies of *Our bodies, ourselves*—a manifesto that challenged women to take control of their own health—and copies of the *Co-evolution quarterly*, a provocative, thoughtful, and generally invigorating magazine that was edited by Kevin Kelly, who would later become one of the senior editors of *Wired* in its heady early days.

In the years since that era, Kaptchuk had done what few of his peers were able to do, which is to cross the "woo" divide and become part of the medical establishment at Harvard, bringing with him not only his extensive knowledge of Asian medicine but his innate Jewish skepticism, some of which he has exercised on the very same beliefs shared by many of the people who elevated his book to the status of a new kind of alternative medical bible. I visited him at home on a snowy afternoon in Cambridge, not knowing what sort of person I was going to see: a venerable old hippie or a buttoned-down academic who had long ago disavowed the quote–unquote naïve views of his past? The answer, thankfully, was neither, though the Ted Kaptchuk who came to the door looked more like a rabbi than an aging tam tam drummer, with a hand-knitted kippah over his long forelocks. When I asked him about his current status of having one foot in the medical establishment and the other in the world of alternative medicine, he said, "I piss everyone off. That's my job."

At one point, I asked him to talk about the formative influences in his past that had given him some insight into the placebo effect. He told me that a decade or so ago, he had been the director of a pain clinic in Boston. Several clients at the clinic told Kaptchuk that they felt much better after talking to an older Jewish staff member named Victor. However, Victor was not supposed to be treating patients, just evaluating them for treatment and referring them to others. So Kaptchuk went to Victor and asked him, "What the hell are you doing with these patients?" Victor's reply was, "Ted, when I was working in the infirmary at Auschwitz, I would get two aspirins a week to treat thousands of people. So I dissolved them in a big bucket, gave everyone a spoonful, and listened to them. That's how I learned to help people."

What Victor learned in the Auschwitz infirmary is something that the medical establishment once understood as indispensable to the art of healing. Indeed, until the mid-twentieth century, injecting art into the mechanics of healing was essential, because until then, very few of the tinctures and extracts in the doctor's traditional black bag had any therapeutic benefit whatsoever. Most of these alleged medicines, which had been passed down from physician to physician for hundreds of years, seem quaint or even obviously absurd now.

One of the items in the standard pharmacopeias, for example, was an odiferous concoction called theriac, used from the time of Mithridates VI of Pontus—sixty-five years before the birth of Christ—up until the 1880s. Containing up to sixty-five secret ingredients—including opium, myrrh, saffron, ginger, cinnamon, and castor bean—the longest-lasting component of the recipe for theriac was the flesh of poisonous snakes. So expensive that often only royalty could afford it, theriac was considered a panacea. It is not overstating to say that the history of medicine is the history of placebos. As some wag observed, the *Materia medica* was a book that got shorter and shorter as medical knowledge increased.

The problem for us in the twenty-first century is that it is too easy to look back at this long history and snicker with derision and a feeling of superiority. In the era of evidence-based medicine, the millennium of placebo-based healing that preceded it seems like a dark age from which humanity has finally awakened. Those centuries of poor sick people, believing they got better because their doctor gave them pills made up from ground-up vipers or popular nostrums like *Revalenta arabica* (another old-school cure-all, this one made of lentils). Those generations of hapless would-be physicians, compiling multi-volume encyclopedias of useless junk, and trying earnestly to treat their long-suffering patients with remedies that were ineffective or even toxic. How far we have come!

Yet bold researchers like Irving Kirsch, who have risked their careers by challenging the comforting assumptions that make billions of dollars a year for big pharma—such as the assumption that drugs which can cause dangerous side-effects are more helpful for mildly depressed people than psychotherapy or exercise—suggest that perhaps we have not come as far as we believe. Indeed, as we look more closely in the margins of the official narratives of medical history, we find signs that the old healers were not as naïve about the tools of their trade as we might think. The third American president, Thomas Jefferson—who kept bookshelves full of pharmacopeias in his library in Monticello—famously wrote to a doctor friend in 1805: "One of the most successful physicians I have ever known, has assured me, that he used more bread pills, drops of coloured water, and powders of hickory ashes, than of all other medicines put together. It was certainly a pious fraud." A "pious fraud" sounds like a paradox, a Jeffersonian Zen koan.

The study of the placebo effect is full of paradoxes like this and the more we learn about the use of placebos in history, the more we realize that many of the old healers were well aware that their patients' belief in them was what triggered the healing, and not the hickory ashes, colored water, or oil of roses. Robert Burton knew this in 1621, when he wrote in *The anatomy of melancholy*:

> A third thing to be required in a patient, is confidence, to be of good cheer, and have sure hope that his physician can help him. Damascen the Arabian requires likewise in the physician himself, that he be confident he can cure him, otherwise his physic will not be effectual, and promise withal that he will certainly help him, make him believe so at least. Galeottus gives this reason, because the form of health is contained in the physician's mind, and as Galen, holds "confidence and hope to be more good than physic," *he cures most in whom most are confident.* Axiocus sick almost to death, at the very sight of Socrates recovered his former health. Paracelsus assigns it for an only cause, why Hippocrates was so fortunate in his cures, not for any extraordinary skill he had; but "because the common people had a most strong conceit of his worth."

In recent years, using brain imaging and the other tools of the modern laboratory, researchers like Tor Wager at Columbia and Fabrizio Benedetti of the University of Turin have explored how our brains and bodies are wired to respond to this "strong conceit" of a physician's worth as a healer.

I think most doctors are aware of this too, though officially, the medical establishment has gone in the direction of attempting to create medicines that could be dispensed by machine without a measurable loss of efficacy. That is a necessary thing too, if not a good one, because these days, we barely get to interact with our doctors, outside of brief, harried office visits and perhaps the occasional email, filtered through a web interface that does not allow for direct personal communication. On examination day, we wait in the waiting room for half an hour after the appointment time, to be led to the examination room by a busy nurse, where we strip off our clothes and wait further. Somewhere, phones are ringing, doors open and shut as other patients get their precious time in the presence of the doctor. The subliminal message is: "You're lucky that the doctor is making time in a solid wall of appointments to deal with your personal issues." I am not blaming doctors; most of them are heroes. However, this is how it is these days, at least in America: the doctor comes in, with forms and print-outs in hand, and quickly assesses the situation. If she is a really good doctor, she strives to make eye contact to reassure you that she is actually in the room, however briefly. The evaluation is made, the expensive tests are ordered, and the doctor is out of the door to the next patient as you stoop to put your clothes on again. At home, you get the phone call from the nurse or the email from the password-protected website with the test results. You get the prescription by mail. The brain's eager placebo machinery latches onto the brand name of the drug—"oh, I hear that one's good"—indicating that you once flicked past a spread in a glossy magazine that consisted of a photograph of clouds, a dog, and a smiling actor playing the role of a formerly depressed person, with a lengthy list of side-effects printed in a font too small to read.

No wonder people spend millions of dollars a year on acupuncture, homeopathy, ear candling, herbs, and other dubious or outright fraudulent forms of alternative medicine. The practitioners of these forms of treatment may be quacks convinced of their own virtue, but at least they are usually not quite so harried and overbooked as real doctors. They ask you how you have felt since the last time they saw you. They express concern for your aches, pains, emotional challenges, and feelings that life is out of balance. They distill from these a story that makes sense and meaning of your cloudy chaos of symptoms. By the standards of so-called evidence-based medicine, these niceties and narratives are virtually irrelevant compared to the all-important question of whether or not a pill or other treatment has proven efficacious under controlled laboratory conditions. However, by the standards of doctoring as it was practiced for hundreds of years, they were regarded as essential to the healing process.

There are many reasons to celebrate what you might call the New Rationalism, including the popularity of professional skeptics like Christopher Hitchens and James Randi, and the new "anti-woo" lines drawn in the sand, like the recent petition signed by hundreds of doctors in Britain demanding that the National Health Service stop wasting money on ineffective homeopathic treatments. In America, this rationalist uprising seems particularly justified in the wake of the tidal wave of nonsense being cynically whipped up by Fox News and the Republican party regarding such issues as the teaching of evolution in the schools, the alleged role of vaccines in causing autism, the alleged threat to marriage posed by millions of gay people who want to marry their lifelong partners, and so on. Faced with that darkness, it seems better to light candles of skepticism.

The problem is, however, that the domain of those seeking to reduce human suffering has now become divided into two mutually exclusive and mutually distrusting camps: those who forget that the action of their precious pharmaceuticals depends in part on the social dynamics of doctor and patient; and those who forget that the real healing power of their herbs and crystals and tinctures of colloidal silver resides somewhere in the patient themselves.

The poet John Keats said that one mark of maturity was what he called "negative capability"—a capacity to be "in uncertainties, mysteries, doubts without any irritable reaching after fact and reason." It strikes me that fully understanding the placebo effect, and getting beyond these seemingly irreconcilable differences in our approach to healing, will require a healthy dose of negative capability on both sides of the alternative versus mainstream medicine divide. I saw that negative capability at work in Ted Kaptchuk, when he told me that he and his wife are both still practicing acupuncturists. I asked him if he is now convinced, by Harvard medical school standards, that the effects of acupuncture are superior to the effects of placebo. "The jury is still out," he said. I asked him how he reconciled that uncertainty with being a member of the medical establishment. "When I practice acupuncture," he said, "I am a perfect T'ang dynasty physician." Another placebo paradox.

10.3 **Science, health, and journalism**

When my article was published on the web, it bore an additional headline, composed by some anonymous editor at Wired.com, of which I would never have approved: "Placebos are getting more effective. Drugmakers are desperate to know why." Understandably, at least one proud, evidence-based blogger with a medical degree took offense at that headline, trashing me and *Wired* for publishing yet another clueless mainstream-media article about the placebo effect. Immediately, several readers of the blog chimed in with extra insults, the thrust of the thread being a kind of self-congratulation about being savvy enough to not be taken in by such obvious tripe as a claim that sugar pills are somehow getting "more effective." Several people cited studies that they were confident I should have been aware of, naming researchers I was obviously unfamiliar with, and so forth, thus proving my lack of even a superficial knowledge of the subject. Very quickly that blog post was linked to other places on the web where someone had linked to my article, delivering the message that there was nothing new to see here, so move along.

The only problem was that in fact I *had* read those papers and cited that research in the text of the piece itself. In other words, it was clear that the author of the blog had not read much past the headline before launching an angry armada in my direction. That did not seem very evidence-based to me, but, rather than taking up arms in a general snit and yelling back, to no one's edification, I simply joined the discussion and pointed out places in the article that might deserve more attention, without trying to humiliate anyone. As a result, several readers actually read the thing and realized that I was not as clueless as had been advertised on the blog. The tone of the discussion shifted to one of mutual respect, and we all ended up learning things.

I recount this incident not to get in the last word but to say that one of the things I learned from this exchange was that sometimes a little too much credence is given to anyone who poses as an annoyed debunker of what Sarah Palin calls "the lamestream media." Yes, coverage of science and medicine in mainstream media is often sorely wanting, amidst a twenty-four-hour deluge of headlines promising new cures for cancer, unprecedented genetic break-throughs, and so on. However, the answer is not always more indignant rage, but more care and attention to nuance. As much as the net can stoke the fires of indignant rage, it can also provide a forum for the collective exploration of nuance.

The traditional role of medical and life-science journalists as guardians of public safety is becoming even more crucial as lay readers' ability to make informed healthcare decisions depends on their being able to grasp increasingly arcane fields of research. At the same time, the democratization of access to health-related information online, and revelations of conflicts of interest in medical journals, have eroded trust in the role of journalists as gatekeepers to potentially life-saving information. Practical opportunities for in-depth reporting are rapidly becoming more scarce. To help readers make wise choices, journalists must invent new ways of engaging them in science and re-establishing the bond of public trust.

A number of advances in the life sciences are likely to come to maturation in the coming years—including personalized medicine, molecular diagnostics, and gene therapy—that draw on sophisticated bodies of technical knowledge not easily translatable into lay terms. Earth-science journalists face similar hurdles in explaining the intricate workings of climate change, with added obstacles introduced by a highly charged political environment and a rancorous international debate on the subject.

Though a poll of voters during the last American national election found that health issues rank as number three (behind the economy and the war in Iraq) on a list of public concerns, the media resources devoted to responsible health coverage are shrinking fast. Medical stories are often reduced to a "lifestyle minute" on broadcast news or a list of bullet points promising "all you need to know" about a complex issue like the safety and effectiveness of antidepressants.

Doing justice to a multilayered subject like the placebo effect—which touches on psychology, pharmacology, social science, clinical trial design, and the economics of globalization—requires a lengthy period of research, multiple interviews, and a high enough word count for the final product to address the various issues at hand. In a collapsing economy, the editorial pressure to produce a stream of headlines promising medical "miracles," buying into facile, prepackaged faux controversies, and oversimplifying complex ideas into tweetable newsblips, is more intense than ever.

In my fourteen years of covering science full-time, I have seen an inexorable drift away from the kind of nuanced, in-depth, long-form storytelling that can at least try to explore the strata of meaning embedded in a phenomenon like the placebo effect. A 6000-word feature in *Wired* used to be relatively standard to cover a knotty issue in depth; articles of that length have become rare. Now, instead, many magazines and websites favor the kind of high-impact, eye-catching charts, illustrations, and multimedia elements that *Wired* editors enthusiastically call "infoporn." I enjoy provocative graphics as much as anyone, but they can so easily mislead readers into feeling like enough information has been delivered to make informed decisions about entire scientific disciplines. I have come to feel like I am defending antiquated ideas of journalistic value against an onslaught of shallow, instant-gratification media.

Being correct is no longer as important as dominating a news cycle, even with notions that turn out to be misguided. All that matters is that "people are talking" or tweeting about your story, even if what they are saying is nonsense. Being willing to champion outrageous ideas and buzzy memes is seen as more bold, and more ultimately valuable to a magazine's brand, than trying to insist on subtlety and deep reporting. In the case of my article, the unknown Wired.com editor's provocative choice of headline about "placebos getting more effective" was outrageous enough to get people reading the piece, and once they started, the inherently fascinating quality of the phenomena associated with the placebo effect held their interest long enough for them to either finish the piece or at least link to it so that it gained a kind of life of its own.

10.4 **No longer "merely the placebo effect"**

For a couple of heady weeks, as links proliferated across Twitter, hip websites like BoingBoing, and other media outlets like the *Washington Post*, I felt like the article was a tuning fork resonating in the key of the zeitgeist. The word "placebo" seemed to be on everyone's lips. I may be fooling myself, but I like to think that the real reason the story struck a nerve was not because of the foolish notion of sugar pills getting stronger, but because of a deep and pervasive hunger for a sense that we have more control over our health than we have been told, as well as a yearning for a model of healthcare that emphasizes interpersonal interaction and caring over quantification and data.

These feelings tap into very ancient needs in us. Another part of the story that did not survive into the final edit was a section where I sketched out theories of the role that the placebo response may have played in the course of evolution. I talked about this with Fabrizio Benedetti, one of the leading placebo researchers, in his office in Turin. Citing the work of pain researcher Patrick Wall, Benedetti spoke about the function of the "pain face," as he put it, which, if I understood him correctly, evolved as a social signal among primates to summon aid when a monkey is hurting and vulnerable. Once the reinforcements have arrived, however, both the pain and the pain face can safely abate. Benedetti speculated that the ebbing of discomfort and inflammation once help is on the way was the primordial beginning of what we call the placebo effect.

Benedetti's book *Placebo effects*, which focuses on placebo phenomena in medicine, was a crucial reference point for me as I wrote the article, but as I interviewed him, he also told me about a more recent book, which made me wish I could read Italian. The title, translated into English, is *The enchanted reality: the placebo effect in everyday life*. In it, Benedetti said, he examines placebo-like effects not only in medicine but also in religion, music, sexual relationships, painting, and cooking. Placebo *cooking*? "Let's say you eat a risotto in San Francisco, and it tastes good," Benedetti explained. "Then you eat the same risotto in Italy. I bet it tastes even better, because there are all these emotional associations and expectations with Italian cooking." In fact, that night I ate a risotto made with black riso venere and fonduta in a charming little trattoria on a side street in Turin. The best risotto I have ever tasted, I am sure of it!

While some may quibble with Benedetti's use of the phrase *placebo effects* outside the context of clinical trials, his notion of searching for placebo-like phenomena in everyday life gets to the way that understanding these phenomena in medicine is changing our notions of how the brain constructs experience from the incoming data of the senses. Our minds are constantly alert and responsive to many subtle sources of information around us, particularly the reactions of others. Have you ever been having a relatively good day when someone came up to you and asked you if you felt OK, because you looked sick or tired? There are few more insidiously efficient ways of ruining someone's day than telling them that they look pale or exhausted. Our minds are in the unconscious business of fulfilling other people's prophecies about us. Since writing the article, I have become a bit more careful about the kinds of casual feedback I give to people I care about. Another way to put it is that placebo responses in the body can transform words into medicine or poison. Our health is partially dependent on the opinions of those around us and the sea of language we swim through every day. Down to the hormones circulating in our bloodstreams and the neurons activated in our brains, we are all in this together.

One of the things that happened after my article came out was that I received reprint requests from several other publications. The most unexpected request came from a magazine for Christian Scientists. I called up the woman who had emailed me from their organization and asked her why she was interested in reprinting an article about drug development and clinical trials. After talking for a while, she admitted that it was because she felt that what placebo researchers are really exploring is the biological pathways by which God heals the sick. Being a Jewish atheist science writer who has been meditating several times a week for years, I told her that while I was happy to grant the reprint permission, I asked her to at least try to keep the word "God" out of the head-line. However, I will admit to feeling in the presence of something truly pro-found when considering the various ways that the mind can help heal (or wound) the body. "We become what we think, having become what we thought," the Buddha is reputed to have said. That does not seem to be much of a stretch from the literal, demonstrable, quantifiable truth of the placebo effect—within certain realistic, evidence-based limits.

In fact, the main thing I learned by writing the article is that the phrases "just the placebo effect" or "merely the placebo effect" are utterly inadequate to describe the reality of what happens when we believe we are in a therapeutic situation. There is nothing mere about it. I no longer use that phrase as most people do, as a way of indicating that whatever phenomenon is being described is of no practical import—the latest instance of deceitful intent acting upon a gullible mind. Now I use the phrase with something like awe, having glimpsed through the prism of the placebo effect, a reflection of the web that unites us all.

Acknowledgement

This chapter was originally published as: Steve Silberman, Placebo effects and science journalism at the mind/body boundary, *The Journal of Mind–Body Regulation,* 1 (2), pp. 44–52, © The Authors, 2011.

Part 4

The placebo lens

Chapter 11

Placebolicious: the many flavors of placebos in Western diets and food cultures

Cory S. Harris and Timothy Johns

11.1 Introduction

In many cultures, food and diet are considered inseparable and essential to both health maintenance and recovery from disease. Like medicines, food simultaneously contains biologically active chemicals and conveys social and cultural meanings that influence individual and collective health (Etkin 1986). Emerging only in the nineteenth and twentieth centuries, a distinction between food and medicine sets Western industrialized societies apart from most of the world's indigenous cultures of the past and present (Etkin and Johns 1998). Yet, even in Westernized societies, items like coffee and dietary supplements straddle the line between food and drug, while diverse social movements and industrial interests disregard this line altogether.

Associated predominantly with medical practice and clinical research, the concepts of placebo and placebo effect extend beyond medicine into other aspects of our daily lives and long-term health. Given the inextricable roles of food and medicine in human health, survival, and evolution (Johns 1999), a search for non-medical placebos logically turns to dietary behavior and food culture—the subject of this chapter. After surveying the various guises of placebo in food and diet, we outline a conceptual model for integrating the many inputs and mind–body interactions contributing to personal dietary habits and responses to food. We then present three case studies, each drawing on different elements and variations of placebo, to illustrate how these complex interactions can impact individual health.

11.2 Placebos on the menu: a survey of placebos in diet and food culture

Placebos serve the same purpose in clinical research, whether in medicine or in nutrition, which is to control for the effects of time and participation in a study. Outside of research, a dietitian is unlikely to employ a pure placebo but likely to recommend interventions lacking clinical evidence of efficacy, interventions that, by some definitions at least, constitute impure placebos. Similarly, many physicians prescribe dietary therapies (e.g., vitamins) in situations without demonstrated or expected efficacy (Raz et al. 2011; Tilburt et al. 2008). Drug-like foods such as coffee and wine, together with their caffeine- and alcohol-free placebo counterparts, not only offer everyday opportunities to experience placebo effects but have long provided a foundational paradigm for placebo research (Fillmore et al. 1994; Hammami et al. 2010; Testa et al. 2006).

Analogies of placebo in diet, however, are often more subtle. An individual's experience of food allergies and intolerances, although founded in immunological and metabolic processes, respectively, also depends on that person's beliefs and expectancies at the conscious and unconscious levels. Food aversions and taboos can likewise provoke physiological responses when challenged, often with no basis in biology but richly embedded within personal and cultural beliefs. Like taboo foods, comfort and ceremonial foods are defined by specific cultural and religious contexts. In many cases, despite unfavorable nutritional (e.g., high-fat) or pharmacological (e.g., intoxicating) profiles, these foods offer a sense of comfort, contentment, tradition, and connectedness that contribute to mental health and well-being. In some cultures, foods may also be magical, sacred, or curative, elevating their spiritual status and psychological impacts (Simoons 1998).

Analogies of placebo in the dieting and health food industries are hard to avoid. From fad diets to hypnotic suggestions, countless people turn to alternative strategies for losing weight—at times with remarkable success, even if only in the short term (Thibault 2011). Product labels advertising "reduced sodium," "no sugar added," "organic," or "natural" can mislead consumers into false perceptions of a food's nutritional value, safety, origin, or environmental footprint. Health foods, from "superfoods" to probiotics, are marketed with reference to disease prevention and healthy aging. These claims are often based in scientific evidence but rarely supported by randomized controlled trials (RCTs) as required for pharmaceuticals. Emerging commercial interest in the marketing of functional foods with approved, evidence-based health claims draws attention back to placebos as controls in clinical research (which is generally more complicated than a sugar pill, but more on that later).

Whether closely or loosely related to medical placebos, foods are much more than the sum of their chemicals. As symbols, they create meaning that our minds and bodies interpret on a physiological level, influencing our food choices and health for better or for worse. Capturing the multi-dimensional nature of our relationships and interactions with food is not easily accomplished through a single lens but instead requires an interdisciplinary approach.

11.3 The list of ingredients: introducing the elements of the "total food effect"

With the exception of clinical trials, direct reference to placebos is rare in nutrition research and related literature. Many social scientists, however, contribute important placebo-related insights on dietary habits, food choice, and nutrition (Booth 1994; Drewnowski and Rolls 2005; Wansink 2004) and implicate concepts of belief, expectancy, conditioning, and context, which align well with medical perspectives. As revealed in previous and subsequent chapters, different conceptualizations of placebos remain relevant beyond the borders of medicine and can be applied to the context of food. Moerman's meaning response is especially germane (Moerman 2002; Chapter 7) as it serves as a proxy for psychological and cognitive factors involved in patient (or consumer) responses to seeking and receiving care (or consuming food).

We adopt a similar but less recognized model, the "total drug effect" (TDE; Figure 11.1a) (Claridge 1970; Helman 2001, 2007) to explore placebo effects in the realm of diet. The TDE model posits that the overall effect of a drug depends not only on the drug's pharmacology but on the interacting attributes of the drug, patient, physician, setting, and context. Although some modifications are required, our adapted model, the "total food effect" (TFE) (Harris and Johns 2011), remains structurally and conceptually compatible with the TDE.

11.3.1 Drug to food

The transition from drug to food is straightforward since they share a common range of attributes. Like drugs, foods take different physical forms, with associated shapes, sizes, colors, flavors, and names. Many of these traits are determined by intrinsic chemistry, from pharmacological activity and digestibility to taste and texture, while others such as names, labels, and prices are culturally assigned. Foods and drugs differ, however, in their chemistries and the meanings, expectations, and sensations they elicit in consumers.

What constitutes a food or a medicine is largely defined by culture and social norms but rooted in biochemical factors such as toxicity, digestibility, and palatability (Moerman 1996). With drugs, pharmacologically active compounds are the critical components. Although present in some foods, usually at much lower levels, these compounds are secondary to nutrients when considering diet. Accordingly, nutritional properties replace pharmacological properties as a

(a)

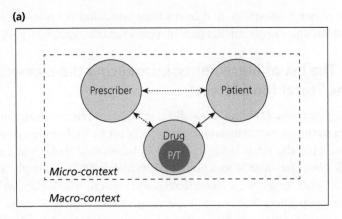

(b)

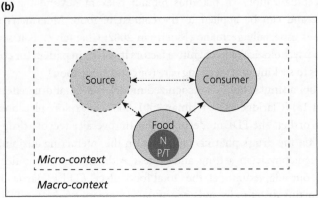

Fig. 11.1 The **(a)** total drug effect model and **(b)** total food effect model. By removing the pharmacological (P), toxicological (T), and/or nutritional (N) components of a drug or food from the model, remaining effects on the patient or consumer can be interpreted as placebo-like and explained through interactions between the remaining elements. The dashed line indicates that the micro-context is distinct from, yet embedded within, the macro-context. The dotted line around the source signifies its potential ambiguity in, or absence from, the total food effect.

Adapted from David Peters, Understanding the Placebo Effect in Complementary Medicine: Theory, Practice and Research, 1st Edition, p. 5, Figure 1.1, Copyright © 2001, with permission from Elsevier.

central component of the TFE (Figure 11.1b). More complex and variable than drug chemistry, food chemistry contributes more variables—and therefore more interactions—to the model. Simple foods like apples, milk, and honey contain thousands of different molecules; the most elaborate pharmaceutical treatment regimen consists of a few dozen at most. The assortment of compounds in a food, of foods in a dish, of dishes in a meal, and of meals in a diet increases this complexity exponentially. Moreover, whereas drugs are manufactured and strictly monitored to ensure chemical consistency, most foods are grown, harvested, processed, and/or cooked in ways that affect their chemistry, resulting in tremendous variability.

11.3.2 Patient to consumer

As persons, the patient receiving treatment and the consumer eating food are one and the same. In addition to physical traits like appearance, people have personalities, experiences, beliefs, and social status that, together with individual chemistry and biology, change with time. Whereas attributes relating to genetics and health are broadly applicable to both medicine and diet, the role of others, such as expectancies and mood, may be more subtle or variable; sadness, for example, may manifest differently at the doctor's office compared to the dinner table.

11.3.3 Prescriber to source

Whether interpreted as a physician, pharmacist, or complementary and alternative medicine (CAM) practitioner, the prescriber plays an integral role in the TDE (Helman 2001, 2007). In all cases, a person links treatment to patient and thus exhibits human characteristics. Attributes affecting patient beliefs, expectations, or treatment outcomes—for example, the person's education, professional acumen, bedside manner, and appearance—are particularly important (Benedetti 2010; Thomas 1987). However, what if no practitioner or prescriber is involved, as when one takes ibuprofen to relieve pain based on previous experience or common knowledge?

Whereas a prescriber may remain pertinent in the context of diet, as when participating in clinical research, consulting a dietician, or nourished by a caregiver, the identity and role of prescriber is often ambiguous or absent. More appropriately, the "source" of a food, meal, or diet may be identified as anyone or anything (e.g., a restaurant, commercial, website) endorsing or providing food or dietary information. The source may also be interpreted as any step in the supply chain linking product to consumer. For consumers focused on the final stages of food production, the role of individual people, from grocers to celebrity chefs, is once again apparent and salient. For those concerned with the food supply chain, the role of specific individuals diminishes compared to that assigned to corporations, technologies, and ideologies. In farming and hunter-gatherer communities, the source may be viewed as soil, sun, and water, as the fruit of one's labor or spiritual forces.

Information about food and diet (in the form of recommendations, health claims, recipes, etc.), provided personally or through popular culture and mass media, can direct choice and impact health outcomes. Attempting to assign such attributes to the source inevitably merges with those of the food, the consumer, and the micro- or macro-context. To reflect this variability and potentially ambiguous contribution to the TFE, the source component is illustrated with a dashed line in Figure 11.1b.

11.3.4 Micro-context

The micro-context of the TDE and that of the TFE require little distinction, characterized by the physical and social setting in which treatment or eating takes place. The type of establishment (or lack thereof) (e.g., highway, forest) and its related traits are central. Beyond structural and sensory elements, the micro-context is further defined by geographical location, time, and weather, as well as the presence and interactions of other people, participating or not, and the social group(s) to which they belong. Together, these combined factors create dynamic, seldom replicated settings that influence consumer psychology and physiology.

11.3.5 Macro-context

The prevailing societal attitudes and values, the socioeconomic and political climate, as well as a region's history, customs, geography, and biological diversity are equally pertinent to the consumption of both food and medicine. Aborting a pregnancy and eating pork respectively present specific medical and nutritional consequences; doing the former within a Catholic society or the latter within an Islamic one, however, may result in additional effects on social, psychological, and physical health. Factors including popular knowledge and prevailing stereotypes about foods and the people who eat them contribute as well. Language is a crucial element of the macro-context, with classification systems organizing medicines, foods, and most everything else into meaningful categories (Bowker and Star 1999; Foucault 2002). Multiple independent classification systems may coexist, each adding labels and layers of meaning to a single item. Eggs are not just part of the "meat and alternatives" food group; they may be a breakfast food, an animal-based food, a taboo food, a nutrient-rich or high-cholesterol food, a yin (or cooling) food in traditional Chinese medicine, or a pungent, heating food in Ayurveda. While classifications are embedded in the macro-context, their pertinence varies from person to person and place to place.

11.3.6 Placebo drugs to placebo foods: limitations

The lack of nutritionally inert foods for experimental use limits comparison between the TDE and TFE models as well as placebo research in nutrition.

Placebo foods, which are almost always active placebos, may designate either pharmacological (e.g., caffeine-free) or nutritional (e.g., calcium-free) inertia. While omitting designated ingredients is easily accomplished (for instance, by not fortifying an otherwise fortified food or omitting the drug from a pill), developing placebo versions of whole foods is more challenging.

Some compounds, like alcohol and caffeine, can be removed through processing without significant impacts on overall food chemistry and sensory quality. Macronutrients can similarly be reduced or removed (for example, fat from dairy products), but rarely without modifying flavor. The extraction of all nutrients, however, not only reduces the food to little more than water (which many consider a nutrient) but fundamentally changes the eating experience of consumers. Liquid foods offer an exception frequently leveraged in food-related research. Still, in contrast to medical placebos, the taste of both the verum and placebo drinks is often masked to prevent unblinding, simplifying the placebo design but limiting the relevance to dietary behaviors (Huijbers et al. 1994; Noe et al. 1998).

Nutritional supplements in the form of pills or powders seem simple to recreate as placebos, but what is an appropriate filler? Lactose, a commonly used filler in pharmaceuticals and placebo pills, is neither nutritionally nor physiologically inert; substituting lactose for another nutrient thus equates to substituting one active drug with another, resulting in active placebos, if not alternative interventions with unexpected direct effects. Adding indigestible fillers, like certain fat substitutes, may (incompletely) simulate the sensory experience of eating but also interfere with nutrient absorption and gastrointestinal function (Wylie-Rosett 2002).

11.4 The main course: integrating the elements of the "total food effect"

How do the components of the model interact and influence a consumer's food-related perceptions, behaviors, and responses? Because the role of the practitioner translates inconsistently into our model, we only briefly explore source–consumer and source–food relationships before focusing on consumer–food interactions and the impact of the micro- and macro-context.

11.4.1 Source–consumer interactions

Placebo research suggests that, when a consumer receives food or dietary advice from a respected individual (the source) inclined to promote better health, the individual's words, attitudes, and behaviors can elicit neurological and physiological responses in the consumer (Benedetti 2010). Relationships with dietitians and personal trainers offer obvious—though seldom studied—opportunities for source–consumer interactions with either positive or negative impacts on consumer outcomes. A role for family relationships, in contrast, is well-supported by empirical evidence. Independent of socioeconomic factors, eating at home or as a family is frequently identified as a positive contributor to diet quality, nutrient intake, and health, especially among children and adolescents (Briefel and Johnson 2004; Patrick and Nicklas 2005; Scaglioni et al. 2008). Alternatively, unhealthy eating environments in the home can promote problematic eating behaviors (Scaglioni et al. 2008).

If the source is not identified as a person but as an enterprise or industry, its attributes and actions may nonetheless impact consumer expectancies, choices, and experiences. Transparency on the part of food retailers is a pertinent example. Nutritional information about menu items—a legislated requirement in an increasing number of countries—may be listed on packaging, posters, pamphlets, or menus, but is often only available online, where it is infrequently accessed and unlikely retained at the point of purchase (Bassett et al. 2008; Roberto et al. 2009). Including caloric information directly on menus offers more promise in terms of calorie control, but only when provided alongside daily intake recommendations. Otherwise, people tend to reduce their caloric intake at first, only to reward themselves shortly thereafter (Roberto et al. 2010).

11.4.2 **Source–food interactions**

The relationship between nutritional and medical practitioners and the interventions they prescribe is based on prior experience as well as information gleaned from training, colleagues, sales representatives, and the media. This relationship not only influences interactions with patients but guides practitioners in selecting from the "menu" of appropriate treatment options once a diagnosis is reached. At least in medicine, a prescriber's knowledge and expectation of therapy can modulate patient outcomes for better or worse (Gracely et al. 1985). While most dietary decisions are in the hands of consumers, comparable situations arise when the source controls what consumers get to eat. If the source has a vested interest in providing safe and nutritious meals, source–food interactions will likely bode well for the TFE (in terms of health). For example, a mother will choose and prepare only the best foods to serve her family—particularly if someone is unwell.

Sources with competing interests, such as profit margins and return business in the private sector (Glanz et al. 2007) or resource availability and food allergies in the public sector (Gregoire 1994), must also be considered. In the food industry, where customer satisfaction and sales prevail, nutritional quality and indirect health consequences usually come second to palatability, convenience, and economy—a trend contributing to the flood of high-calorie, low-cost foods and increasing global rates of obesity and metabolic disorders (Drewnowski and Darmon 2005).

By manipulating the attributes of the food, from shape and color to packaging and branding, the source influences food chemistry as well as consumer beliefs and expectations. Cooks do not just select their ingredients but measure, mix, and prepare them. A food producer's chosen practices of farming, processing, storage, and transport not only affect nutrient content but food safety (Bhat 2008). Strategically designed by industry to meet strict regulatory guidelines and marketing goals, food labels selectively draw attention toward desired attributes and away from undesired ones. Even though labels list some nutritional information, many consumers ignore or cannot apply it appropriately (Cowburn and Stockley 2005).

11.4.3 The patient-drug and consumer-food relationships

Pharmacology and metabolism

Individual responses to diet are rooted in food chemistry and human biology. Many foods contain biologically active non-nutrients that can exert powerful effects on consumer health. Like drugs, these substances (as well as most nutrients) must pass through the digestive system into the blood and liver before they serve their eventual function or reach their site of biological activity. This depends on, among other things, the transport, metabolism, and clearance of ingested chemicals—processes that are largely predetermined by consumer genetics, age, weight, overall health, and external factors including diet. Here are but a few examples of food–consumer interactions at the level of pharmacology and metabolism: genetics underlie the reduced capacity to metabolize alcohol and lactose in certain ethnic populations (Edenberg 2007; Swallow 2003); a full stomach slows the absorption of alcohol and the ensuing onset of cognitive impairment (Millar et al. 1992); substances in garlic and grapefruit inhibit drug metabolism, transport, and, consequently, bioavailability (Diaconu et al. 2011; Gallicano et al. 2003).

Nutrition

Unlike medicines, nutrients are essential to growth, development, health maintenance, and everyday bodily function. The body has thus evolved specific mechanisms to monitor and regulate nutrient availability, use, and storage, primarily through neuroendocrine pathways that also control hunger and appetite (Cummings and Overduin 2007). Deficiency or excess of any nutrient is, in itself, a health concern only remedied by increasing or decreasing the availability of the particular nutrient(s).

When consumed in excess, macronutrients are stored or excreted with long-term impacts on weight and risk of diet-related chronic disease (Hung et al. 2003; Pecoits-Filho 2007). In contrast, excesses of vitamins and minerals can lead to acute and severe toxicity requiring immediate medical attention. With the exception of rare genetic disorders impairing nutrient uptake, metabolism, or clearance, nutrient deficiencies rarely develop due to consumer biology but, instead, to economic, social, political, geographical, and ideological factors, which are equally pertinent to situations of over-nutrition (Tanumihardjo et al. 2007).

Looking briefly at these examples through the TFE model, nutrient content dominates consumer–food interactions. Removing the nutrient component from the model renders the long-term prognosis for nutrient deficient individuals as poor, regardless of any positive psychosocial benefits the food may offer. The opposite argument generally holds for nutrient poisoning and over-nutrition—consumers would benefit from the removal of the nutrient in excess. In cases of over-nutrition, however, the lack of energy-dense carbohydrates and fats can also alter taste and texture as well as hormonal and reward stimuli that contribute to chronic overeating (Smeets et al. 2011; Stubbs 2001). Accordingly, any ensuing reduction in food intake is soon followed by renewed urges.

Flavor

In addition to nutrition and pharmacology, food and drug chemistry determines taste, odor, texture, and color as gustatory, olfactory, somatosensory, auditory, visual, and trigeminal inputs that together determine individual flavor perception. With sensory systems adaptively inclined toward obtaining nutrients and avoiding poisons, we innately prefer sweet and salty, an indication of nutrient-rich foods, over sour and bitter (Birch 1999)—tastes tightly bound to the evolution of modern medicine (Johns 1999). Several genes are implicated in flavor perception, particularly with regard to taste sensitivity. Smoking and exposure to other toxins also impacts on perception of chemical stimuli, as can personal health, particularly with regards to the respiratory and olfactory systems. Upon perceiving flavor-related stimuli, consumers respond and behave in accordance with not only their sensitivity but their prior experience with the food or its qualities as well as their personal dietary habits, preferences, and traditions (Lindemann 2001; Logue 2004).

A fertile field of research, flavor perception is rife with placebo-like effects. However, since a comprehensive review is beyond the scope of this chapter, we briefly examine two contributing factors—taste and color—to highlight the interacting influences of biology and culture on diet.

Taste

TAS2R38 is a well-characterized gene that encodes a bitter taste receptor broadly tuned to perceive sulfur-containing compounds commonly found in broccoli, related vegetables, green tea, and soya. Recognized as a genetic trait before the identification of TAS2R28, the capacity to sense bitter-tasting chemicals distinguished individuals, based on sensitivity, into groups of super-, medium-, or non-tasters (Bartoshuk et al. 1994). Research investigating whether this variation relates to individual food preferences, dietary habits, and physical health has yielded inconsistent results. Whereas sensitivity to bitter and sweet taste, the texture of fat, and the astringency of alcohol associates well with taster phenoltype, TAS2R38 haplotype is seldom associated with dietary habits, anthropometric measurements, or disease risk (Gorovic et al. 2011; Navarro-Allende et al. 2008; Ooi et al. 2010; Timpson et al. 2005). As a result, many researchers conclude that psychological and cultural factors outweigh genetically determined taste perception with regard to personal food choices (Gorovic et al. 2011; Navarro-Allende et al. 2008; Ooi et al. 2010).

Color

Although a chemical-based trait, color is perceived prior to consuming a food (or drug) and requires no direct biochemical interaction to wield its meaningful power. The stimulant effect of red pills and the sedative effect of blue pills, discussed in previous chapters, exemplify the potency of color on patient responses. When it comes to food, color shapes consumer perceptions of flavor and quality through learned associations and expectations derived from previous experience. For example, whereas British people tend to associate red- and blue-colored drinks with cherry and raspberry, respectively, Taiwanese people more likely identify red as cranberry and blue as mint (Shankar et al. 2010). In addition to prejudicing flavor expectations, color alters flavor perception; green-colored cherry-flavored drinks, for instance, are sometimes reported to taste like lime (DuBose et al. 1980). Red liquids are sometimes (Johnson and Clydesdale 1982), but not always (Strugnell 1997), perceived as sweeter than clear liquids of equal sugar content and the odors of colored solutions are perceived as more intense than those of equally-scented clear solutions (Zellner and Whitten 1999).

Within the wine-drinking community, red denotes distinct qualities calling for specific terminology. In experimental settings, however, untrained wine tasters almost unanimously describe artificially red-colored white wine as a red wine based on its aromatic qualities (Morrot et al. 2001). Wine experts perform better but remain susceptible to "placebo" red wine, less accurately judging the attributes of white wine illuminated by red light (Ross et al. 2008) or colored with red dye and presented in clear glassware (Parr et al. 2002).

Shape and format

The physical appearance of food influences consumption to a great degree. To safeguard against spoiled or unsanitary products at the grocery store, we seek perfect-looking foods that, perhaps counterproductive to one`s motive, probably reflect the use of pesticides, waxes, or preservatives rather than nutritional quality or flavor. At the dinner table, we want to eat what looks good. However, if deemed unappetizing, the sight of food can eradicate appetite or even cause illness.

While we know that shape and format of medical treatments (or placebos) can influence patient outcomes (de Craen et al. 2000; Linde et al. 2010), the influence of food shape and format on consumer preferences, behaviors, and responses has received little experimental attention outside of the industry. The effects of liquid versus solid food on appetite and satiety represent an exception, though evidence remains equivocal. Despite reports that liquids trigger satiation pathways less effectively than solids, leading to the recent admonition of sweetened beverages for their putative role in rising rates of obesity, other evidence indicates that liquid nutrients are equally or more satiating than solids (Almiron-Roig et al. 2003). This variability is not surprising given that hunger, appetite, and satiation are regulated not only through activation of specific chemoreceptors in the gastrointestinal system but the integration of various physiological, sensory, and cognitive stimuli.

Food and nutrient format potentially affects consumer beliefs and decisions. Sugar-based candies, for example, appear in countless shapes and textures with roughly the same list of ingredients. Moreover, the term "sugar," along with its negative connotations for health, refers specifically to sucrose on food label ingredient lists. As a result, other forms are regularly added to foods: the more obvious brown, confectioner's, granulated, invert, maple, raw, and white sugars, as well as the less transparent processing variants (e.g., corn syrup, evaporated cane juice). Consumers inclined to read the list likely consider such ingredients, however interpreted, in making food choices.

Quantity and size

How does quantity affect food consumption, dietary habits, and the TFE? Analogous to pill number in medicine, serving size influences food consumption, at times contributing to health risks such as overeating. Numerous studies, both laboratory and free-living, demonstrate that increased serving size results in increased energy intake (Ello-Martin et al. 2005; Fisher and Kral 2008). In other words, you eat more popcorn at the movies if you buy a large instead of a small size, regardless of what you ate for dinner. Here, cognitive attention and visual difficulty in judging portion size from larger containers are but two of the factors at play; the social environment and associated behavioral norms add another level of complexity. Increasing the number and variety of offered food items (e.g., popcorn, candies, nachos) similarly leads to higher energy intake (Cohen 2008).

Research on nutritional supplements (though not typically considered food) suggests that, as with placebo pills (de Craen et al. 1999), more is better—at least through the eyes of many consumers. Whereas the immunosupportive effects of vitamin C are well substantiated, increased dietary intake, even at doses more than ten times the daily recommended value, fails to consistently reduce the duration or severity of colds in clinical research[1] (Douglas et al. 2007). Still, despite the conclusion from a recent systematic review that "routine mega-dose prophylaxis is not rationally justified for community use," (Douglas et al. 2007) a great many people continue increasing their consumption of vitamin C in search of relief or protection from cold-like symptoms.

Price and labels

Food traits such as brand and price offer both sensory and social cues that consumers associate with quality, value, and even effects on health. Language and imagery presented on product labels, packaging, advertisements, and in the media foster learned and socially and culturally contrived associations that affect consumer behavior. Using placebo-based paradigms, researchers have reported both "brand" and "price" effects in the treatment of headache (Branthwaite and Cooper 1981) and pain (Waber et al. 2008), respectively. Interestingly, some of this research was inspired by studies on the effects of marketing on cognitive performance following consumption of an energy drink—a food!

By manipulating consumer expectations of quality without the use of placebos, the authors found that a person's ability to solve puzzles was not only affected by price but by previous brand exposure, self-reported expectancies, as well as the provision and strength of supporting materials (Shiv et al. 2005). The influence of discounted price was lost when individuals were reminded of popular price–quality beliefs, indicating a role for unconscious processing. Notably, regular-priced drinks only improved performance if accompanied by strongly supportive statements that also increased self-reported alertness but not motivation (the product claims to "boost alertness" with no reference to motivation) (Shiv et al. 2005).

Because consumers perceive lower-priced items—foods, drugs, or other—as lesser in quality, they judge them as such (Gerstner 1985; Roe and Munroe

1989). If the same wine is presented in separate bottles marked with different prices, people generally say the more expensive one is better (Plassman et al. 2008). Furthermore, a drink labeled as a preferred brand can taste better and activate the brain differentially to the same unlabeled drink (Allison and Uhl 1964; McClure et al. 2004), while meat tastes better when labeled "75% lean" rather than "25% fat" (Levin and Gaeth 1988).

Consumer experience

Many of the examples discussed so far involve interactions between food traits and consumer psychology; how people interpret a food's taste, color, size, price, and labels affects how they perceive, choose to eat, and respond to it. These interactions are highly dependent on personal experience and implicate both unconscious and conscious learning processes. Classical conditioned (Pavlovian) responses (an underlying mechanism of many placebo effects) are well documented in the realm of diet; conditioned taste aversions and, of course, salivating at the sight or smell of food (Klosterhalfen et al. 2000) are two clear examples. Personal experience also shapes response expectancies. With exposure to any stimulus, the experience becomes integrated into memories, attitudes, and expectations about the stimulus and subsequently influences the experience of future exposures (Kirsch 1999). In terms of diet, people experience the various sensory qualities and satiating or pharmacological/toxicological effects of different foods all the time. This intimate, ongoing interaction between diet, mind, and body—past, present, and future—forms the foundation of personal food preferences and aversions, ultimately manifesting as choices and habits that determine nutritional and health status.

As Takarangi and Loftus explain in Chapter 12 of this book, memory is imperfect and highly susceptible to suggestion. False memories, whether good or bad, can alter people's attitudes about food as well as their subsequent decisions and actions (Bernstein and Loftus 2009). Geared to answer questions of psychology rather than nutrition, most relevant research has focused on foods like hard-boiled eggs, asparagus, and dill pickles, without concern for dietary implications. According to one study, however, people may avoid a fattening food if convinced they had a negative experience with it as a child (Bernstein et al. 2005). Unfortunately, the avoidance effect was only observed for infrequently encountered high-fat foods (Bernstein et al. 2005), suggesting that daily dietary habits are harder to break through means of suggestion.

Second-hand knowledge

The manipulation of memory illustrates that, in addition to personal experience, consumer beliefs and expectations are also shaped by suggestion. Information gleaned from family, friends, social networks, and the media, whether true or false, leads to (perceived) consumer knowledge, enhanced awareness, and modified behaviors. The role of direct-to-consumer advertising by the pharmaceutical industry on patient treatment preferences in the United States serves as a good example from the medical milieu (Datti and Carter 2006; Mintzes et al. 2003). Increasingly, information pertaining to food safety and health benefits similarly results in higher market demand but seldom out-competes the sway of information about palatability and cost.

11.4.4 **The impacts of the micro-context**

Filled with staff, furniture, appliances, and other sensory stimuli symbolic of food and cooking, kitchens and dining rooms are inherently associated with eating. To create the desired dining experience for their customers, most restaurant owners pay meticulous attention to floor plan, décor, lighting, and music. Though not for commercial purposes, many home owners invest in the design and décor of their dining rooms for similar reasons of culture, comfort, and cleanliness. However, does the eating environment affect diet and nutrition?

In medicine, elements of the healthcare facility influence both patients and staff (Rubin 1998), with a variety of physical and social factors contributing to health outcomes (Table 11.1). Evidence likewise supports the existence of micro-context effects in diet, but the majority of research has focused on external influences and food consumption. The mere sight, proximity, or variety of food increases energy intake, as does watching television or a movie while eating (Wansink 2004). Lighting also alters calorie consumption as well as taste perception; darkness confuses subjective satiety leading to greater food intake and inaccurate estimates of consumed calories (Scheibehenne et al. 2010; Wansink 2004). Alternatively, without vision, attention to other senses increases and, as promoted by restaurants premised on fine dining in complete darkness, leads to enriched taste experiences. Perhaps an analog of medicine's high-tech, cutting-edge interventions associated with powerful placebo-like effects (Kaptchuk et al. 2000; Moerman 2011), "dark" restaurants may more appropriately owe their success to their modernity and the social and cultural esteem of the experience.

The impact of the social environment on diet depends on individual preference and the context of eating. Whereas medicine is mostly private in Western cultures (but social in others), eating is almost always a social activity with shared relations, experiences, and cultures as a common point of reference. Indeed, eating socially or alone influences nutritional quality and energy consumption differently for different people, perhaps due to social pressures that arbitrate personal behavior (Wansink 2004).

Table 11.1 Examples of how micro-context traits impact on the health of patients and healthcare staff

Feature	Effect on patient health	Effect on staff health
Private vs. shared room	↓ Infection (Shirani et al. 1986)	↓ Stress (Chaudhury et al. 2006)
No window	↑ Disorientation (Keep et al. 1980)	
	↑ Delusions (Keep et al. 1980)	
Sunny rooms and views	↓ Length of stay (Beauchemin and Hays 1996)	↑ Job satisfaction (Mroczek et al. 2005)
	↓ Mortality after myocardial infarction (Beauchemin and Hays 1998)	↑ Well-being (Leather 1998)
	↓ Use of analgesics (Ulrich 1984)	
Disruptive noise	↑ Stress (Hilton 1985)	↑ Stress (Choiniere 2010; Ryherd et al. 2008)
	↓ Sleep (Richardson et al. 2007)	↓ Communication (Shapiro and Berland 1972)
	↓ Preterm infant development (Brown 2009)	
Controlled noise	↓ Pulse amplitude (Hagerman et al. 2005)	↑ Speech intelligibility
	↓ Re-hospitalization of coronary care patients (Hagerman et al. 2005)	↓ Pressure and strain (Blomkvist et al. 2005)

Reproduced from Cory Harris and Timothy Johns, The total food effect: exploring placebo analogies in diet and food culture, *The Journal of Mind–Body Regulation*, 1(3), pp. 154, Table 1, © The Authors, 2011.

11.4.5 **The impacts of the macro-context**

Most culture-dependent meanings ascribed to color, format, number, and price are rooted in the macro-context. Geographical, economic, and cultural determinants of accessing, experiencing, and interpreting food are also relevant examples. As illustrated by the explosion of corn-based products in North American diets, agricultural subsidies shape national and global food markets by manipulating the availability and price of selected foods. Cultural norms dictate what types of food are acceptable and how they should be presented:

- Serving fish without the head is more appealing to some people but also reduces nutritional value.
- The production and sale of genetically modified foods is well-established in North America but not tolerated in Europe.
- Highly nutritious and abundant, insects are considered taboo in some cultures but staples or delicacies in others.

11.5 **A sampling of desserts: three case studies**

The following case studies explore how interactions between food, consumer, source, setting, and context contribute to consumer responses in three distinct scenarios. While each focuses on a different type of food and a distinct variation on placebo, all illustrate the potency of top–down effects in the way people feel and act after eating.

11.5.1 **Case study 1: drug-like foods—alcohol and behavior**

Alcohol has been known, enjoyed, and abused by humans for millennia. Because alcohol (ethanol) provides calories and most alcoholic beverages contain other nutrients and biologically active chemicals, the TFE of such drinks extends beyond the intoxicating effects of the alcohol itself. For simplicity, however, this case study focuses on consumer–food–source interactions that contribute to alcohol's effects on consumer physiology, cognition, and, most specifically, social behavior.

Different types of "booze," from beer to wine to distilled spirits, owe their specific qualities to their ingredients and production processes, which collectively contribute to personal preferences and popular acceptability. The ethanol in all drinks, however, is identical in all ways except perhaps quantity. It exerts well-established dose–response effects throughout the body, most notably the central nervous system. Like the previously noted effects of price and labeling on consumer perceptions of wine and beer, respectively, food traits suggestive of alcohol content can elicit strong placebo-like responses in consumers.

The pharmacokinetics and pharmacodynamics of alcohol depend on consumer genetics, body size and composition, liver and kidney function, diet and drinking habits, among other factors. Modulating consumer responses to alcohol through bottom–up processes, these biological and lifestyle traits underlie why, for example, healthy, big, muscular, or well-fed people tend to tolerate alcohol better than people who are unhealthy, small, chubby, or fasted. In contrast, consumer beliefs and expectations about alcohol generate top–down effects. Because virtually everyone has first- or second-hand experience with alcohol and its effects, people expect that drinking will make them feel and act in a particular manner. As Kirsch describes in Chapter 2, such response expectancies often translate into experience.

With the help of placebo alcohol controls, social scientists have repeatedly demonstrated that people who believe they consumed alcohol are prone to exhibiting some—but not all—symptoms and behaviors typical of inebriation.[2] For example, male consumers of placebo alcohol show signs consistent with sexual arousal, including altered heart rate, skin temperature, and penile tumescence (Briddell et al. 1978; Lang et al. 1980; Lansky and Wilson 1981). People who think they are under the influence are also more likely to engage in social (mis)behaviors commonly associated with alcohol, from increased risk taking and decreased sexual inhibition (McMillen et al. 1989; George and Marlatt 1986; George et al. 2000) to increased aggression and interest in viewing violent imagery (Cherek et al. 1985; George et al. 1989; Lang et al. 1975). Interestingly, certain responses to placebo alcohol (e.g., increased cravings) do not follow surreptitiously administered alcohol (Hull and Bond 1986), whereas non-social behaviors and cognitive functions appear to be impervious to placebo but not real alcohol (Assefi and Garry 2003; Hull and Bond 1986).

In these studies, the "source" (i.e., the researcher) is central to the TFE, manipulating consumer expectations by deceptively suggesting or concealing alcohol content. Because many experiments were conducted in real or simulated social environments, similar source-driven interactions are likely whenever someone manipulates consumer beliefs about alcohol content. Unexpectedly, the role of the scientist, the context of the research, and the use of placebo controls reveal that consumers compensate for anticipated cognitive impairment through vigilant attention to situational cues (Testa et al. 2006); a demonstration of top–down control over alcohol's actions on cognitive function.

Both physical and social setting can also alter drinking habits and the experienced effects of alcohol. For example, wine seems to taste better when consumed under red or blue rather than green or white ambient lighting (Oberfeld et al. 2009). Compared to drinking alone, drinking among others generally increases alcohol intake, affective responses, and feelings of euphoria through mechanisms of shared experience and reinforced expectations (Lindman 1982; Pliner and Cappel 1974; Wigmore et al. 1991).

Due to alcohol's pervasiveness in human culture across time and geography, its macro-context bears heavily on individual alcohol consumption. Whereas some cultures consider alcohol taboo, others celebrate and incorporate it into their social, religious, and everyday traditions. Today, depending on where one resides, the production, marketing, sale, purchase, and/or consumption of alcohol may be regulated by law, shaping not only availability and accessibility but also the cultural roles and symbolic meanings of alcohol as well as the legal and social consequences of drunkenness. Other factors, such as the prevalence of alcoholism and related social ills and the influence of public and private sectors can similarly affect popular alcohol-related attitudes and expectations.

11.5.2 Case study 2: dairy and lactose intolerances

Common notions of lactose intolerance (LI) among many practitioners and the general public reflect a simple set of consumer–food interactions that lead to an uncomfortable physiological response: if a person does not produce adequate amounts of lactase to break down the lactose they consume, a condition known as lactase non-persistence (LNP) will likely result in him or her experiencing gastrointestinal symptoms such as abdominal pain, bloating, and flatulence after eating dairy. Indeed, LI is diagnosed when a patient is deemed LNP following a lactose challenge *and* subsequently experiences symptoms. The relationship between lactase levels, dairy consumption, and symptom manifestation, however, is rarely so straightforward. Whereas individuals with LNP do not always experience symptoms after eating lactose, those with adequate lactase activity are not always symptom-free (Vesa et al. 1996). Moreover, regardless of lactase status, people present with gastrointestinal symptoms following consumption of placebo (lactose-free) lactose challenges. In fact, a meta-analysis of twenty-one studies with LNP individuals given placebo or lactose doses typically found in meals indicates that lactose is not a major cause of symptoms (Savaiano et al. 2006).

Whether or not someone responds negatively to eating dairy products depends on numerous interacting traits within the TFE model. Lactose content is the primary food trait responsible for LI but varies widely between dairy products, from negligible or low in most cheeses to high in evaporated and condensed milk. Other food substances, for example allergens or toxins, can cause similar symptomology that is easily misattributed to lactose. The physical and sensory qualities of dairy products, as well as conditioned or expectancy-driven responses, evoke associations with lactose regardless of lactose content.

In addition to genetics and age, a consumer's intestinal microflora influence lactose digestion by providing lactase activity but also symptom development by fermenting undigested lactose and releasing hydrogen gas, which can lead to bloating and flatulence. Regular consumption of lactose (e.g., one glass of milk a day) drastically improves lactose digestion, even among individuals with LNP (Hertzler and Savaiano 1996). Consumer experience, beliefs, and expectations relating to dairy products or one's ability to tolerate lactose exert powerful yet often overlooked top–down effects on both acute physiological responses and long-term dietary habits and nutrition. Despite consistent evidence that LI sufferers can generally consume a moderate amount of lactose (e.g., one cup of milk) and remain asymptomatic (Suarez et al. 1997), many believe they must exclude all types of dairy product from their diets. In North America, where dairy products are the primary source of dietary calcium, these diets pose a risk to bone health if alternative sources of calcium are not found (Buchowski et al. 2002; Fleming and Heimbach 1994).

The words and actions of practitioners (the source), together with the clinical context, affect consumer beliefs, expectations, and potentially symptoms during the diagnostic process and, depending on prognosis, future responses to or avoidance of dairy products. Beyond influencing the types, quality, and availability of dairy products, the macro-context similarly impacts on consumer and clinician psychology. That LI is widespread, more so among certain populations, is common knowledge. When a consumer presents with irregular or nonspecific gastrointestinal problems, LI is thus presumed a likely cause, particularly if the consumer belongs to a high-risk group. This knowledge, together with consumer or practitioner experiences, may bias beliefs and even self- or clinical diagnosis. The prevalence of LI, however, is lower than popular estimates, which are based on rates of LNP rather than LI (LNP paired with symptoms). Clinical research, for example, consistently demonstrates that many maldigesters show few symptoms after lactose challenges equivalent to one liter of milk (Casellas et al. 2010).

Indeed, there is a significant gap in the evidence linking LNP to symptom development in clinical research on LI. Whereas bottom–up processes only bridge this gap in places, consumer psychology offers an overarching explanatory model warranting more thorough investigation.

11.5.3 Case study 3: ceremonial foods—the host and Holy Communion

To serve as comparison and to illustrate the influence of ceremony on health, let us first consider an example from the medical literature (Kaptchuk et al. 2010). In a non-deceptive, open-label trial for the treatment of irritable bowel syndrome (IBS), patients were randomized to receive open-label placebo pills or no treatment for three weeks while receiving the same quality, frequency, and duration of care. Uniquely, prior to randomization, patients met with a practitioner who explained that a placebo pill was inert and that: "1) the placebo effect is powerful, 2) the body can automatically respond to taking placebo pills like Pavlov's dogs who salivated when they heard a bell, 3) a positive attitude helps but is not necessary, and 4) taking the pills faithfully is critical." Using four different subjective measures of IBS symptomology and quality of life, both treatment groups improved but patients taking placebos reported significantly greater improvements (Kaptchuk et al. 2010).

With no pharmacological component and both groups exposed to the same context and doctor–patient interactions, we can interpret these results through a simplified TDE model. Physically, the blue and maroon placebo capsules were filled with an inert substance and issued in a labeled container by a practitioner in a healthcare setting. From the patient perspective, these traits alone could have triggered conscious and unconscious responses. The ceremony of receiving and taking medicine, together with associated expectations of benefit, contributed to patient improvement, at least in part.

For Christians, the breaking of the bread is essential to celebrating Holy Communion (the Eucharist or Lord's supper). For Catholics, the bread (host or sacrament) is traditionally a small, thin, round wafer with little taste or color, negligible nutritional value, and no pharmacological activity. Symbolically, however, the communion bread is the body of Christ and the act of eating it brings one in direct connection with Him. Moreover, the beliefs and expectations surrounding Communion are shared between the congregant (patient), priest (practitioner), congregation (micro-context), and greater Christian community (macro-context). Communion is taken in church with the host distributed by appropriate representatives then consumed following traditional practices. Interestingly, both the IBS trial and the breaking of the bread contain elements of operant conditioning; patients may report improvements to please researchers and churchgoers may take communion to avoid criticism or shame.

As suggested by the IBS trial, despite the lack of interactions between food chemistry and consumer, eating or not eating the bread can influence spiritual and mental health, if not physical health as well. Additionally, like the no-treatment group of the IBS placebo study (Kaptchuk et al. 2010), practicing Christians attending church, but unable to eat the sacrament, would benefit from other interactions (e.g., praying) but perhaps not as much as those who took Communion.

11.6 *"Cheque please!"*—closing remarks

The TFE approach is subject to several caveats and limitations. Beyond the practical and conceptual problems with nutritionally inert foods, adapting the model from medicine to diet resulted in new ambiguities and complications (Harris and Johns 2011). Briefly, the majority of constraints relate to complexity and time. In many scenarios, the number and complexity of interactions contributing to the TFE limit experimental utility, since collecting the necessary data and controlling for the necessary variables may be unfeasible. The ambiguity of the "source" component can add even more variables, while increasing the time frame of the investigation will definitely do so. Whereas the vast majority of evidence presented here involves only acute effects, the most significant impacts of diet on health are long term. Researchers study these long-term effects by epidemiological approaches, at least correlatively, but have difficulty untangling the factors at the level of individual foods and consumers. Temporal effects are further complicated by the quantity and frequency of food consumption, which, unlike medicines, are not prescribed in doses for specific periods of time or easily tracked for reliable reporting. Despite these constraints, the TFE offers a holistic lens through which to integrate and explore often segregated bottom–up and top–down influences on diet, and particularly placebo effects.

The examples discussed throughout this chapter reveal various types of placebo-like effects and placebogenic mechanisms. For example, unconsciously learned food aversions are typically rooted in conditioning, drunken behavior following placebo alcohol stems from response expectancies, and the consumption of larger portions from larger bowls or fewer calories from calorie-labeled menus reflects cognitive effects—the same core mechanisms behind medical placebo effects. Analogies of placebos in food and nutrition, however, reveal novel variations on conventional forms and relational structures.

Food labels present a unique permutation of the placebo paradigm where, despite receiving accurate information, consumers often under- or overestimate their nutrient intake due to a limited understanding of food labels and nutritional recommendations. Artificial sweeteners and fat substitutes are designed to simulate calorie-rich foods in every way except their "active" components, which in this case are associated with *negative* health outcomes (Hung et al. 2003). Here, people *knowingly* consume these placebo foods expecting to reduce their risk of developing chronic conditions such as diabetes, obesity, cancer, and cardiovascular disease, while enjoying the pleasures of indulgence. However, lacking the specific stimuli to activate the brain's reward circuitry, low-calorie alternatives often fail to provide the same sensory experience as the real thing. Perceived LI offers yet another variation where consumers who falsely underestimate their ability to tolerate dairy products not only react to lactose but avoid such products altogether—responses with negative impacts on their quality of life and, potentially, nutrition and health.

Like medicine, where placebo drugs are more effective in some circumstances than others (Benedetti 2009), certain aspects of diet appear more or less responsive to placebo-like interactions. Placebo effects are insignificant with regards to nutrient deficiencies but often robust in trials on diet-related problems such as IBS and LI (Casellas et al. 2010; Enck and Klosterhalfen 2005; Kaptchuk et al. 2010) as well as food-based intervention studies for the common cold (Carr et al. 1981) and postmenopausal hot flushes (Nahas et al. 2007). Moreover, food-related placebo effects may be subjective or objective (e.g., flavor perception vs. caloric intake) and elicit short- or long-term responses (e.g., improved cognitive performance vs. conditioned taste aversions).

With so much in common, perhaps placebo effects in medicine and diet share a common neurobiology. From a neurological standpoint, relieving (or suppressing) discomfort and gaining reward are not very different. When people want to suppress hunger-related discomfort, they simultaneously want the reward of food, which in itself is a means of relieving hunger. The mesolimbic dopaminergic system—the brain's motivation and reward center—drives the seeking behaviors and rewards associated with eating, sex, gambling, and euphoric or addictive drugs. Thanks to evidence derived almost exclusively from placebo research, we also know that expectations of treatment and improvement can activate the mesolimbic dopamine system of patients afflicted with pain, depression, and Parkinson's disease (Benedetti 2010; de la Fuente-Fernandez et al. 2006; Zubieta and Stohler 2009).[3] With expectancies appearing prominently in many diet-related behaviors and placebo effects, dopamine likely plays a pivotal role. Involvement of the opioid and cannabinoid systems, both implicated in placebo analgesia (Benedetti 2006; Benedetti et al. 2011) and eating patterns (Davis et al. 2011; Pagotto et al. 2006) also warrants investigation. Given the integrated inputs mediating dietary behaviors and consequences, other neurotransmitters and signaling pathways are likely to be involved as well.

While neuroimaging promises to shed more light on the mechanisms governing both eating habits and placebo effects, no single discipline can capture and interpret the complex relationships between people and food. As with placebo science, untangling the multilayered interactions that determine how eating affects personal and collective health requires interdisciplinary approaches.

The conceptual extension of placebo from medicine to diet offers mutual benefit to both domains. Whereas the TFE provides a novel explanatory model for investigating and interpreting food-related behaviors and responses, the insights gained inform placebo science (and related disciplines), clinical practice, and research, as well as industry and public health policy. The study of placebo-related phenomena in diet also affords new experimental models and stimulates innovative questions and avenues of research.

Acknowledgments

This chapter was originally published as: Cory Harris and Timothy Johns, The total food effect: exploring placebo analogies in diet and food culture, *The Journal of Mind–Body Regulation*, 1 (3), pp. 143–160, © The Authors, 2011.

We thank the Raz Lab for the workshop and creative exchanges that informed this essay.

Notes

1 Vitamin C supplementation for prophylaxis may be justified in people exposed to severe physical activity and to cold environments. Prophylactic use in the normal population resulted in mildly reduced duration but use as treatment had no effect (Douglas et al. 2007).

2 Note that the evidence cited in the section's case study stems from research with healthy social drinkers and cannot be assumed transferable to heavy drinkers and alcoholics.

3 Note that motivation and reward associated with sickness and relief is probably more similar to those of hunger and thirst than sex or gambling, since failure to act can be harmful to health and survival (Benedetti 2010).

References

Allison, R. I. and Uhl, K. P. (1964). Influence of beer brand identification of taste perception. *Journal of Marketing Research*, **1**(3), 36–39.

Almiron-Roig, E., Chen, Y., and Drewnowski, A. (2003). Liquid calories and the failure of satiety: how good is the evidence? *Obesity Reviews*, **4**(4), 201–212.

Assefi, S. L. and Garry, M. (2003). Absolut® memory distortions: alcohol placebos influence the misinformation effect. *Psychological Science*, **14**(1), 77–80.

Bartoshuk, L. M., Duffy, V. B., and Miller, I. J. (1994). PTC/PROP tasting: anatomy, psychophysics, and sex effects. *Physiology & Behavior*, **56**(6), 1165–1171.

Bassett, M. T., Dumanovsky, T., Huang, C., et al. (2008). Purchasing behavior and calorie information at fast-food chains in New York City, 2007. *American Journal of Public Health*, **98**(8), 1457–1459.

Beauchemin, K. M. and Hays, P. (1996). Sunny hospital rooms expedite recovery from severe and refractory depressions. *Journal of Affective Disorders*, **40**(1–2), 49–51.

Beauchemin, K. M. and Hays, P. (1998). Dying in the dark: sunshine, gender and outcomes in myocardial infarction. *Journal of the Royal Society of Medicine*, **91**(7), 352–354.

Benedetti, F. (2006). Placebo analgesia. *Neurological Sciences*, **2**(Suppl. 2), S100–102.

Benedetti, F. (2009). *Placebo effects: understanding the mechanisms in health and disease.* Oxford/ New York: Oxford University Press.

Benedetti, F. (2010). *The patient's brain: the neuroscience behind the doctor–patient relationship.* New York, NY: Oxford University Press.

Benedetti, F., Amanzio, M., Rosato, R., and Blanchard, C. (2011). Nonopioid placebo analgesia is mediated by CB1 cannabinoid receptors. *Nature Medicine*, **17**(10), 1228–1230.

Bernstein, D. M., Laney, C., Morris, E. K., and Loftus, E. F. (2005). False beliefs about fattening foods can have healthy consequences. *Proceedings of the National Academy of Sciences of the United States of America*, **102**(39), 13724–13731.

Bernstein, D. M. and Loftus, E. F. (2009). The consequences of false memories for food preferences and choices. *Perspectives on Psychological Science*, **4**(2), 135–138.

Bhat, R. V. (2008). Human health problems associated with current agricultural food production. *Asia Pacific Journal of Clinical Nutrition*, **17**(Suppl. 1), 91–94.

Birch, L. L. (1999). Development of food preferences. *Annual Review of Nutrition*, **19**, 41–62.

Blomkvist, V., Eriksen, C. A., Theorell, T., Ulrich, R., and Rasmanis, G. (2005). Acoustics and psychosocial environment in intensive coronary care. *Occupational and Environmental Medicine*, **62**(3), 62:e1. DOI:10.1136/oem.2004.017632

Booth, D. A. (1994). *Psychology of nutrition.* London/Bristol, PA: Taylor and Francis.

Bowker, G. C. and Star, S. L. (1999). *Sorting things out: classification and its consequences.* Cambridge, MA: MIT Press.

Branthwaite, A. and Cooper, P. (1981). Analgesic effects of branding in treatment of head-aches. *British Medical Journal*, **282**(6276), 1576–1578.

Briddell, D. W., Rimm, D. C., Caddy, G. R., Krawitz, G., Sholis, D., and Wunderlin, R. J. (1978). Effects of alcohol and cognitive set on sexual arousal to deviant stimuli. *Journal of Abnormal Psychology*, **87**(4), 418.

Briefel, R. R. and Johnson, C. L. (2004). Secular trends in dietary intake in the United States. *Annual Review of Nutrition*, **24**, 401–431.

Brown, G. (2009). NICU noise and the preterm infant. *Neonatal Network*, **28**(3), 165–173.

Buchowski, M. S., Semenya, J., and Johnson, A. O. (2002). Dietary calcium intake in lactose maldigesting intolerant and tolerant African-American women. *Journal of the American College of Nutrition*, **21**(1), 47–54.

Carr, A. B., Einstein, R., Lai, L. Y., Martin, N. G., and Starmer, G. A. (1981). Vitamin C and the common cold: a second MZ Cotwin control study. *Acta Geneticae Medicae et Gemellologiae*, **30**(4), 249–255.

Casellas, F., Aparici, A., Casaus, M., Rodriguez, P., and Malagelada, J. R. (2010). Subjective perception of lactose intolerance does not always indicate lactose malabsorption. *Clinical Hastroenterology and Hepatology*, **8**(7), 581–586.

Chaudhury, H., Mahmood, A., and Valente, M. (2006). Nurses' perception of single-occupancy versus multioccupancy rooms in acute care environments: an exploratory comparative assessment. *Applied Nursing Research*, **19**(3), 118–125.

Cherek, D. R., Steinberg, J. L., and Manno, B. R. (1985). Effects of alcohol on human aggressive behavior. *Journal of Studies on Alcohol*, **46**(4), 321–328.

Choiniere, D. B. (2010). The effects of hospital noise. *Nursing Administration Quarterly*, **34**(4), 327–333.

Claridge, G. S. (1970). *Drugs and human behaviour.* London: Allen Lane.

Cohen, D. A. (2008). Obesity and the built environment: changes in environmental cues cause energy imbalances. *International Journal of Obesity*, **32**(Suppl. 7), S137–142.

Cowburn, G. and Stockley, L. (2005). Consumer understanding and use of nutrition labelling: a systematic review. *Public Health Nutrition*, **8**(1), 21–28.

Cummings, D. E. and Overduin, J. (2007). Gastrointestinal regulation of food intake. *Journal of Clinical Investigation*, **117**(1), 13–23.

Datti, B. and Carter, M. W. (2006). The effect of direct-to-consumer advertising on prescription drug use by older adults. *Drugs & Aging*, **23**(1), 71–81.

Davis, C., Zai, C., Levitan, R. D., et al. (2011). Opiates, overeating and obesity: a psychogenetic analysis. *International Journal of Obesity*, **35**, 1347–1354.

de Craen, A. J., Moerman, D. E., Heisterkamp, S. H., Tytgat, G. N., Tijssen, J. G., and Kleijnen, J. (1999). Placebo effect in the treatment of duodenal ulcer. *British Journal of Clinical Pharmacology*, **48**(6), 853–860.

de Craen, A. J., Tijssen, J. G., de Gans, J., and Kleijnen, J. (2000). Placebo effect in the acute treatment of migraine: subcutaneous placebos are better than oral placebos. *Journal of Neurology*, **247**(3), 183–188.

de la Fuente-Fernandez, R., Lidstone, S., and Stoessl, A. J. (2006). Placebo effect and dopamine release. *Journal of Neural Transmission*, **70**(Suppl.), 415–418.

Diaconu, C. H., Cuciureanu, M., Vlase, L., and Cuciureanu, R. (2011). Food-drug interactions: grapefruit juice. *Revista Medico*, **115**(1), 245–250.

Douglas, R. M., Hemila, H., Chalker, E., and Treacy, B. (2007). Vitamin C for preventing and treating the common cold. *Cochrane Database of Systematic Reviews*, **3**, CD000980.

Drewnowski, A. and Darmon, N. (2005). The economics of obesity: dietary energy density and energy cost. *American Journal of Clinical Nutrition*, **82**(1), 265S–273S.

Drewnowski, A. and Rolls, B. J. (2005). How to modify the food environment. *Journal of Nutrition*, **135**(4), 898–899.

DuBose, C. N., Cardello, A.V., and Maller, O. (1980). Effects of colorants and flavorants on identification, perceived flavor intensity, and hedonic quality of fruit-flavored beverages and cake. *Journal of Food Science*, **48**(5), 1393–1399.

Edenberg, H. J. (2007). The genetics of alcohol metabolism: role of alcohol dehydrogenase and aldehyde dehydrogenase variants. *Alcohol Research & Health*, **30**(1), 5–13.

Ello-Martin, J. A., Ledikwe, J. H., and Rolls, B. J. (2005). The influence of food portion size and energy density on energy intake: implications for weight management. *American Journal of Clinical Nutrition*, **82**(1 Suppl.), 236S–241S.

Enck, P. and Klosterhalfen, S. (2005). The placebo response in functional bowel disorders: perspectives and putative mechanisms. *Neurogastroenterology and Motility*, **17**(3), 325–331.

Etkin, N. L. (1986). Multidisciplinary perspectives in the interpretation of plants used on indigenous medicine and diet. In: *Plants in indigenous medicine and diet: biobehavioral approaches* (ed. N. L. Etkin). Bedford Hills, New York: Redgrave Publishing Company, pp. 2–29.

Etkin, N. L. and Johns, T. (1998). "Pharmafoods" and "nutraceuticals": paradigm shifts in biotherapeutics. In: *Plants for food and medicine* (eds. H. D. V. Prendergast, N. L. Etkin, D. R. Harris, and P. J. Houghton). Kew: Royal Botanic Gardens, pp. 3–16.

Fillmore, M. T., Mulvihill, L. E., and Vogel-Sprott, M. (1994). The expected drug and its expected effect interact to determine placebo responses to alcohol and caffeine. *Psychopharmacology*, **115**(3), 383–388.

Fisher, J. O. and Kral, T. V. (2008). Super-size me: portion size effects on young children's eating. *Physiology & Behavior*, **94**(1), 39–47.

Fleming, K. H. and Heimbach, J. T. (1994). Consumption of calcium in the U.S.: food sources and intake levels. *Journal of Nutrition*, **124**(8 Suppl.), 1426S–1430S.

Foucault, M. (2002). *The order of things: an archaeology of the human sciences*: Taylor and Francis, New York.

Gallicano, K., Foster, B., and Choudhri, S. (2003). Effect of short-term administration of garlic supplements on single-dose ritonavir pharmacokinetics in healthy volunteers. *British Journal of Clinical Pharmacology*, **55**(2), 199–202.

George, W. H., Dermen, K. H., and Nochajski, T. H. (1989). Expectancy set, self-reported expectancies and predispositional traits: predicting interest in violence and erotica. *Journal of Studies on Alcohol*, **50**(6), 541–551.

George, W. H. and Marlatt, G. A. (1986). The effects of alcohol and anger on interest in violence, erotica, and deviance. *Journal of Abnormal Psychology*, **95**(2), 150.

George, W. H., Stoner, S. A., Norris, J., Lopez, P. A., and Lehman, G. L. (2000). Alcohol expectancies and sexuality: a self-fulfilling prophecy analysis of dyadic perceptions and behavior. *Journal of Studies on Alcohol*, **61**(1), 168–176.

Gerstner, E. (1985). Do higher prices signal higher quality? *Journal of Marketing Research*, **XXII**, 209–215.

Glanz, K., Resnicow, K., Seymour, J., et al. (2007). How major restaurant chains plan their menus: the role of profit, demand, and health. *American Journal of Preventive Medicine*, **32**(5), 383–388.

Gorovic, N., Afzal, S., Tjonneland, A., et al. (2011). Genetic variation in the hTAS2R38 taste receptor and brassica vegetable intake. *Scandinavian Journal of Clinical and Laboratory Investigation*, **71**(4), 274–279.

Gracely, R. H., Dubner, R., Deeter, W. R., and Wolskee, P. J. (1985). Clinicians' expectations influence placebo analgesia. *Lancet*, **1**(8419), 43.

Gregoire, M. B. (1994). Competencies for district school nutrition directors/supervisors. *School Foodservice Research Review*, **18**(2), 89–100.

Hagerman, I., Rasmanis, G., Blomkvist, V., Ulrich, R., Eriksen, C. A., and Theorell, T. (2005). Influence of intensive coronary care acoustics on the quality of care and physiological state of patients. *International Journal of Cardiology*, **98**(2), 267–270.

Hammami, M. M., Al-Gaai, E. A., Alvi, S., and Hammami, M. B. (2010). Interaction between drug and placebo effects: a cross-over balanced placebo design trial. *Trials*, **11**, 110.

Harris, C. S. and Johns, T. (2011). The total effect: exploring placebo analogies in diet and food culture. *Journal of Mind–Body Regulation*, **1**(3), 143–160.

Helman, C. (2001). Placebos and nocebos: the cultural construction of belief. In: *Understanding the placebo effect in complementary medicine: theory, practice and research* (ed. D. Peters). Edinburgh: Harcourt Publishers Limited, pp. 3–16.

Helman, C. (2007). *Culture, health and illness* (5th edn.). London: Hodder Arnold.

Hertzler, S. R. and Savaiano, D. A. (1996). Colonic adaptation to daily lactose feeding in lactose maldigesters reduces lactose intolerance. *American Journal of Clinical Nutrition*, **64**(2), 232–236

Hilton, B. A. (1985). Noise in acute patient care areas. *Research in Nursing & Health*, **8**(3), 283–291.

Huijbers, G. B., Colen, A. A., Jansen, J. J., Kardinaal, A. F., Vlieg-Boerstra, B. J., and Martens, B. P. (1994). Masking foods for food challenge: practical aspects of masking foods for a double-blind, placebo-controlled food challenge. *Journal of the American Dietetic Association*, **94**(6), 645–649.

Hull, J. G. and Bond, C. F. (1986). Social and behavioral consequences of alcohol consumption and expectancy: a meta-analysis. *Psychological Bulletin*, **99**(3), 347.

Hung, T., Sievenpiper, J. L., Marchie, A., Kendall, C. W., and Jenkins, D. J. (2003). Fat versus carbohydrate in insulin resistance, obesity, diabetes and cardiovascular disease. *Current Opinion in Clinical Nutrition and Metabolic Care*, **6**(2), 165–176.

Johns, T. (1999). The chemical ecology of human ingestive behaviors. *Annual Review of Anthropology*, **28**, 27–50.

Johnson, J. and Clydesdale, F. M. (1982). Perceived sweetness and redness in coloured sucrose solutions. *Journal of Food Science*, **47**, 747–752.

Kaptchuk, T. J., Friedlander, E., Kelley, J. M., et al. (2010). Placebos without deception: a randomized controlled trial in irritable bowel syndrome. *PLoS One*, **5**(12), e15591.

Kaptchuk, T. J., Goldman, P., Stone, D. A., and Stason, W. B. (2000). Do medical devices have enhanced placebo effects? *Journal of Clinical Epidemiology*, **53**(8), 786–792.

Keep, P., James, J., and Inman, M. (1980). Windows in the intensive therapy unit. *Anaesthesia*, **35**(3), 257–262.

Kirsch, I. (1999). *How expectancies shape experience* (1st edn.). Washington, DC: American Psychological Association.

Klosterhalfen, S., Ruttgers, A., Krumrey, E., et al. (2000). Pavlovian conditioning of taste aversion using a motion sickness paradigm. *Psychosomatic Medicine*, **62**(5), 671–677.

Lang, A. R., Goeckner, D. J., Adesso, V. J., and Marlatt, G. A. (1975). Effects of alcohol on aggression in male social drinkers. *Journal of Abnormal Psychology*, **84**(5), 508.

Lang, A. R., Searles, J., Lauerman, R., and Adesso, V. J. (1980). Expectancy, alcohol, and sex guilt as determinants of interest in and reaction to sexual stimuli. *Journal of Abnormal Psychology*, **89**(5), 644.

Lansky, D. and Wilson, G. T. (1981). Alcohol, expectations, and sexual arousal in males: an information processing analysis. *Journal of Abnormal Psychology*, **90**(1), 35.

Leather, P. (1998). Windows in the workplace: sunlight, view, and occupational stress. *Environment and Behavior*, **30**(6), 739–762.

Levin, I. P. and Gaeth, G. J. (1988). How consumers are affected by the framing of attribute information before and after consuming the product. *Journal of Consumer Research*, **15**(3), 374–378.

Linde, K., Niemann, K., and Meissner, K. (2010). Are sham acupuncture interventions more effective than (other) placebos? A re-analysis of data from the Cochrane review on placebo effects. *Forsch Komplementmed*, **17**, 259–264.

Lindemann, B. (2001). Receptors and transduction in taste. *Nature*, **413**(6852), 219–225.

Lindman, R. (1982). Social and solitary drinking: effects on consumption and mood in male social drinkers. *Physiology & Behavior*, **28**(6), 1093–1095.

Logue, A. W. (2004). *The psychology of eating and drinking* (3rd edn.). New York: Brunner-Routledge.

McClure, S. M., Li, J., Tomlin, D., Cypert, K. S., Montague, L. M., and Montague, P. R. (2004). Neural correlates of behavioral preference for culturally familiar drinks. *Neuron*, **44**(2), 379–387.

McMillen, D. L., Smith, S. M., and Wells-Parker, E. (1989). The effects of alcohol, expectancy, and sensation seeking on driving risk taking. *Addictive Behaviors*, **14**(4), 477–483.

Millar, K., Hammersley, R. H., and Finnigan, F. (1992). Reduction of alcohol-induced performance impairment by prior ingestion of food. *British Journal of Psychology*, **83** (Pt. 2), 261–278.

Mintzes, B., Barer, M. L., Kravitz, R. L., et al. (2003). How does direct-to-consumer advertising (DTCA) affect prescribing? A survey in primary care environments with and without legal DTCA. *Canadian Medical Association Journal*, **169**(5), 405–412.

Moerman, D. E. (1996). An analysis of the food plants and drug plants of native North America. *Journal of Ethnopharmacology*, **52**(1), 1–22.

Moerman, D. E. (2002). *Meaning, medicine and the "placebo effect."* Cambridge/New York: Cambridge University Press.

Moerman, D. (2011). Examining a powerful healing effect through a cultural lens, and finding meaning. *The Journal of Mind–Body Regulation*, **1**(2), 63–72.

Morrot, G., Brochet, F., and Dubourdieu, D. (2001). The color of odors. *Brain and Language*, **79**(2), 309–320.

Mroczek, J., Mikitarian, G., Vieira, E. K., and Rotarius, T. (2005). Hospital design and staff perceptions: an exploratory analysis. *The Health Care Manager*, **24**(3), 233–244.

Nahas, E. A., Nahas-Neto, J., Orsatti, F. L., Carvalho, E. P., Oliveira, M. L., and Dias, R. (2007). Efficacy and safety of a soy isoflavone extract in postmenopausal women: a randomized, double-blind, and placebo-controlled study. *Maturitas*, **58**(3), 249–258.

Navarro-Allende, A., Khataan, N., and El-Sohemy, A. (2008). Impact of genetic and environmental determinants of taste with food preferences in older adults. *Journal of Nutrition for the Elderly*, **27**(3–4), 267–276.

Noe, D., Bartemucci, L., Mariani, N., and Cantari, D. (1998). Practical aspects of preparation of foods for double-blind, placebo-controlled food challenge. *Allergy*, **53**(46 Suppl.), 75–77.

Oberfeld, D., Hecht, H., Allendorf, U., and Wickelmaier, F. (2009). Ambient lighting modifies the flavor of wine. *Journal of Sensory Studies*, **24**(6), 797–832.

Ooi, S. X., Lee, P. L., Law, H. Y., and Say, Y. H. (2010). Bitter receptor gene (TAS2R38) P49A genotypes and their associations with aversion to vegetables and sweet/fat foods in Malaysian subjects. *Asia Pacific Journal of Clinical Nutrition*, **19**(4), 491–498.

Pagotto, U., Marsicano, G., Cota, D., Lutz, B., and Pasquali, R. (2006). The emerging role of the endocannabinoid system in endocrine regulation and energy balance. *Endocrine Reviews*, **27**(1), 73–100.

Parr, W. V., Heatherbell, D., and White, K. G. (2002). Demystifying wine expertise: olfactory threshold, perceptual skill and semantic memory in expert and novice wine judges. *Chemical Senses*, **27**(8), 747–755.

Patrick, H. and Nicklas, T. A. (2005). A review of family and social determinants of children's eating patterns and diet quality. *Journal of the American College of Nutrition*, **24**(2), 83–92.

Pecoits-Filho, R. (2007). Dietary protein intake and kidney disease in Western diet. *Contributions to Nephrology*, **155**, 102–112.

Plassmann, H., O'Doherty, J., Shiv, B., and Rangel, A. (2008). Marketing actions can modulate neural representations of experienced pleasantness. *Proceedings of the National Academy of Sciences*, **105**(3), 1050–1054.

Pliner, P. and Cappell, H. (1974). Modification of affective consequences of alcohol: a comparison of social and solitary drinking. *Journal of Abnormal Psychology*, **83**, 418–425.

Raz, A., Campbell, N., Guindi, D., Holcroft, C., Dery, C., and Cukier, O. (2011). Placebos in clinical practice: comparing attitudes, beliefs, and patterns of use between academic psychiatrists and nonpsychiatrists. *Canadian Journal of Psychiatry*, **56**(4), 198–208.

Richardson, A., Allsop, M., Coghill, E., and Turnock, C. (2007). Earplugs and eye masks: do they improve critical care patients' sleep? *Nursing in Critical Care*, **12**(6), 278–286.

Roberto, C. A., Larsen, P. D., Agnew, H., Baik, J., and Brownell, K. D. (2010). Evaluating the impact of menu labeling on food choices and intake. *American Journal of Public Health*, **100**(2), 312–318.

Roberto, C. A., Schwartz, M. B., and Brownell, K. D. (2009). Rationale and evidence for menu-labeling legislation. *American Journal of Preventive Medicine*, **37**(6), 546–551.

Roe, A. R. and Munroe, K. B. (1989). The effect of price, brand name, and store name on buyers' perceptions of product quality: an integrative review. *Journal of Marketing Research*, **XXVI**, 351–357.

Ross, C. F., Bohlscheid, J., and Weller, K. (2008). Influence of visual masking technique on the assessment of two red wines by trained and consumer assessors. *Journal of Food Science*, **73**(6), S279–285.

Rubin, H. R. (1998). Status report—an investigation to determine whether the built environment affects patients' medical outcomes. *Journal of Healthcare Design*, **10**, 11–13.

Ryherd, E. E., Waye, K. P., and Ljungkvist, L. (2008). Characterizing noise and perceived work environment in a neurological intensive care unit. *Journal of the Acoustical Society of America*, **123**(2), 747–756.

Savaiano, D. A., Boushey, C. J., and McCabe, G. P. (2006). Lactose intolerance symptoms assessed by meta-analysis: a grain of truth that leads to exaggeration. *Journal of Nutrition*, **136**(4), 1107–1113.

Scaglioni, S., Salvioni, M., and Galimberti, C. (2008). Influence of parental attitudes in the development of children eating behaviour. *British Journal of Nutrition*, **99**(Suppl. 1), S22–25.

Scheibehenne, B., Todd, P. M., and Wansink, B. (2010). Dining in the dark. The importance of visual cues for food consumption and satiety. *Appetite*, **55**(3), 710–713.

Shankar, M. U., Levitan, C. A., and Spence, C. (2010). Grape expectations: the role of cognitive influences in color–flavor interactions. *Consciousness and Cognition*, **19**(1), 380–390.

Shapiro, R. A. and Berland, T. (1972). Noise in the operating room. *The New England journal of Medicine*, **287**(24), 1236–1238.

Shirani, K. Z., McManus, A. T., Vaughan, G. M., McManus, W. F., Pruitt, B. A., Jr., and Mason, A. D., Jr. (1986). Effects of environment on infection in burn patients. *Archives of Surgery*, **121**(1), 31–36.

Shiv, B., Carmon, Z., and Areily, D. (2005). Placebo effects of marketing actions: consumers may get what they pay for. *Journal of Marketing Research*, **XLII**, 383–393.

Simoons, F. J. (1998). *Plants of life, plants of death*. Madison: University of Wisconsin Press.

Smeets, P. A., Weijzen, P., de Graaf, C., and Viergever, M. A. (2011). Consumption of caloric and non-caloric versions of a soft drink differentially affects brain activation during tasting. *NeuroImage*, **54**(2), 1367–1374.

Strugnell, C. (1997). Colour and its role in sweetness perception. *Appetite*, **28**, 85.

Stubbs, R. J. (2001). The effect of ingesting olestra-based foods on feeding behavior and energy balance in humans. *Critical Reviews in Food Science and Nutrition*, **41**(5), 363–386.

Suarez, F. L., Savaiano, D., Arbisi, P., and Levitt, M. D. (1997). Tolerance to the daily ingestion of two cups of milk by individuals claiming lactose intolerance. *American Journal of Clinical Nutrition*, **65**(5), 1502–1506.

Swallow, D. M. (2003). Genetics of lactase persistence and lactose intolerance. *Annual Review of Genetics*, **37**, 197–219.

Tanumihardjo, S. A., Anderson, C., Kaufer-Horwitz, M., et al. (2007). Poverty, obesity, and malnutrition: an international perspective recognizing the paradox. *Journal of the American Dietetic Association*, **107**(11), 1966–1972.

Testa, M., Fillmore, M. T., Norris, J., et al. (2006). Understanding alcohol expectancy effects: revisiting the placebo condition. *Alcoholism, Clinical and Experimental Research*, **30**(2), 339–348.

Thibault, L. (2011). The total food effect: an original view on foods' placebo effects. *Journal of Mind-Body Regulation*, **1**(3), 171–172.

Thomas, K. B. (1987). General practice consultations: is there any point in being positive? *British Medical Journal*, **294**(6581), 1200–1202.

Tilburt, J. C., Emanuel, E. J., Kaptchuk, T. J., Curlin, F. A., and Miller, F. G. (2008). Prescribing "placebo treatments": results of national survey of US internists and rheumatologists. *British Medical Journal*, **337**, a1938.

Timpson, N. J., Christensen, M., Lawlor, D. A., et al. (2005). TAS2R38 (phenylthiocarbamide) haplotypes, coronary heart disease traits, and eating behavior in the British Women's Heart and Health Study. *American Journal of Clinical Nutrition*, **81**(5), 1005–1011.

Ulrich, R. S. (1984). View through a window may influence recovery from surgery. *Science*, **224**(4647), 420–421.

Vesa, T., Korpela, R., and Sahi, T. (1996). Tolerance to small amounts of lactose in lactose maldigesters. *American Journal of Clinical Nutrition*, **64**(2), 197–201.

Waber, R. L., Shiv, B., Carmon, Z., and Ariely, D. (2008). Commercial features of placebo and therapeutic efficacy. *Journal of the American Medical Association*, **299**(9), 1016–1017.

Wansink, B. (2004). Environmental factors that increase the food intake and consumption volume of unknowing consumers. *Annual Review of Nutrition*, **24**, 455–479.

Wigmore, S. W. and Hinson, R. E. (1991). The influence of setting on consumption in the balanced placebo design. *British Journal of Addiction*, **86**(2), 205–215.

Wylie-Rosett, J. (2002). Fat substitutes and health: an advisory from the Nutrition Committee of the American Heart Association. *Circulation*, **105**(23), 2800–2804.

Zellner, D. A. and Whitten, L.A. (1999). The effect of color intensity and appropriateness on color-induced odor enhancement. *American Journal of Psychology*, **112**(4), 585–614.

Zubieta, J. K. and Stohler, C. S. (2009). Neurobiological mechanisms of placebo responses. *Annals of the New York Academy of Sciences*, **1156**, 198–210.

Chapter 12

Suggestion, placebos, and false memories

Melanie K. T. Takarangi and Elizabeth F. Loftus

12.1 Introduction

The importance of social science perspectives on the placebo effect has been highlighted throughout this volume. In this chapter, we focus on the role of suggestion in creating the placebo effect, and liken this process to the development of false memories under suggestive conditions. We know from decades of memory research that people can often come to falsely believe that some part of an event, or even an entire event, really happened. We first consider research demonstrating memory distortion—in response to a variety of suggestive techniques—for an event people witnessed, or one in which they were involved. The placebo effect involves a different sort of suggestion; namely, that an inert substance produces specific outcomes. We consider the use of placebos to alter social behaviors, and describe recent research combining placebo and memory distortion paradigms. Finally, we consider areas of potential overlap between placebos and false memories, including individual differences and ethical implications. Taken together, this chapter highlights the importance of understanding placebo effects in non-medical domains, and encourages further thinking and research in areas where suggestibility is a common theme.

12.2 The malleability of memory

Despite its intuitive appeal as a metaphor, our memories are not stored like digital movie files on a smartphone. We are unable to pinpoint a particular file and play it back unedited. Instead, when we retrieve a memory, we reconstruct the details, as if we were a movie editor splicing together different clips. However, unlike the movie director, we lack both knowledge of what really happened, and precision in our ability to construct a coherent story. Indeed, the memories we ultimately retrieve may contain parts of the original experience, assumptions about how things are or were, and new information we learned since the event took place. In other words, our memories are vulnerable to suggestion and distortion (see Schacter 2001).

Traditionally, there have been two types of false memory studies: those that demonstrate how memories can be changed by external suggestions and those that demonstrate spontaneous false memories in the absence of explicit suggestion (e.g., Gerrie et al. 2006; Roediger and McDermott 1995). Our focus here is on the former type. External suggestions can take many forms, including post-event information such as leading questions (Loftus and Palmer 1974) and conversations with co-witnesses (Wright et al. 2000). In some cases, such suggestions have led people to remember complete, detailed events that never happened (Loftus and Pickrell 1995). Moreover, these memories can have consequences for future behavior (Bernstein and Loftus 2009).

12.3 **Suggestions about what we have seen**

Research on memory accuracy for witnessed events is particularly important when a witness is required to give evidence about what they saw. In such cases, there are many opportunities for suggestive influences or "misinformation"—other witnesses, media reports, police interviews, and so on. Research on the role of suggestion in distorting memory dates back to the 1970s, when researchers developed a popular three-stage procedure for studying suggestion and memory (Loftus et al. 1978). First, subjects watch a simulated event that typically calls for eyewitness testimony. Examples include crimes such as shoplifting, burglary, and wallet-snatching (Loftus 1991; Okado and Stark 2005; Takarangi et al. 2006). After a delay, subjects are exposed to some suggestive post-event information (PEI) about the event. Finally, subjects answer questions about what they saw. Several decades of research using this paradigm demonstrates that witnesses are often likely to recall PEI as being part of the original event (see Loftus 2005). Suggested details, or PEI, may be introduced into memory via leading questioning. In one example, Loftus and Palmer (1974) asked people to watch a traffic accident film clip and then to estimate how fast the cars were traveling. The wording of the question was suggestive: some subjects were asked "How fast were the cars going when they *smashed into* each other?," while for others, the verb was "hit," "collided," bumped," or "contacted." Importantly, subjects' speed estimates were higher when the question contained the word *smashed* rather than *hit*. In a follow-up study, subjects who heard the word *smashed* were more likely to say (inaccurately) that they had seen broken glass at the scene, than subjects who heard the word *hit*. Suggested and altered details may also be introduced into people's memory by exposure to new and misleading information about the event that subjects witnessed (e.g., Loftus et al. 1978). Suggestive PEI is often contained within a narrative; for example, some subjects may be told inaccurately that "the shoplifter stole a chemistry book" when they saw him steal a mathematics book.

More recently, researchers have investigated how suggestions from "co-witnesses" can influence memory for a shared witnessed event (French et al. 2008; Gabbert et al. 2003; Wright et al. 2000). In these studies, pairs of subjects ostensibly witness the same event, discuss the event together, and later are individually asked about their memory of the event. Suggestion is introduced by having the pairs discuss, among other things, particular details that the experimenter knows them to have seen differently. For example, one subject may have seen the shoplifter steal a chemistry book, while the other subject saw him steal a mathematics book. This research has consistently found that people often incorporate elements of each other's memory reports into their own memory after discussion.

Across hundreds of studies on the misinformation effect, subjects have remembered stop signs as yield signs, the Eiffel Tower as the Leaning Tower of Pisa, a white instead of a blue vehicle in a crime scene, and criminal accomplices that were not present. Taken together, these studies show that our recollections are susceptible to distortion when we are questioned in a suggestive fashion, or when we talk to other people. These results have practical implications because there is substantial evidence that real eyewitnesses are likely to talk to one another (e.g., Paterson and Kemp 2006), that criminal justice professionals ask leading questions (e.g., Powell et al. 2005), and that other sources of "misinformation"—such as the media—can have distortive effects on memory (Austin and Strange 2012).

12.4 Suggestions about what we have done

Just as eyewitness memory has clear criminal justice implications, notable cases of false confessions and recovered memories have drawn attention to the role of suggestibility in altering memory for our own autobiography (e.g., Gudjonsson 2003; Loftus and Ketcham 1994). In subsequent sections, we review some of the key suggestive influences on autobiographical memories.

12.4.1 Imagination exercises

In the laboratory, researchers have used several methods to study how imagination acts as a form of suggestion. Goff and Roediger (1998) demonstrated that imagination techniques can lead to false memories for simple actions. In their paradigm, subjects perform, imagine doing, or only see (or hear) a series of action statements (e.g., "flip the coin"). During a subsequent session, subjects imagine some of the actions they did not previously perform and later answer questions about what actions they actually performed during the initial session. Typically, the more times subjects imagine an unperformed action, the more likely they are to remember having performed it. This finding extends to unlikely actions, such as kissing a toy frog and proposing marriage to a Pepsi machine (Seamon et al. 2006; Thomas and Loftus 2002).

Garry et al. (1996) examined the influence of imagination on memory for more complex childhood autobiographical experiences. In this paradigm, subjects first indicate the likelihood that certain events ("broke a window with your hand") happened to them during childhood. Later, they imagine experiencing some of these events and then respond again to the original event list. Results demonstrate *imagination inflation*: people tend to become more confident they have experienced events that they only imagined (see also Sharman and Barnier 2008; Sharman and Scoboria 2009).

Taken together, this research shows that the imagination can be a powerful form of suggestion; increasing confidence that a false autobiographical event occurred. However, it can also lead directly to a false memory. For example, using imagination techniques, Mazzoni and Memon (2003) convinced subjects that they had a fictitious minor medical procedure as a child. Moreover, the mechanisms underlying imagination as suggestion appear to extend to other tasks. Subjects show increased confidence in a false event when they are asked to simply paraphrase that event, or explain how it might have occurred (Sharman et al. 2004, 2005).

12.4.2 Corroboration

Corroboration of a false event by another person can be a powerful suggestion. In fact, the mere claim that another person has witnessed wrongdoing can lead a subject to falsely confess that wrongdoing. In an early example, Kassin and Kiechel (1996) examined how corroboration might lead to distorted memory. They accused subjects of damaging a computer by pressing the wrong key. Although innocent subjects tended to initially deny the charge, when a confederate who said she had witnessed the key-press corroborated the accusation, many subjects signed a confession, internalized guilt for the act, and confabulated details consistent with the belief that they had pressed the key. Subsequent research has shown that subjects are willing to confess even in the face of negative consequences, such as paying to repair the computer, or having to re-enter data (Horselenberg et al. 2003; Redlich and Goodman 2003).

Nash and Wade (2008) took corroboration one step further; they were interested in whether visual evidence of wrongdoing would increase the likelihood of confession. Subjects participated in a gambling task, which involved them taking money in and out of a monopoly-style "bank" after winning or losing on quiz questions. Afterwards, subjects were accused of stealing money from the bank; some were told that incriminating video evidence existed, while others were shown doctored video evidence of them appearing to steal the money. Subjects who saw the video were more likely to confess to and internalize the act, and to confabulate details about the act than subjects who were only told about the evidence.

To summarize, this body of research shows that corroborative evidence that supports a false event can induce people to accept guilt for an act they did not commit, and even to develop memories to support their guilty feelings. Different forms of suggestion can also work together. Using Goff and Roediger's (1998) paradigm described in the previous "Imagination exercises" section, Nash et al. (2009) showed some subjects doctored video images of themselves watching a research assistant perform some of the actions. Both imagination and exposure to the videos separately led subjects to falsely remember actually performing actions; the combination of both led to more false memories.

12.4.3 Social contagion

Recently, suggestive "co-witness" effects have been extended to personally relevant and socially shared autobiographical memories. Barnier et al. (2008) asked subjects to share memories of recent personal events (e.g., school graduation dance) with a confederate, who then described their own (supposed) memory of the same event. Then, as the subject and confederate took turns recounting the salient points of their recall partner's memory, the confederate introduced false information about the subject's memory. Finally, subjects individually recalled their own memories. Importantly, during this phase, many subjects described information introduced by the confederate, and information from the confederates' memories, as part of their memory. Thus, as with witnessed events, discussing an autobiographical experience with other people can alter memory for that experience.

12.4.4 Implantation studies

The research presented so far has demonstrated conclusively that people can, and often do, claim to remember suggested details of a witnessed or personally experienced event. However, can suggestion cause people to remember a wholly false event? More than a decade of research shows the answer to this question is yes: it is possible to plant wholly false memories into people's minds using a combination of suggestive influences.

In the original "lost in the mall" implantation study, Loftus and Pickrell (1995) presented subjects with a booklet containing one-paragraph stories about three true childhood events, and one mildly traumatic false event: being lost in a shopping mall at about the age of five. A parent, older sibling, or other close relative, who verified that the subject had not actually been lost, provided details of the true events. Subjects read each story in the booklet, and wrote everything that they could remember about the events. In two follow-up interviews, the researchers provided portions of the original events as retrieval cues. Not surprisingly, subjects were reasonably good at remembering true events. However, over the three interviews, approximately 25% of subjects also came to remember being lost in a shopping mall (either wholly or partially), and some even gave specific details about the event.

In subsequent studies using similar manipulations, people have come to remember unlikely experiences like spilling punch on the bride's parents at a family wedding, and potentially traumatic experiences like being hospitalized overnight, being attacked by a dog, or having a serious indoor or outdoor accident (Hyman and Pentland 1996; Hyman et al. 1995; Porter et al. 1999). Importantly, these false memories can be detailed, emotional, consequential, and confidently held (see Loftus and Bernstein 2005).

Other memory implantation researchers have replicated the suggestive techniques used by therapists specializing in "memory recovery work." For example, Scoboria et al. (2002) found that subjects were more susceptible to misleading information when hypnotized. Mazzoni et al. (1999) used dream interpretation to encourage subjects to falsely believe that they had been lost as young children. Spanos et al. (1999) planted false infant memories (seeing a colored mobile hanging over their crib on the day after birth) by hypnotizing and age-regressing subjects to the day after their birth or having them participate in a "guided mnemonic restructuring" procedure.

12.4.5 Photographs and other visual aids

More recently, researchers have examined other, novel suggestive techniques for planting false memories. In a clever twist on the lost in the mall procedure, Wade et al. (2002) used family photographs depicting childhood events. Again, one event was false: a doctored image of the subject taking a ride in a hot air balloon. Over three interviews, subjects worked on remembering the events based simply on the photographs. When subjects had recalled all they remembered about the events, the experimenter led them through a guided imagery phase, instructing them to imagine for example, the balloon, the weather, what it would have felt like to be in the balloon, what they could see, and so on. By the end of the study, 50% of subjects had remembered at least some details about the hot air balloon ride.

However, because we are relatively unlikely to reminisce using doctored photographs, Lindsay et al. (2004) wondered whether real photographs could also produce false memories. They asked subjects to remember three childhood events from three different school years: two true events from grades 5 to 6 and 3 to 4, and a false event from grades 1 to 2. The false event described the time that the subject put Slime (the children's toy) in their teacher's desk drawer, only to be caught out and punished. Some subjects read narratives describing each event, while other subjects read narratives accompanied by their class photo from the year in which the event occurred. By the end of the study, 78% of narrative + photo subjects recalled details about the Slime episode compared to 45% of the subjects who only read the narrative.

In another example of visual aids as suggestions, Braun et al. (2002) had subjects rate their confidence that a list of events had happened to them during childhood, before and after exposure to a mock advertisement. Embedded in the list of events was the target event—shaking hands with Bugs Bunny at Disneyland—an impossible event because as a Warner Brothers character, subjects would never encounter Bugs Bunny at Disneyland. Subjects saw a potential advertisement and rated it on several attitude dimensions. Some subjects saw an advertisement that described the target event, while others saw an unrelated control advertisement. Subjects who saw the "Bugs" advertisement became more confident that they had shaken hands with him, and were more likely to say that they *remembered* shaking hands compared with subjects who did not see the target advertisement. In a follow-up study, Grinley (2002) showed that the increase in subjects' confidence translated into vivid memories full of sensory detail, such as hugging Bugs, shaking his hand, and hearing him utter his famous words "What's up, Doc?".

12.4.6 Feedback

Researchers have also used false computer feedback to suggest to subjects that they had certain experiences as children or adolescents. In one study, Bernstein et al. (2005a) asked subjects to complete a number of questionnaires, including a "personality questionnaire" and a "food history inventory." When subjects returned one week later, the researchers told them that the computer had generated—based on their questionnaire responses—a personalized profile of their early childhood experiences with food. All subjects received three identical pieces of feedback true of many children (e.g., "eating chocolate birthday cake made you happy") and one piece of critical feedback: either "you got sick after eating a hard-boiled egg" or "you felt ill after eating a dill pickle." Later on, subjects completed the food history inventory again, showing an increased confidence that the targeted food event had happened to them. Researchers have used this paradigm to successfully plant false memories for various negative (and positive) food experiences (see Bernstein et al. 2005b; Laney et al. 2008a; Scoboria et al. 2008), and recently, to plant memories for a bad experience with the Disney character Pluto (Berkowitz et al. 2008). In this study, after being exposed to false feedback about their childhood experiences and some bogus information, roughly a third of subjects reported that they remembered or at least believed they had experienced the target event—"had your ear licked by Pluto."

Taken together, the "implantation" research shows that a variety of different suggestions can produce entirely false memories, either alone or in combination with other techniques such as imagination, false narratives, true and false photos, fake advertisements, and false feedback. However, this research raises an important follow-up question: do false beliefs and memories have consequences for behavior? The food false memory literature has begun to address this question. For example, Bernstein et al. (2005a) asked subjects to imagine themselves at an afternoon barbeque party and rate the likelihood of consuming a long list of foods and beverages. Subjects who had developed a memory of being sick after eating dill pickles reported less preference for and willingness to eat them, compared to control subjects who had not received false feedback. Moreover, subjects who believed that they became sick from eating hard-boiled eggs rated not only their likelihood of eating this food lower than control subjects did, but also their likelihood of eating related foods, such as egg salad.

The food preference consequences of these memory distortions extend to positive food memories. Laney et al. (2008a) found that subjects who falsely remembered that they had loved asparagus the first time they tried it as a child said they would be more likely to eat sautéed asparagus in a restaurant and would pay more for a pound of asparagus at the grocery store. There are similar results with other foods, including strawberry ice-cream and peach yogurt, and at even longer-term follow-up (Geraerts et al. 2008; Laney et al. 2008b; Scoboria et al. 2008). Moreover, the behavioral consequences of false food memories include actual eating behavior. For example, Geraerts et al. (2008) found that four months after the memory suggestion, subjects with a memory of being sick following egg salad actually ate fewer egg-salad sandwiches compared to control subjects and subjects who resisted the original suggestion.

Taken together, the literature shows that false memories can affect the decisions people make in the future about how to behave. In other words, false memories are not just problematic in themselves; they have practical consequences as well.

12.5 **Placebo suggestions**

In this chapter thus far, we have reviewed research showing that plying people with certain kinds of suggestive information can make them believe that they experienced things that never happened, and that these false memories can have consequences. Importantly, not only can people be led to believe that they experienced events that did not occur, but they can also be led to experience feelings and symptoms that they would not otherwise feel, via the placebo effect. Again, these false experiences have behavioral consequences. In the following section, we discuss the placebo effect, its similarity to the kinds of suggestion that can alter memory, and circumstances in which placebos may act as a form of suggestion that changes both memory and behavior.

12.5.1 The placebo effect

The placebo effect occurs when an inert substance produces genuine physiological or psychological changes (Kirsch 1985; Marlatt and Rohsenow 1980; Stewart-Williams 2004; Stewart-Williams and Podd 2004). Usually, administration of a substance intended to aid well-being is accompanied by an explanation of that substance's expected effects, but of course, in the case of a placebo substance, this explanation is bogus and acts as a suggestion about what people should expect to experience as a result of taking the substance. Put simply, placebos are suggestions. Before discussing what placebos can tell us about memory suggestibility, we first consider how placebos are used in other domains.

12.5.2 Placebos and health

The use of placebos in medical treatment dates back to ancient times. Civilizations such as the Assyrians, Greeks, and Egyptians often used placebos as "drug treatments" (Shapiro and Shapiro 1997a, b). As recently as the 1930s and 1940s, physicians used placebos regularly (Spiro 1997); even today 62% of physicians believe that administering placebos is ethical (Tilburt et al. 2008). Is there an empirical justification for administering placebos? Evidence—particularly in the case of depression—suggests that the answer to this question may be yes (see Chapter 2). Using meta-analysis, Kirsch et al. (2008) found that the benefit of selective serotonin reuptake inhibitors (SSRIs) as antidepressants, over placebos, did not meet the necessary criteria of clinical significance specified by the National Institute of Clinical Excellence (United Kingdom). Other studies have shown placebo effects for other conditions including angina and congestive heart failure, asthma, herpes simplex, duodenal ulcer, and Parkinson's disease (Benson and Friedman 1996; see also Price et al. 2008).

Researchers typically use the balanced placebo design (BPD; Marlatt and Rohsenow 1980) to distinguish the physiological and psychological effects of a substance. Subjects are either told that they are taking a particular substance (e.g., a drug) or a placebo, and this information is either true or false. The BPD also allows researchers to study factors related to a treatment's administration that are not part of the treatment itself but may contribute to treatment effectiveness. For example, research using placebo analgesia has shown that "open" administration (i.e., in full view of the patient) is more effective than "hidden" administration (e.g., by an automatic pump device) of the same substance (see Price et al. 2008 for a review).

However, the placebo effect is not restricted to treatment *benefits*. Loftus and Fries (2008) investigated whether, when people believe that a substance or medical procedure might cause unpleasant symptoms, they are more likely to develop these symptoms, than if they never knew about the symptoms. Participants were scleroderma patients enrolled in a clinical trial. Known side-effects of the drug cocktail (propanolol and alpha-methyldopa) included upset stomach, tearfulness, dizziness, and headache. Before beginning the trial, patients received either a standard informed consent message or a "special message." Both messages informed patients of possible drug side-effects, and listed the known side-effects, plus additional implausible and fictitious ones (ringing in ears, burning sensation in feet). The "special message" warned patients that "simply mentioning possible annoying symptoms causes some people to experience these symptoms—even when no drug is taken at all" and advised them to try and reduce their expectancy about the side-effects. Not surprisingly, both patients who received the drug cocktail and patients who received a placebo experienced side-effects, including the fictitious ones. However, the special message reduced the reported side-effects and also decreased somewhat the use of medications to treat those unlikely symptoms.

12.5.3 Placebos and social behavior

Placebo effects are not limited to the medical domain. They have become popular as a tool for studying expectations about social behaviors, particularly antisocial or undesirable behaviors such as substance misuse. For example, people have particular expectations about how alcohol will make them feel (more relaxed, positive, and sociable), and these expectations are known to be a factor in maintaining drinking (Cooper 1994; Labrie et al. 2007). Thus, when people *believe* they are drinking alcohol, they should be more likely to engage in social behaviors consistent with expectations, and to use such expectations as an excuse to engage in or explain away otherwise undesirable behavior (Hull and Bond 1986; Marlatt and Rohsenow 1980). Indeed, when people consume placebo alcohol they show decreased sexual inhibition (George and Marlatt 1986; George et al. 2000; Lansky and Wilson 1981), increased risk taking (McMillan et al. 1989), and increased aggression (Cherek et al. 1985; Lang et al. 1975) and interest in viewing violent and erotic material (George et al. 1989). Research shows similarly robust expectancy effects for nicotine placebos and smoking behavior (e.g., Kelemen and Kaighobadi 2007; Wesnes et al. 1983). More recently however, attention has turned to the question of whether placebos affect non-social behavior like attention and memory.

12.5.4 **Placebos and non-social behavior**

We know that physiologically, alcohol consumption impairs cognitive functions such as fine motor skills, reaction time, and visual attention (Gustafson 1986; Mackay et al. 2002; Rohrbaugh et al. 1988). However, alcohol placebos do not typically affect these same behaviors (see Hull and Bond 1986 for a review). In one example, Clifasefi et al. (2006) investigated how alcohol and alcohol placebos affected inattentional blindness (IB)—a failure to detect unexpected salient objects that appear in one's visual field. They told half their subjects that they were receiving alcohol, and half that they were receiving a placebo. This information was either true or false. All subjects participated in Simons and Chabris' (1999) classic IB paradigm: they watched a video clip of two teams passing basketballs back and forth, and monitored the number of passes occurring within a certain team. During this clip, a woman dressed in a gorilla suit walks into the middle of the screen, stops and beats her chest, then walks away. Generally, many subjects fail to notice the gorilla. Importantly, Clifasefi et al. (2006) found that intoxicated subjects (regardless of what they were told) were twice as likely to show "blindness" than sober subjects, but there was no placebo effect: alcohol expectancies did not affect whether or not people noticed the gorilla.

Similarly, there is no evidence that placebos affect objective or explicit memory (such as memory for word lists). For example, Kelemen and Kaighobadi (2007) compared nicotine versus a nicotine placebo. Although subjects who received the placebo reported hunger suppression, self-reported alertness, and concentration (in line with their expectations about nicotine), the placebo did not affect memory performance. In other words, although subjects reported experiencing cognitive effects, these effects did not translate to actual performance. In another example, Kvavilashvili and Ellis (1999) examined how bogus "memory enhancing" or "memory impairing" drugs influenced free recall. Their subjects reported effects in line with their beliefs about the substance (i.e., better or worse memory) but the placebo only affected performance in the "impairment" condition: these subjects recalled fewer words and made more errors. Why would social behavior be different to cognitive behavior? One possibility is that some cognitive behaviors are simply not within the capabilities of the person and thus no amount of expectancy could produce them (Kirsch and Lynn 1999). For example, if you think you are going to do worse on a task, you may act out the expectancy by decreasing effort or motivation, but you would need to be capable of actually having a better memory in order to act out the expectancy of a better memory.

Van Oorsouw and Merckelbach (2007) also examined the influence of bogus memory drugs on memory accuracy for an emotional event (a violent and emotive segment of the film *American History X)*. Contrary to previous research, subjects who expected the drug to improve their memories recalled more accurate information than subjects who expected the drug to impair or do nothing to their memories. Methodological differences may explain this discrepancy in results: subjects were told that the researchers were interested in the efficacy of memory drugs, and given an inadvertent opportunity to rehearse the event before the memory test. Thus, memory improvement could have resulted from increased effort at encoding (before the administration of the drug), combined with the drug suggestion.

In summary then, placebos do not appear to have a robust effect on non-social cognitive behaviors. Indeed, another critical difference between social and non-social behaviors is that people are unlikely to have strong pre-existing expectations about how placebos affect specific cognitive abilities (Goldman et al. 1987; Kvavilashvili and Ellis 1999). Moreover, people may not be concerned with explaining away certain cognitive behaviors in the same way that they might want to excuse risky or taboo social behavior (Hull and Bond 1986; Kvavilashvili and Ellis 1999). However, what happens when the suggestion of a cognitive placebo is combined with some other, socially derived, suggestion? In the next section, we consider what placebos can tell us about memory suggestibility.

12.6 **The placebo effect and susceptibility to misinformation**

In the previous sections, we discussed how suggestive influences can lead to memory distortion, and how a placebo can act as a suggestion, creating expectancies about the effects of a particular substance. Can placebos, then, act as a counter (or as an additive) suggestion to certain types of memory tasks? A limited line of research has examined this question.

People do not necessarily have pre-existing views about how placebos affect specific cognitive abilities. However, Assefi and Garry (2003) reasoned that when memory tasks have a social component, we might expect the same pattern of placebo effects found for social behaviors. As previously discussed, misleading suggestions often come from an external (social) source. Thus, if people believe they have consumed alcohol, they might—in line with expectancies about alcohol's influence—distrust their memories for an event they witnessed while intoxicated, and therefore be less likely to question or scrutinize misleading external suggestions. To test this hypothesis, Assefi and Garry told half their subjects that they were receiving a vodka tonic drink (Told Alcohol) and the other subjects that they were receiving a plain tonic drink (Told Tonic). In fact, all subjects received flat tonic. Subjects then took part in a standard misinformation effect procedure.

Subjects' memory for items about which they received no misleading information was generally accurate, regardless of what they were told about their beverage. However, in line with predictions, Told Alcohol subjects were more likely than Told Tonic subjects to capitulate to misleading suggestions. In other words, although an alcohol placebo did not affect the cognitive task of remembering the event in the absence of social influence, there was a placebo effect for the social component of memory in this paradigm: subjects' susceptibility to misinformation. Interestingly, in this instance, subjects who are acting on one source of suggestion (expectations associated with alcohol) actually become more susceptible to another source of suggestion (the misleading narrative). The two forms of suggestion, according to these data, appear to act in concert.

If memory distortion is malleable, perhaps placebos might also be a means of investigating whether people can "resist" other suggestive influences. For example, could a placebo *decrease* susceptibility to misinformation? To test this question, Clifasefi et al. (2007) adopted a similar procedure to Kvavilash-vili and Ellis (1999), administering a bogus cognitive-enhancing drug ("R273") to subjects as part of a fake drug trial. Clifasefi et al. (2007) were stringent in establishing the believability of the placebo story (subjects saw a drug company researcher dressed in a white lab coat, learned about R273's positive effects on military radar operators, and saw the drugs being prepared). Clifasefi et al. (2007) told half of the subjects that they would receive R273 (Told Drug) and half that they would receive the inactive version of the drug (Told Inactive). In fact, both groups received lime-flavored baking soda dissolved in water. After consuming the drug, subjects completed the standard misinformation effect procedure, and rated how R273 had affected them. Importantly, Told Drug subjects reported enhanced senses, better concentration, better memory, and quicker responses. These data suggest that the measures taken to create expectancies about the drug were successful. Again, all subjects' memory for items about which they were not misled was generally accurate. However, Told Drug subjects were more likely than Told Inactive subjects to resist misleading suggestion. In fact, subjects who believed that they had taken R273 did not show a misinformation effect. Thus, although a cognitive-enhancing placebo did not affect memory in the absence of suggestion (control items), as with the alcohol study, the placebo suggestion did affect subjects' susceptibility to misinformation. In this case, the placebo decreased memory distortion.

Taken together, these studies show that although, strictly speaking, placebos that aim to decrease or increase memory performance do not work, placebo manipulations do appear to affect social aspects of memory. How is the expectancy of enhanced cognitive ability actually enacted though? Recall that earlier we suggested that such enhancement would need to be within the capabilities of the person. To investigate the mechanism, Parker et al. (2008) conducted a partial replication of the R273 study. They found that Told Drug subjects appeared to use more cognitive effort during the memory test than their Told Inactive counterparts. That is, Told Drug subjects tended to slow down their responding to the test, suggesting that they were deliberating more carefully over their memories. Thus, as a result of capitulating to one suggestion (the placebo), people avoided another (the misleading information), and their memories were more accurate.

To further test this monitoring explanation for memory-enhancing placebos, Parker et al. (2011) examined how R273 affected performance on a memory task that requires ongoing monitoring: prospective memory (PM). PM is the intention to perform future actions and a common memory failure, though not one that necessarily occurs in the face of external suggestion (Einstein and McDaniel 2004). Critically, a person must first bring an intended action to mind, without any explicit request to remember it; second, they must perform the action at the correct time, while faced with other distractions (McDaniel and Einstein 2000). An example is remembering to pass on an urgent message to a colleague when you next see them, while carrying on with work as usual. In a laboratory parallel to PM in the real world, subjects perform an ongoing task (e.g., word categorization), while attempting to remember to perform another one-off task (e.g., press a certain key when they see a certain cue word or word fragment) (see Einstein et al. 2005). Evidence from research using this paradigm shows that people can vary their cognitive effort while completing the task, according to specific circumstances, such as task importance.

Parker et al. (2011) hypothesized that people's expectations about their cognitive abilities might influence monitoring in the PM task. That is, if people have perceived control over their monitoring ability, they should perform this task more effectively. To test their hypothesis, Parker et al. combined the PM paradigm with the R273 suggestion. Indeed, when people were under the influence of a cognitive-enhancing drug placebo, they were more likely to perform the one-off target task. However, this improvement was only found when subjects had to engage in effortful monitoring. These results suggest that subjects who believed they were taking R273 developed expectancies about the drug that led them to be more motivated, or to use more cognitive effort, in the PM task, compared to the Told Inactive subjects.

12.7 **False memories and placebo effects**

In the chapter thus far, we have considered the history of suggestion in terms of planting false memories, planting expectancies about the effects of a placebo substance, and the small body of research that has considered a combination of suggestive placebo and memory techniques. We have alluded to areas of overlap between memory distortions and placebo effects, and—as described elsewhere within this volume—with hypnosis. Several of these areas warrant further discussion.

12.7.1 **Individual differences in suggestibility**

It is possible that individual differences (e.g., in personality) that underlie placebo responsiveness are also associated with vulnerability to memory distortion. That is, those people who are susceptible to developing false memories might also be those most affected by a placebo, or by hypnosis. Is there any empirical support for this proposition? We review the evidence next.

First, are these suggestive outcomes related to one another? Research presented in this chapter suggests that placebo suggestions can work in tandem with other kinds of suggestion to produce memory distortion. Moreover, both placebo and false memory responses appear to have *some* relationship with hypnotizability: the placebo response is weakly related to hypnotic susceptibility, and hypnotizability seems to be related to a person's ability to create more memories and more complex memories. There is also some evidence that highly hypnotizable people are prone to false memory development (see Barnier and McConkey 1992; Lynn and Nash 1994).

Second, are there individual differences that predict suggestive responding? Recent research suggests that distorted memories arising from misinformation are associated with cognitive deficiencies, including intelligence and perceptual and general memory abilities (Zhu et al. 2010a). However, research on personality types related to false memory development has produced mixed findings. For example, some research shows that people who score high on a measure of dissociation (Dissociative Experiences Scale version C; DES-C), are more likely to experience memory distortions than people with less dissociative tendencies (Candel et al. 2003; Hyman and Billings 1998; Merckelbach et al. 1999; Ost et al. 1997, 2005; Porter et al. 2000). However, other studies have not found this relationship (Eisen et al. 2002; Hekkanen and McEvoy 2002; Horselenberg et al. 2000; Platt et al. 1998; Wade 2004; Wilkinson and Hyman 1998). Research has shown that people high in self-monitoring (a strong tendency towards wanting to please other people; Snyder 1974) are both more and less likely to develop false memories (Gudjonsson 1995; Ost et al. 2002, 2005).

Neither Porter et al. (2000) nor Wade (2004) found a relationship between personality and false memory development. However, introverts (low scorers on extroversion) interviewed by more extroverted interviewers were most likely to develop a false memory. Recent research has revealed that the combination of cognitive and personality factors may be important. Among people low in cognitive abilities, personality characteristics such as co-operativeness, reward dependence, and self-directedness, appear to increase susceptibility to misinformation (Zhu et al. 2010b).

The relationship between individual differences and susceptibility to placebos seems similarly unreliable (see Chapter 2, this volume). Thus, it may be unlikely that a group of "placebo responders" can be reliably identified. By contrast, hypnotic suggestibility appears to be more trait-like (Kirsch 2010). This discrepancy may point to key differences between memory distortions, placebos, and hypnosis. For example, even though hypnosis may be experienced as involuntary, it may in fact be more effortful than responding to the more automatic placebo effect. Following this line of thinking, we might therefore expect more similar characteristics to underlie susceptibility to placebos and memory distortions. We know that memory distortions often occur as a byproduct of the automatic nature of the source-monitoring process (Lindsay 2008). Indeed, when people switch from an automatic to a more controlled monitoring process, they are better able to resist suggestion.

On balance however, perhaps it is not useful to think about suggestion as trait-like; maybe no individual difference predictor of suggestibility exists. Indeed, situational factors may be more important. In this chapter, we discussed a range of situational influences that work—both in isolation and in tandem— to produce false memories. However, some false memories do not arise from suggestion (Mazzoni 2002). People who are susceptible to a naturally occurring false memory may not be susceptible to suggestion per se. However, individual characteristics may influence motivation to believe different kinds of things. For example, prestige-enhancing memory distortions like remembering getting a higher grade than you did would be more likely in someone concerned with academic performance and grades.

In summary, a similar mechanism *may* underlie the suggestion that is common to placebo effects, memory distortion, and hypnosis. However, more work is required to establish whether the same kinds of people are indeed susceptible to all three, for example, by directly comparing these methods of suggestion within the same study. As such, further investigation into individual differences and susceptibility to suggestion would be a fruitful route for future research and represents one method of reasonably marrying false memory work and placebo work in a way that would enhance thinking about both topics.

12.7.2 **Ethical issues**

Another area of overlap between memory distortions and placebo effects is a methodological one: deception plays a key role both in creating false memories and, arguably, in placebo effects. The planning and delivery of memory implantation studies requires careful consideration of the nature of the target memory and debriefing procedures. One ethical debate relating to implantation research is whether people should believe things (a) only if they are true or (b) also if it is beneficial for them to do so. There is a third possibility though: that people can believe a falsehood if it is not harmful for them to do so and if such research will help us to understand the mechanisms underlying harmful false memories. However, these ethical issues become more complex in a medical setting. Indeed, the ethical limitations of medical placebo research restrict researchers' ability to gather empirical data. False memory research (and psychological techniques in general) may be a domain in which placebo-related questions can be addressed without fewer restrictions. Research on bogus cognitive-enhancing drugs is one example; such research, which could be extended to include other outcome measures, allows researchers to investigate underlying mechanisms and predictors of a placebo response.

References

Assefi, S. and Garry, M. (2003). Absolute memory distortions: alcohol placebos influence the misinformation effect. *Psychological Science*, **14**, 77–80.

Austin, J. and Strange, D. (2012). Television produces more false recognition for news than newspapers. *Psychology of Popular Media Culture*, **3**, 167–175.

Barnier, A. J. and McConkey, K. M. (1992). Reports of real and false memories: the relevance of hypnosis, hypnotizability, and context of memory test. *Journal of Abnormal Psychology*, **101**, 521–527.

Barnier, A. J., Sutton, J., Harris, C. B., and Wilson, R. A. (2008). A conceptual and empirical framework for the social distribution of cognition: the case of memory. *Cognitive Systems Research*, **9**, 33–51.

Benson, H. and Friedman, R. (1996). Harnessing the power of the placebo effect and renaming it "Remembered Wellness." *Annual Review of Medicine*, **47**, 193–199.

Berkowitz, S. R., Laney, C., Morris, E. K., Garry, M., and Loftus, E. F. (2008). Pluto behaving badly: false beliefs and their consequences. *American Journal of Psychology*, **121**, 643–660.

Bernstein, D. M. and Loftus, E. F. (2009). The consequences of false memories for food preferences and choices. *Perspectives on Psychological Science*, **4**, 135–139.

Bernstein, D. M., Laney, C., Morris, E. K., and Loftus, E. F. (2005a). False memories about food can lead to food avoidance. *Social Cognition*, **23**, 10–33.

Bernstein, D. M., Laney, C., Morris, E. K., and Loftus, E. F. (2005b). False beliefs about fattening foods can have healthy consequences. *Proceedings of the National Academy of Sciences, USA*, **102**, 13724–13731.

Braun, K. A., Ellis, R., and Loftus, E. F. (2002). Make my memory: how advertising can change our memories of the past. *Psychology and Marketing*, **19**, 1–23.

Candel, I., Merckelbach, H., and Kuijpers, M. (2003). Dissociative experiences are related to commissions in emotional memory. *Behaviour Research and Therapy*, **41**, 719–725.

Cherek, D. R., Steinberg, J. L., and Manno, B. R. (1985). Effects of alcohol on human aggressive behaviour. *Journal of Studies on Alcohol*, **46**, 321–328.

Clifasefi, S., Garry, M., Harper, D., Sharman, S. J., and Sutherland, R. (2007). Psychotropic placebos create resistance to the misinformation effect. *Psychonomic Bulletin & Review*, **12**, 112–117.

Clifasefi, S. L., Takarangi, M. K. T., and Bergman, J. S. (2006). Blind drunk: the effects of alcohol on inattentional blindness. *Applied Cognitive Psychology*, **20**, 697–704.

Cooper, M. L. (1994). Motivations for alcohol use among adolescents: development and validation of a four-factor model. *Psychological Assessment*, **6**, 117–128.

Einstein, G. O. and McDaniel, M. A. (2004). Remembering to remember. In: *A guide for successful aging* (eds. G. O. Einstein and M. A. McDaniel). New Haven: Yale University Press.

Einstein, G. O., McDaniel, M. A., Thomas, R., et al. (2005). Multiple processes in prospective memory retrieval: factors determining monitoring versus spontaneous retrieval. *Journal of Experimental Psychology: General*, **134**, 327–342.

Eisen, M. L., Morgan, D. M., and Mickes, L. (2002). Individual differences in eyewitness memory: examining relations between acquiescence, attention, and resistance to misleading information. *Personality and Individual Differences*, **33**(4), 553–571.

French, L., Garry, M., and Mori, K. (2008). You say tomato? Collaborative remembering leads to more false memories for intimate couples than for strangers. *Memory*, **16**(3), 262–273.

Gabbert, F., Memon, A., and Allan, K. (2003). Memory conformity: can eyewitnesses influence each other's memories for an event? *Applied Cognitive Psychology*, **17**(5), 533–543.

Garry, M., Manning, C. G., Loftus, E. F., and Sherman, S. J. (1996). Imagination inflation: imagining a childhood event inflates confidence that it occurred. *Psychonomic Bulletin and Review*, **3**, 208–214.

George, W. H. and Marlatt, G. A. (1986). The effects of alcohol and anger on interest in violence, erotica, and deviance. *Journal of Abnormal Psychology*, **95**, 150–158.

George, W. H., Dermen, K. H., and Nochajski, T. H. (1989). Expectancy set, self-reported expectancies and predispositional traits: predicting interest in violence and erotica. *Journal of Studies on Alcohol and Drugs*, **50**, 541–551.

George, W. H., Stoner, S. A., Norris, J., Lopez, P. A., and Lehman, G. L. (2000). Alcohol expectancies and sexuality: a self-fulfilling prophecy analysis of dyadic perceptions and behaviour. *Journal of Studies on Alcohol*, **61**, 168–176.

Geraerts, E., Bernstein, D. M., Merckelbach, H., Linders, C., Raymaekers, L., and Loftus, E. F. (2008). Lasting false beliefs and their behavioral consequences. *Psychological Science*, **19**, 749–753.

Gerrie, M. P., Belcher, L. E., and Garry, M. (2006). "Mind the gap": false memories for missing aspects of events. *Applied Cognitive Psychology*, **20**, 689–696.

Goff, L. M. and Roediger, H. L. III (1998). Imagination inflation for action events: repeated imaginings lead to illusory recollections. *Memory & Cognition*, **26**, 20–33.

Goldman, M. S., Brown, S. A., and Christiansen, B. A. (1987). Expectancy theory: thinking about drinking. In: *Psychological theories of drinking and alcoholism* (eds. H. T. Blane and K. E. Leonard). New York: Guilford Press.

Grinley, M. J. (2002). *Effects of advertising on semantic and episodic memory.* Unpublished master's thesis, University of Washington.

Gudjonsson, G. (1995). I'll help you boys as much as I can—how eagerness to please can result in a false confession. *Journal of Forensic Psychiatry*, 6(2), 333–342.

Gudjonsson, G. H. (2003). *The psychology of interrogations and confessions: a handbook.* New York: John Wiley & Sons.

Gustafson, R. (1986). Visual attentional span as a function of a small dose of alcohol. *Perceptual and Motor Skills*, 63, 367–370.

Hekkanen, S. T. and McEvoy, C. (2002). False memories and source monitoring problems: criterion differences. *Applied Cognitive Psychology*, 16, 73–85.

Horselenberg, R., Merckelbach, H., and Josephs, S. (2003). Individual differences and false confessions: a conceptual replication of Kassin and Kiechel (1996). *Psychology, Crime and Law*, 9, 1–8.

Horselenberg, R., Merckelbach, H., Muris, P., Rassin, E., Silsenaar, M., and Spann, V. (2000). Imagining fictitious childhood events: the role of individual differences in imagination inflation. *Clinical Psychology & Psychotherapy*, 7(2), 128–137.

Hull, J. G. and Bond, C. F. (1986). Social and behavioral consequences of alcohol consumption and expectancy: a meta-analysis. *Psychological Bulletin*, 99, 347–360.

Hyman, I. E. Jr. and Billings, F. J. (1998). Individual differences and the creation of false childhood memories. *Memory*, 6, 1–20.

Hyman, I. E. and Pentland, J. (1996). The role of mental imagery in the creation of false childhood memories. *Journal of Memory and Language*, 35, 101–117.

Hyman, I. E. Jr., Husband, T. H., and Billings, F. J. (1995). False memories of childhood experiences. *Applied Cognitive Psychology*, 9, 181–197.

Kassin, S. M. and Kiechel, K. L. (1996). The social psychology of false confessions: compliance, internalization, and confabulation. *Psychological Science*, 7(3), 125–128.

Kelemen, W. L. and Kaighobadi, F. (2007). Expectancy and pharmacology influence the subjective effects of nicotine using a balanced-placebo design. *Experimental Clinical Psychopharamcology*, 15, 93–101.

Kirsch, I. (1985). Response expectancy as a determinant of experience and behaviour. *American Psychologist*, 40, 1189–1202.

Kirsch, I. (2010). *The emperor's new drugs: exploding the antidepressant myth.* New York, NY: Basic Books.

Kirsch, I. and Lynn, S. J. (1999). Automaticity in clinical psychology. *American Psychologist*, 54, 504–515.

Kirsch, I., Deacon, B. J., Nuedo-Medina, T. B., Scoboria, A., Moore, T. J., and Johnson, B. T. (2008). Initial severity and antidepressant benefits: a meta-analysis of data submitted to the Food and Drug Administration. *Public Library of Science Medicine*, 5(2), e45. DOI:10.1371/journal.pmed.0050045

Kvavilashvili, L. and Ellis, J. A. (1999). The effects of positive and negative placebos on human memory performances. *Memory*, 7, 421–437.

Labrie, J. W., Hummer, J. F., and Pedersen, E. R. (2007). Reasons for drinking in the college student context: the differential role and risk of the social motivator. *Journal of Studies on Alcohol and Drugs*, 68, 393–398.

Laney, C., Morris, E. K., Bernstein, D. M., Wakefield, B. M., and Loftus, E. F. (2008a). Asparagus, a love story: healthier eating could be just a false memory away. *Experimental Psychology*, 55, 291–300.

Laney, C., Bowman-Fowler, N., Nelson, K. J., Bernstein, D. M., and Loftus, E. F. (2008b). The persistence of false beliefs. *Acta Psychologica*, 129, 190–197.

Lang, A. R., Goeckner, D. T., Adesso, V. J., and Marlatt, G. A. (1975). Effects of alcohol on aggression in male social drinkers. *Journal of Abnormal Psychology*, 84, 508–518.

Lansky, D. and Wilson, G. T. (1981). Alcohol, expectations, and sexual arousal in males: an information processing analysis. *Journal of Abnormal Psychology*, 90, 35–45.

Lindsay, D. S. (2008). Source monitoring. In: *Learning and memory: a comprehensive reference. Vol. 2: Cognitive psychology of memory* (ed. H. L. Roediger, III). Oxford: Elsevier.

Lindsay, D. S., Hagen, L., Read, J. D., Wade, K. A., and Garry, M. (2004). True photographs and false memories. *Psychological Science*, 15, 149–154.

Loftus, E. F. (1991). Made in memory: distortions in recollection after misleading information. In: *The psychology of learning and motivation: advances in research and theory* (ed. G. H. Bower). San Diego: Academic Press.

Loftus, E. F. (2005). A 30-year investigation of the malleability of memory. *Learning and Memory*, 12, 361–366.

Loftus, E. F. and Bernstein, D. M. (2005). Rich false memories: the royal road to success. In: *Experimental cognitive psychology and its applications: festschrift in honor of Lyle Bourne, Walter Kintsch, and Thomas Landauer* (ed. A. Healy). Washington DC: APA Press.

Loftus, E. F. and Fries, J. (2008). The potential perils of informed consent. *McGill Journal of Medicine*, 11, 217–218.

Loftus, E. F. and Ketcham, K. (1994). *The myth of repressed memory*. New York: St. Martin's Press.

Loftus, E. F. and Palmer, J. C. (1974). Reconstruction of automobile destruction. *Journal of Verbal Learning and Verbal Behavior*, 13, 585–589.

Loftus, E. F. and Pickrell, J. E. (1995). The formation of false memories. *Psychiatric Annals*, 25, 720–725.

Loftus, E. F., Miller, D. G., and Burns, H. J. (1978). Semantic integration of verbal information into a visual memory. *Journal of Experimental Psychology: Human Learning & Memory*, 4, 19–31.

Lynn, S. J. and Nash, M. R. (1994). Truth in memory: ramifications for psychotherapy and hypnotherapy. *American Journal of Clinical Hypnosis*, 36, 194–208.

Mackay, M., Tiplady, B., and Scholey, A. B. (2002). Interactions between alcohol and caffeine in relation to psychomotor speed and accuracy. *Human Psychopharmacology: Clinical & Experimental*, 17, 151–156.

Marlatt, G. A. and Rohsenow, D. J. (1980). Cognitive processes in alcohol use: expectancy and the balanced placebo design. In: *Advances in substance abuse (vol. 1)* (ed. N. K. Mello). Greenwich, CT, USA: JAI Press.

Mazzoni, G. (2002). Naturally occurring and suggestion-dependent memory distortions: the convergence of disparate research traditions. *European Psychologist*, 7, 17–30.

Mazzoni, G. A. L. and Memon, A. (2003). Imagination can create false autobiographical memories. *Psychological Science*, 14, 186–188.

Mazzoni, G. A. L., Loftus, E. F., Seitz, A., and Lynn, S. J. (1999). Changing beliefs and memories through dream interpretation. *Applied Cognitive Psychology*, 13, 125–144.

McDaniel, M. A. and Einstein, G. O. (2000). Strategic and automatic processes in prospective memory retrieval: a multiprocess framework. *Applied Cognitive Psychology*, 14, 127–144.

McMillan, D. L., Smith, S. M., and Wells-Parker, E. (1989). The effects of alcohol, expectancy and sensation seeking on driving risk taking. *Addictive Behaviors*, 14, 477–483.

Merckelbach, H., Muris, P., and Rassin, E. (1999). Fantasy proneness and cognitive failures as correlates of dissociative experiences. *Personality and Individual Differences*, 26, 961–967.

Nash, R. A. and Wade, K. A. (2008). Innocent but proven guilty: eliciting internalized false confessions using doctored-video evidence. *Applied Cognitive Psychology*, 23, 624–637.

Nash, R. A., Wade, K. A., and Lindsay, D. S. (2009). Digitally manipulating memory: effects of doctored videos and imagination in distorting beliefs and memories. *Memory & Cognition*, 37(4), 441–424.

Okado, Y. and Stark, C. E. L. (2005). Neural activity during encoding predicts false memories created by misinformation. *Learning and Memory*, 12, 3–11.

Ost, J., Fellows, B. J., and Bull, R. (1997). Individual differences and the suggestibility of human memory. *Contemporary Hypnosis*, 14, 132–137.

Ost, J., Foster, S., Costall, A., and Bull, R. (2005). False reports of childhood events in appropriate interviews. *Memory*, 13, 700–710.

Ost, J., Vrij, A., Costall, A., and Bull, R. (2002). Crashing memories and reality monitoring: distinguishing between perceptions, imaginations and false memories. *Applied Cognitive Psychology*, 16, 125–134.

Parker, S., Garry, M., Einstein, G. O., and McDaniel, M. A. (2011). A sham drug improves a demanding prospective memory task. *Memory*, 19, 606–612.

Parker, S., Garry, M., Engle, R. W., Harper, D. N., and Clifasefi, S. L. (2008). Psychotropic placebos reduce the misinformation effect by increasing monitoring at test. *Memory*, 16, 410–419.

Paterson, H. M. and Kemp, R. I. (2006). Co-witnesses talk: a survey of eyewitness discussion. *Psychology, Crime, & Law*, 12(2), 181–191.

Platt, R. D., Lacey, S. C., Lobst, A. D., and Finkelman, D. (1998). Absorption, dissociation and fantasy-proneness as predictors of memory distortion in autobiographical and laboratory-generated memories. *Applied Cognitive Psychology*, 12, S77–S89.

Porter, H. G., Birt, A. R., Yuille, J. C., and Lehman, D. R. (2000). Negotiating false memories: interviewer and rememberer characteristics relate to memory distortion. *Psychological Science*, 11(6), 507–510.

Porter, S., Yuille, J. C., and Lehman, D. R. (1999). The nature of real, implanted, and fabricated memories for emotional childhood events: implications for the recovered memory debate. *Law and Human Behavior*, 23, 517–537.

Powell, M. B., Fisher, R. P., and Wright, R. (2005). Investigative interviewing. In: *Psychology and law: an empirical perspective* (eds. N. Brewer and K. D. Williams). New York: Guilford Press.

Price, D. D., Finniss, D. G., and Benedetti, F. (2008). A comprehensive review of the placebo effect: recent advances and current thought. *Annual Review of Psychology*, **59**, 565–590.

Redlich, A. D. and Goodman, G. S. (2003). Taking responsibility for an act not committed: the influence of age and suggestibility. *Law and Human Behavior*, **27**, 141–156. DOI: 10.1023/A:1022543012851

Roediger III, H. L. and McDermott, K. B. (1995). Creating false memories: remembering words not presented in lists. *Journal of Experimental Psychology: Learning, Memory, and Cognition*, **21**, 803–814.

Rohrbaugh, J. W., Stapleton, J. M., Parasuraman, R., et al. (1988). Alcohol intoxication reduces visual sustained attention. *Psychopharmacology*, **96**, 442–446.

Schacter, D. L. (2001). *The seven sins of memory: how the mind forgets and remembers.* Boston: Houghton Mifflin.

Scoboria, A., Mazzoni, G., and Jarry, J. L. (2008). Suggesting childhood food illness results in reduced eating behavior. *Acta Psychologica*, **128**, 304–309.

Scorboria, A., Mazzoni, G. A. L., Kirsch, I., and Milling, L. S. (2002). Immediate and persisting effects of misleading questions and hypnosis on memory reports. *Journal of Experimental Psychology: Applied*, **8**, 26–32.

Seamon, J. G., Philbin, M. M., and Harrison, L. G. (2006). Do you remember proposing marriage to the Pepsi machine? False recollections from a campus walk. *Psychonomic Bulletin & Review*, **13**(5), 752–756.

Shapiro, A. K. and Shapiro, E. (1997a). *The powerful placebo: from ancient priest to modern physician.* Baltimore: The John Hopkins University Press.

Shapiro, A. K. and Shapiro, E. (1997b). The placebo: is it much ado about nothing? In: *The placebo effect: an interdisciplinary exploration* (ed. A. E. Harrington). Cambridge, USA: Harvard University Press.

Sharman, S. J. and Barnier, A. J. (2008). Imagining nice and nasty events in childhood or adulthood: recent positive events show the most imagination inflation. *Acta Psychologica*, **129**(2), 228–233.

Sharman, S. J. and Scoboria, A. (2009). Imagination equally influences false memories of high and low plausibility events. *Applied Cognitive Psychology*, **23**(6), 813–827.

Sharman, S. J., Garry, M., and Beuke, C. J. (2004). Imagination or exposure causes imagination inflation. *American Journal of Psychology*, **117**, 157–168.

Sharman, S. J., Manning, C. G., and Garry, M. (2005). Explain this: explaining childhood events inflates confidence for those events. *Applied Cognitive Psychology*, **19**(1), 67–74.

Simons, D. J. and Chabris, C. F. (1999). Gorillas in our midst: sustained inattentional blindness for dynamic events. *Perception*, **28**, 1059–1074.

Snyder, M. (1974). Self-monitoring of expressive behaviour. *Journal of Personality and Social Psychology*, **30**, 526–537.

Spanos, N. P., Burgess, C. A., Burgess, M. F., Samuels, C., and Blois, W. O. (1999). Creating memories of infancy with hypnotic and non-hypnotic procedures. *Applied Cognitive Psychology*, **3**, 201–218.

Spiro, H. (1997). Clinical reflections on the placebo phenomenon. In: *The placebo effect: an interdisciplinary exploration* (ed. A. Harrington). Cambridge, USA: Harvard University Press.

Stewart-Williams, S. (2004). The placebo puzzle: putting together the pieces. *Health Psychology*, **23**, 198–206.

Stewart-Williams, S. and Podd, J. (2004). The placebo effect: dissolving the expectancy versus conditioning debate. *Psychological Bulletin*, **130**, 324–340.

Takarangi, M. K. T., Parker, S., and Garry, M. (2006). Modernising the misinformation effect: the development of a new stimulus set. *Applied Cognitive Psychology*, **20**, 583–590.

Thomas, A. K. and Loftus, E. F. (2002). Creating bizarre false memories through imagination. *Memory & Cognition*, **30**, 423–431.

Tilburt, J. C., Emanuel, E. J., Kaptchuk, T. J., Curlin, F. A., and Miller, F. G. (2008). Prescribing "placebo treatments": results of a national survey of US internists and rheumatologists. *British Medical Journal*, **337**, 1–5.

Van Oorsouw, K. and Merckelbach, H. (2007). Expectancies and memory for an emotional film fragment: a placebo study. *American Journal of Psychology*, **120**, 287–301.

Wade, K. A. (2004). *Factors that influence source monitoring do not necessarily influence false childhood memories*. Unpublished doctoral thesis, Victoria University, Wellington, New Zealand.

Wade, K. A., Garry, M., Read, J. D., and Lindsay, S. A. (2002). A picture is worth a thousand lies. *Psychonomic Bulletin and Review*, **9**, 597–603.

Wesnes, K., Revell, A. D., and Warburton, D. M. (1983). Work and stress as motives for smoking. In: *Smoking and the lung* (eds.G. Cimming and G. Bonsignore). New York: Plenum.

Wilkinson, C. and Hyman, I. E. Jr. (1998). Individual differences related to two types of memory errors: word lists may not generalize to autobiographical memory. *Applied Cognitive Psychology*, **12**, S29–246.

Wright, D. B., Self, G., and Justice, C. (2000). Memory conformity: exploring misinformation effects when presented by another person. *British Journal of Psychology*, **91**, 189–202.

Zhu, B., Chen, C., Loftus, E. F., et al. (2010a). Individual differences in false memory from misinformation: cognitive factors. *Memory*, **18**, 543–555.

Zhu, B, Chen, C.,Loftus, E. F., et al. (2010b). Individual differences in false memory from misinformation: personality characteristics. *Personality and Individual Differences*, **48**, 889–894.

Chapter 13

Fetish as placebo: the social history of a sexual idea

Edward Shorter

13.1 **Introduction**

Until the stunning success of the novel *Fifty shades of grey*, the whole question of fetish and role playing, formerly known as sadomasochism, belonged to the chronicles of the sexual byways (James 2011). Yet by early 2013, sales of *Fifty shades* had exceeded 30 million copies, and it had become one of the best-selling novels of modern times (Wembridge 2012). The desires that *Fifty shades* has awakened (and that have become part of modern culture) thus stride to the very middle of the intersection between sexuality and medicine—medicine in the sense of assessing to what extent deeply felt desires represent biology, and to what extent they represent "placebo," or non-biological, culturally modeled sexual aspirations. (In actual fact, fetish is a non-theme in *Fifty shades*, and the trilogy, of which *Fifty shades of grey* is the first volume, is centered solely around the theme of role playing.)

Why placebo? The analogy from psychopharmacology to social science is clear: in both cases, placebo modifies a biological rhythm through suggestion. In trials of psychopharmacologic agents, placebo evokes a subjective response so convincing as to be mistaken, by the patient, for evidence of drug action. Placebo pharmacology has real effects, in other words, and it is often difficult to distinguish them from true pharmacologic effects. As Louis Lasagna, the dean of American psychopharmacologists, wrote in 1971, "One reason the placebo is important in regard to clinical trials is that it has been shown to have an amazing ability to mimic the 'active' drugs in its effects" (1971, p. 45).

Similarly in culture, the placebo effect of an idea evokes a subjective response so strong as to be taken as evidence of the action of biology. There has been no biological change in response to cultural suggestion, yet the impact on individuals is so powerful as to feel "biological." This chapter traces such a subjective individual response in the impact of sexual fetish upon the subjectivity of sexually active individuals: people feel their response to fetish so intensely as to believe that the very parenchyma of the brain itself has always generated such a response. Yet fetish seems not to possess a biology of its own, and the strong attraction within the fetish subculture to such themes as latex and leather must rest upon suggestion, upon placebo in other words, rather than upon biology.

13.2 **The biology of sexuality**

Human sexuality possesses a biology of its own that is as old as time (Shorter 2005). We are accustomed to thinking of the basic sexual orientations—heterosexuality, male homosexuality, and female lesbianism—as individual choices strongly influenced by social convention. Until recently, the doctrine has prevailed within the social sciences that sexual orientation is the product of an unconscious choice made early in childhood. Psychoanalytic doctrine insisted for many years that unsuccessful efforts to pass through the anal stage of child development to the genital stage resulted in paranoia, and in same-sex attraction. In 1905, in his book *Three essays on sexual theory*, Freud said:

> Psychoanalysis postulates the independence from gender of the free disposition to choose male and female objects, as this is observed in childhood, in primitive societies and in early historic times . . . For inverts [homosexuals] we see unquestionably the predominance of archaic constitutions and primitive psychic mechanisms. The force of the narcissistic object choice and the clinging to the erotic significance of the anal zone are the essential characteristics (1942, p. 44–45n).

A latter-day version of the psychoanalytic argument emphasizes "social construction" in the making of gender and sexuality: society chooses for us our sexual roles and orientations. David Greenberg, for example, argues that in the distant European past, "homosexuality was part of a criminal subculture, not a gay one" (1988, p. 309).

Today, both Freud and social construction have come under fire. Recent "essentialist" views ascribe to sexual orientation a powerful biological component, possibly genetic in nature, possibly uterine, and fixed before the child is even born. It is not accidental that a majority of gay men and lesbian women report their earliest sexual fantasies as homoerotic in nature (Savin-Williams 1997). At a street fair in San Francisco in 1999, researchers quizzed a random group of 720 adults about sexual orientation: lesbian women had significantly longer index fingers than did non-lesbian women (finger length is determined *in utero* by fetal androgens). Few gay men and women believe that their sexuality is not biologically ordained (Williams et al. 2000).

In the debate between the biological determinists and the social constructionists, the former have landed some telling blows. Today, the notion that homosexuality is socially constructed evokes derision in the gay community, and the scientific evidence as well seems to point to a powerful somatic impetus to sexual orientation beginning early in life. The three great sexual orientations of gay, lesbian, and straight are thus likely biological orientations. Homosexuality and lesbianism have been documented since the Ancient Greeks (Shorter 2005), and "bisexuals" are thought to be mainly homosexual men and women who have not yet declared themselves.

13.3 **Overlays: changes to biological orientations**

Changes to these three great orientations that have occurred across the ages may therefore be interpreted as "overlays," riders on the great steeds that surge beneath. The steeds themselves gallop across the centuries, yet their riders may change, or—not to push this metaphor too far—the number, clothing, and position of the riders may change as well. Here culture plays a role.

Among obvious overlays are differences in age at marriage: some societies tolerate wide differences among the partners and find May–December unions quite acceptable; for other societies, such couplings are odious, given the probability that vastly older husbands will predecease their wives, leaving them as widows dependent upon the commonweal for support. Our own society has little tolerance for large age differences between the spouses; in eighteenth-century France, this was quite acceptable, the woman often older than the man to reduce her years at risk from childbearing (Van Gennep 1972). Hence, age differences are an overlay.

Male attraction to female beauty, especially facial beauty, may be seen as an overlay, rather than the product of biological male attraction to beauty or, as social constructionists might have it, the cultural glorification of a certain kind of female attractiveness promoted in the media. Peasant proverbs are full of injunctions about not marrying beautiful women, who are imagined to spend their days primping and sparing their hands rather than pitching into the arduous regimen of farm work. In the French province of Franche-Comté, the ability of future wives to sustain a regimen of grueling work certainly trumped beauty. Among the folk sayings were: "You can't eat beauty with a spoon" and "It's better to be able to say, 'Hey, ugly, what's for dinner,' than 'Tell me, my lovely, do we have anything to eat tonight?'" (Perron 1892, p. 85).

Of course, many men and women, at various points in time and within different societies, have delected the beauty of the opposite sex, and made it a criterion of partner choice. However others, also numerous, have not, and physical beauty may be viewed as an overlay to the three powerful sexual orientations as they storm forward in time.

Fetish, too, is an overlay.

13.4 **Fetish as an overlay**

Right up front, one must distinguish between fetish and role playing. Fetish is spurring sexual appetites to redoubled frenzy through external inanimate objects, such as underwear, fur, leather, or latex: the list of fetishes that have emerged over the years is long (Steele 1996). Fetish does not mean an object that *substitutes* for intercourse. One is truly in sexual Sunday school with the *Diagnostic and statistical manual* (DSM) series of the American Psychiatric Association (APA). The third edition, which appeared in 1980 and greatly changed psychiatric diagnosis, insisted, in the "Fetishism" section, that "The essential feature is the use of nonliving objects (fetishes) as a repeatedly preferred or exclusive method of achieving sexual excitement." Even worse, it states "Once established, the disorder tends to be chronic"(!) (APA 1980, p. 268). The most recent, fourth edition is scarcely different (APA 2000, especially p. 569–570). Yet in the worldwide fetish communities, there would be agreement that fetish is a healthy enhancer, not a pathological substitute.

Role playing means the voluntary exchange of power in a sexual situation, so that the person who has voluntarily agreed to surrender power is called the "sub" or the "bottom," and he or she whom mutual agreement has placed in charge is called the "top" or the "dominant." These voluntary agreements to transfer power for fixed periods of time and under tightly specified conditions were referred to in the past as "SM," for "sadomasochism," or "BDSM," for "bondage-domination-sadism-masochism," which is the customary internet term. Today, mainly for the sake of optics, the whole bundle of "topping" and "bottoming" is called "role playing," and is seen as different, in that it is consensual (as opposed to classic psychological sadism or delight in the infliction of suffering upon an unwilling individual).

The overlap between fetish and role playing is substantial but not complete. Many fetishists delight in the pleasure of leather or latex in sexual situations, without wishing to dominate their partners or be dominated by them. Similarly, many sadomasochists are content to role play without the slightest fetishistic adornment. Fetish and role playing are, in other words, quite different domains of sexual activity, although a Venn diagram would show a certain overlap that has never been quantified in survey research.

Fetish and role playing are both overlays on the three great sexualities, although their chronology is somewhat different. It is indeed their brief historic existence that qualifies both fetish and role playing as placebo-like adornments of biology, rather than possessing a biology of their own. The logic is that if they were brain-driven, they would have become manifest, historically, far earlier in time. Voluntary sadomasochism does seem to have quite a rich history, while fetish is very recent. It is indeed this very recency that confers upon fetish, in particular, its placebo quality: a culturally derived behavior that is so meaningful to the participants that it feels to them as though it must be driven by biology—but is not.

13.5 **Fetish and role playing in history**

Among the earliest cases of role playing in history is that of an anonymous Italian male, a friend of the fifteenth-century scholar Giovanni Pico della Mirandola, who told Pico that he enjoyed being flogged by his wife. The friend said that it was "a taste I acquired as child," meaning that he experienced it at a deep sensual level. "Moreover," said Pico, the friend "was in other aspects not a wicked man and recognized and detested this ailment of his" (Pico Della Mirandola 1946, p. 413).[1] Over the years, the frequency of references to flogging and the like accelerates, so that by the late seventeenth century, in England, it was quite commonplace: in London, there was a male club, the "Flogging Cullies" (cull meaning testicles), in which the members paid women to come in and flagellate them (Norton 1992, p. 68).

Yet in these years, fetish was quite absent. The works of the Marquis de Sade in the late eighteenth century revel in the most orgiastic scenes of sadomasochism imaginable (Le Brun and Pauvert 1986).[2] Yet one scans in vain such Sadean classics as *Juliette*, history's first dominatrix, for any reference to leather or other fetish. The participants are usually entirely clothed, or entirely naked, and the fact that most scenes seem to end with all the participants dead suggests that allegory rather than eros may have been what Sade had mainly in mind. Yet fetish is absent from Sade, without question.

Fetish makes an early eruption into history with Leopold von Sacher-Masoch's *Venus in fur* in 1870—and the fetish that Sacher-Masoch launched was not leather but fur (Figure 13.1). The hero, the young Severin, tells the dominatrix Wanda that, "Nothing is so calculated to inflame my passion as the tyranny, the cruelty . . . of a beautiful woman. But I can't imagine this woman . . . without fur" (Sacher-Masoch [1870] 1996, p. 46). Severin adores the SM part, of Wanda whacking him, but her array of fur clearly adds to his pleasure. History's first fetish was thus fur.

Sacher-Masoch, it must be said, perceived his own fondness for fetish as profoundly biological, something deeply "natural:"

> I saw in sensuality something holy, indeed the only holy thing, in which for a woman
> and her beauty there was something godlike, the most important task of life being the
> perpetuation of humankind; that, above all, is her calling . . . I saw in the woman the
> personification of nature, the Isis, and the man as her high priest, her slave ([1870]
> 1996, p. 47).

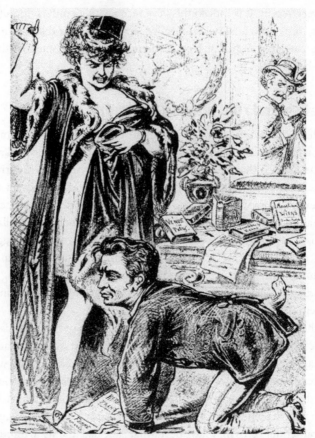

Fig. 13.1 Sacher-Masoch introduces fetish to role playing. This 1890 caricature by Austrian artist Carl von Stur shows him being disciplined by the dominatrix "Wanda" from *Venus in fur*, with a copy of the volume among the books on the table behind him. "Seine Muse" (His Muse) by Carl von Stur (1840–1905). Chalk lithograph, 1890, AKG 1537279.

No question of social construction here; for Sacher-Masoch, it was the inner nature of man and woman that spoke.

In these early days of fetish in the nineteenth century, the gamut of potential fetishes stretched much wider than today. Marion Delorme's guide to "All kinds of fetishes," published in German in Paris around 1900, listed as fetishes "beautiful feet of women, combs, wigs, underwear, and red hair" (cited in Hayn and Gotendorf 1913, p. 285). Yet fur dominated the scene until at least the First World War. In October 1909, James Joyce offered to buy Nora a splendid sable set including a cap, stole, and muff. "Would you like that?" he asked hopefully (Ellman 1975, p. 172).

Yet by the years between the two world wars, fur was replaced by leather as fetish object number one. It is this rapidity of transition that enhances the overlay aspect of such "fashion perceived as biology" behavior that is the essence of cultural fetish. We go from zero to sixty within little more than a decade, the players all the while under the impression that their behavior is profoundly biological, rooted within the very fiber of their being. (An internet fetish image featuring a dominatrix is erroneously captioned, "Leather: helping men behave for centuries" (Flickr)). In England, the initial eruption of leather occurs in the first decade before the First World War: for example, a 1909 pamphlet was entitled "Figure-training and deportment by means of the discipline of tight corsets, narrow high-heeled boots, and clinging kid gloves." A magazine called *London Life*, appearing between 1923 and 1940, spotlighted fetishistic females wearing high-heel shoes and boots (Steele 1996, p. 51, 70–71). It is in these years that the image of the dominatrix, dressed head to toe in leather, begins to sharpen. The Kinsey Collection in Bloomington, Indiana, the world's foremost archive of erotica, offers the first images of a dominatrix in the 1920s, showing, for example in Berlin, one leather-clad domme alongside another domme in fur; a second image from 1928 reveals a booted domme topping a man (Figure 13.2) (see Shorter 2005, p. 224).

These images were, of course, designed to stoke the male pornographic imagination. How curious that their appearance historically should have been so sudden, and so recent. Yet can anyone doubt that the men who frequented the prostitutes offering these services in such big cities as London, Paris, and Berlin between the world wars believed themselves in the grip of a demonic biological force? They were responding to cultural suggestions that they perceived as biological, the very definition of a cultural placebo.

Why does culture encourage fetish in these years and not much earlier? The blossoming of fetish after 1870 coincided with a substantial widening of the entire palette of sexual offerings that separated the, in fact, rather erotic Victorians from their predecessors, for whom religious doctrine limited them substantially to the missionary position. In my 2005 book *Written in the flesh* I have attempted to document these years as the epoch of the "great breakout," the unfettering of all kinds of sexuality and the eroticizing of all parts of the body—deep kissing, the anus, the adoration of the long limbs—in what one might think of as the "sensualizing of sexuality" (Shorter 2005, p. 109–147). It was precisely in aid of this kind of sensualization that such exquisite touches as fetish started to appear.

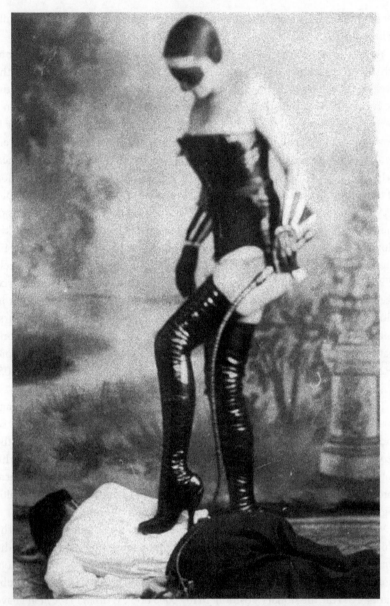

Fig. 13.2 Leather clothing begins to supplant fur as a fetish after the First World War. Early depiction of a leather-clad dominatrix, 1928 gelatin silver print.

© 1928, The Kinsey Institute for Research in Sex, Gender, and Reproduction, KI-DC:65706.

13.6 **The fetish overlay upon the three great sexualities**

The eruption of fetish into the world of heterosexuality has been amply documented. Of interest is that this eruption occurred somewhat later into the world of gay males and still later, yet with the same ineluctable force, into the lives of lesbian women.

The predominant public image of gay males until the 1960s had been that of effeminacy, the drag queen, and the "nance." This changed abruptly in the 1960s with the arrival of the male "clone," the hypermasculine gay male stud, who wore leather straps across an otherwise naked torso, a heavy belt, and black boots. The iconic figure of the macho man was, of course, a fetish figure (see Figure 13.3). It permeated the urban gay male subculture (see Levine 1998). One journalist said of Christopher Street in Manhattan in 1978, "The universal stance is a studied masculinity. There are no limp wrists, no giggles, no indiscreet hip swiveling . . . This is macho country" (Kleinberg 1978, p. 6). Iconic for macho country (aka Manhattan) was a leather bar that John Preston, in his classic novel *Mr. Benson* about the gay SM scene, calls "The Ramrod." "The Ramrod was as full of men as I had hoped," writes the protagonist. "They formed a veritable sea of black leather" (Preston [1983] 1992, p. 42). The protagonist in the novel is just gasping for contact with these leather-covered gods, and feels himself the embodiment of the sexuality of gay men since time immemorial. Yet the scene was a decade old, at best.

As the gay leather scene was in full swing, the lesbian leather scene was just emerging. In 1978, writer Pat Califia and academic Gayle Rubin founded a lesbian SM group in San Francisco called Samois, after the estate of the fictional "Anne Marie" in the Story of O. Samois was situated at that point in the Venn diagram where leather and role playing crossed over. Samois became known for its 1981 SM sampler *Coming to power*, republished in 1983 with worldwide distribution (Samois 1983), and for the sequel *The second coming: a leatherdyke reader*, published in 1996 (Califia and Sweeney 1996). Samois has not been entirely uncontroversial within the lesbian community, yet it certainly anchors the existence of leather fetish as an important overlay within the great stream of lesbian sexuality that has flowed across the ages.

13.7 **Conclusion**

In the end, what do we learn from this exercise? What is the intersection between *Fifty shades* and modern psychopharmacology?

The concept of placebo in medicine makes sense only in the context of active treatment. Before the rise of modern pharmacology, when few effective drugs existed, all agents were, more or less, sugar pills: the rows of alkaloids and tonics

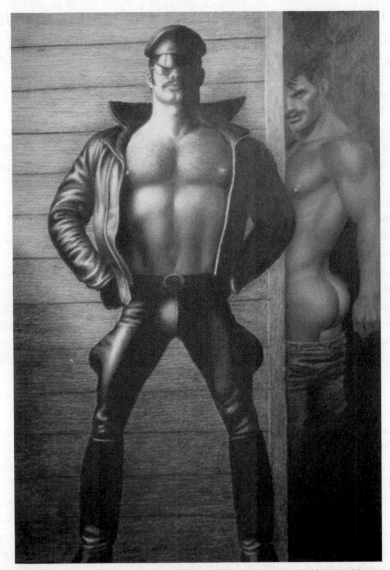

Fig. 13.3 The hypermasculine leatherman celebrated by artist Tom of Finland becomes an icon for the gay community around 1970.

TOM OF FINLAND (Touko Laaksonen, Finnish, 1920–1991), Untitled, 1980, Color pencil on paper, ToFF #80.02, © 1980, Tom of Finland Foundation.

put out by the "long-line" drug houses had little impact on the course of disease. All were placebos, in the sense that agents with a genuine pharmacological effect were few on the ground. The therapeutic revolution of the 1950s changed this dramatically, by creating powerful new classes of chemotherapeutic agents, such as the phenothiazines in psychiatry (Shorter 2009). Only at that point did it make sense to separate a placebo effect from a treatment effect in order to ascertain just how useful the new agents were.

Similarly, in cultural studies of placebo, it makes little sense to talk about a placebo effect in the absence of an underlying brain biology. In the social construction school, all is society and biology counts for little, and if society is responsible for almost all behavior, it is idle to postulate the existence of placebo-style suggestion. All the signals that influence behavior originate from society, not from the brain. The notion that some signals are so powerful that individuals believe they must be biological in origin is pointless who cares, if brain and body have little influence on behavior?

Only the existence of biological thinking about behavior makes the concept of the cultural placebo relevant. *Fifty shades* functions as a kind of cultural placebo because the desires it awakens have been created as much by culture as by biology. Most of the millions of readers of the novel and its sequelae were not born into this world as sadomasochists! Only in understanding where they come from does it become important to talk about pseudo-neural suggestion as a source of behavior, because we have at the same time the genuine neural influencing of behavior. This is the interesting thing about sexuality: that it mixes together the cultural and the biological. Only if we have genuine brain-driven sexuality can we talk about non-brain sexual effects, or placebo effects that feel just as real to the participants as do the brain-driven effects. From the subjective viewpoint of the players, brain effects and suggestive effects are identical and indistinguishable. It is only the social scientists, just as the pharmacologists, who wish to sort them out.

Notes

1 The volume contains a parallel Italian translation, "Un abitudine contratta da bambino."
2 See Volumes 8 and 9 for "Juliette."

References

American Psychiatric Association (1980). *Diagnostic and statistical manual of mental disorders* (3rd edn.). Washington, DC: APA.

American Psychiatric Association (2000). *Diagnostic and statistical manual of mental disorders* (revised 4th edn.). Washington, DC: APA.

Califia, P. and Sweeney, R. (1996). *The second coming: a leatherdyke reader*. Los Angeles: Alyson.

Ellman, R. (1975). *Selected letters of James Joyce*. New York: Viking Press.

Flickr. *Baine61* [online]. Accessed 2012.

Freud, S. (1942). Drei abhandlungen zur sexualtheorie (1905). In: *Gesammelte werke* (ed. S. Freud). London: Imago Publishing Co.

Greenberg, D. F. (1988). *The construction of homosexuality.* Chicago: University of Chicago Press.

Hayn, H. and Gotendorf, A. N. (1913). *Bibliotheca Germanorum erotica et curiosa.* Munich: Muller.

James, E. L. (2011). *Fifty shades of grey.* New York: Random House.

Kleinberg, S. (1978). "Where have all the sissies gone?" *Christopher Street,* 2(9), 4–12.

Lasagna, L. (1971). Decision processes in establishing the efficacy and safety of psychotropic agents. In: *Principles and problems in establishing the efficacy of psychotropic agents* (eds. L. Bouthilet, J. Levine, and B. C. Schiele). Washington, DC: National Institute of Mental Health.

Le Brun, A. and Pauvert, J. J. (1986). *Œuvres complètes du marquis de Sade.* Paris: Pauvert.

Levine, M. P. (1998). *Gay macho: the life and death of the homosexual clone.* New York: New York University Press.

Norton, R. (1992). *Mother Clap's Molly House: the gay subculture in England 1700--1830.* London: GMP.

Perron, C. (1892). *Les Franc-Comtois . . .* Besançon: Abel Cariage.

Pico Della Mirandola, G. (1946 reprint). *Disputationes adversus astrologiam divinatricem . . . A cura di Eugenio Garin (1495).* Florence: Vallecchi.

Preston, J. ([1983] 1992). *Mr. Benson.* New York: Badboy Edition.

Sacher-Masoch, L. ([1870] 1996). *Venus im pelz.* Köln: Könemann.

Samois (1983). *Coming to power: writings and graphics on lesbian S/M.* Boston: Alyson.

Savin-Williams, R. C. (1997). *". . . And then I became gay": young men's stories.* New York: Routledge.

Shorter, E. (2005). *Written in the flesh: a history of desire:* Toronto: University of Toronto Press.

Shorter, E. (2009). *Before Prozac: the troubled history of mood disorders in psychiatry.* New York: Oxford University Press.

Steele, V. (1996). *Fetish: fashion, sex and power.* New York: Oxford University Press.

Van Gennep, A. (1972). *Manuel de folklore français contemporain.* Paris: Auguste Picard.

Wembridge, M. (2012). Potter whipped by Shades of Grey. *Financial Times,* August 2, p. 12.

Williams, T. J., Pepitone, M. E., Christensen, S. E., et al. (2000). Finger-length ratios and sexual orientation. *Nature,* 404, 455–456. DOI: 10.1038/35006555.

Chapter 14

"Take two and vote in the morning": reflections on the political placebo effect

Michael Orsini and Paul Saurette

14.1 Introduction

The use of medical metaphors in politics is a well-honed rhetorical strategy. We talk of "diagnosing" political and social problems; of public policy prescribing a "plan of treatment" to solve social ills; of governments having to "give the public some tough medicine"; of politicians "sugar coating" the pills that the public does not want to swallow. Sometimes these metaphors help to clarify the political world. Other times, however, the rhetorical comparison masks more than it reveals.

This chapter asks whether the idea of a "political placebo"—or more precisely, a "political placebo effect"—is a useful concept to introduce to the social sciences. Up to this point, the idea of a "political placebo" has been used only haphazardly and mostly in journalistic writing and with little conceptual clarity. In these circles, it has been employed as little more than a shorthand description for political rhetoric or empty promises which, in offering the policy equivalent of useless sugar pills, are nothing more than placeholders for procrastination or manipulative attempts to sell snake oil to the masses.

This common usage, however, misinterprets the very idea of a placebo effect as it has been used in the medical and scientific context and thus misrepresents the ways in which the concept of a political placebo effect might be relevant to our understanding of the political landscape. To be clear, the medical and scientific descriptions of a placebo effect are clearly not a description of a state in which a doctor lies to a patient and prescribes her/him a "solution" that has no effect whatsoever, other than to preserve a doctor's authority or interests. Rather, the most persuasive theories about placebo effects describe it as a situation in which certain actions and words undertaken by medical or scientific authorities lead to an observable effect in the patient, but one that is different from the effects (or lack of effects) that would have been predicted on the basis of the dominant scientific and medical models. As Harrington (2006, p. 181) describes it, there are at least three definitions of the placebo effect in circulation:

a) a short-term and illusory impression of improved health that some patients experience when they take an inert substance that looks like real medicine (e.g., a sugar pill);

b) the non-specific effects of medical treatment that, in clinical trials, must be controlled in order for researchers to assess the specific effects of new interventions, especially drugs;

c) a powerful mind–body phenomenon with a specific "real" biology all its own that medicine should study and exploit.

Despite common assumptions that the third definition is the most enlightened of the three, Harrington explains that the first two remain influential and have yet to be displaced by the third. While each of these definitions "is thoroughly incompatible with the others," each "nevertheless enjoys some authority in society today" (Harrington 2006, p. 182).

Rather than reproduce the disagreements in the scholarly community about how to define the placebo effect in medicine, this chapter focuses on outlining the main relevant characteristics of what we believe is the strongest definition in order to develop a concept of a political placebo effect. We argue that it is profoundly inaccurate to use the concept of a political placebo effect to describe those banal and frequent situations where politicians intentionally mislead the public or try to avoid solving problems by offering solutions or claims that they clearly know will have no impact on the political problem that has been "diagnosed" or on the issue that has been identified as requiring urgent action. Instead, we suggest that political placebo effects should refer to situations in which primarily mental stimuli (e.g., language, concepts, and policy ideas) have important and observable effects other than those captured by the dominant, predictive, rational actor theories, but which might be understandable on the basis of theories that explore the multifaceted effects of structures of meaning, emotions, and the complex interaction between mind and body. Moreover, we want to argue that such a reconceptualization could help us to reflect more thoughtfully about many types of political events and situations.

Fully exploring these contentions is beyond the scope of a single chapter and we have had to forego many interesting questions and avenues of exploration in the interests of space. As such, the modest goal of this chapter is, first, to sketch the main parameters of a redefined concept of the political placebo effect and then, second, to illustrate how this might help us to interpret contemporary politics by using the concept of a political placebo effect to analyze, albeit briefly, two recent political events. To do so, we begin by outlining the traditional medical understandings of the placebo effect to set the context correctly. Following this, we outline three characteristics of new medical definitions of the placebo effect and suggest the ways in which these inform our concept of a political placebo effect. Then, we offer brief and necessarily partial analyses of two political events using this concept and show how this provides a different interpretation than many dominant political science perspectives. We finally close with a short conclusion.

14.2 **Traditional perspectives on the placebo effect**

For many citizens of modern, industrialized societies, medicine is the archetypical and most concretely experienced example of the practical role that science plays in our everyday life. Viewed as a site where legitimate scientific knowledge is used to objectively diagnose illness and prescribe reliable and effective solutions, it is generally regarded as a profoundly evidence-based practice in which the direct causal effects of various treatments are well established and clear. Yet, there are many phenomena that science can observe but cannot precisely explain. Common reactions to such cases (by researchers, doctors, and the public at large) range from grandfatherly dismissals of the phenomenon as irrelevant (i.e., if the occurrences seem "random" or direct, specific causes cannot be identified as mandated by the scientific method and are assumed to be nonexistent and/or inexplicable and thus unworthy of study) to the outright rejection of them as being the figments of people's imaginations. This latter reaction, and the serious consequences that result, can be seen in the medical community's historic and ongoing tendency to disregard and belittle a variety of alternative therapies and traditional medicines of various forms; to dismiss women's health concerns as merely "in one's head" (see Dumit 2006); and to refuse to recognize a range of what have come to be known as "contested illnesses," such as multiple chemical sensitivity, fibromyalgia, and chronic fatigue syndrome (see Brown et al. 2004).

This context is particularly relevant when considering the genealogy of the traditional medical definition of the placebo effect. At its most basic, the term "placebo" is used to describe an intervention of some type—whether it be a sugar pill, a saline injection, or a physical procedure—that is believed to be "inert" and have no direct, specific, causal impact on the condition of interest. What makes the placebo such an interesting phenomenon, however, is not simply that it is a widely used tool to create control groups in medical research but, rather, that there is an observable phenomenon called the 'placebo effect'.

A conventional definition of the placebo effect describes the fact that, under certain conditions, the administration of supposedly inert and non-causal treatments is accompanied by measurable changes in the patient in ways that cannot be explained by current scientific knowledge. The placebo effect is a highly variable phenomenon that is quite dependent on the context in which it is observed and administered. Its existence and strength varies considerably between cultures, individuals, and time and it is not easily predicted since, despite significant effort, researchers have not identified reliable "placebo responder" characteristics.

Given the broader context already described, it is perhaps not surprising that the medical community has traditionally responded to this effect quite ambivalently. On the one hand, the behavior of medical practitioners seems to suggest that many believe that the placebo effect is an important reality, since studies indicate that many doctors prescribe vitamins, pills, or anti-biotics (even in cases where no evidence exists that they will have a physical or chemical impact) because they believe that there are real and positive (even if inexplicable) health benefits to this practice.[1] On the other hand, however, the placebo effect has been largely dismissed as a legitimate type of therapy in itself.[2] In fact, the very term "placebo" (from the Latin meaning "to please") highlights its contested validity by suggesting that placebos are merely given to "please" the patient and are not worthy of serious scientific investigation.

If this were all there was to the current state of thinking on placebos and the placebo effect, it would be of little interest to those of us who study the political world. At worst, it would be a catch-all phrase to group a series of political phe-nomena that are inexplicable through a set of universal natural laws of human behavior and interaction. Even at best, it would merely describe the nature of knowledge in the social sciences. As many theories in the social sciences have shown, certain aspects of the social world (i.e., the fact that it is made up of interactions between at least semi-conscious beings who demonstrate vastly different responses to similar stimuli across individuals, cultures, and temporal periods) make it profoundly resistant to many of the dominant epistemological strands in the hard sciences (e.g., assumptions about the existence of enduring laws of nature; the use of certainty, repeatability, and predictability as markers of reliable evidence).

Over the last decade or so, however, an increasing number of fields of medical and scientific inquiry have begun to offer complex and thoughtful perspectives on phenomena such as the placebo effect. Exploring these developments, and their relevance for a concept of a political placebo effect, is therefore the focus of the next section.

14.3 New perspectives on placebos and the implications for politics

Given space constraints, we have chosen to focus on three broad themes in the scientific literature that are most relevant for our attempt to develop a useful and valid concept of the placebo for political contexts.

14.3.1 Mind–body interplay

It is increasingly clear that placebo effects "are not mysterious, random and inexplicable. They are examples of the increasingly well-demonstrated (but only incompletely understood) complex interplay between the mind and the body" (Harrington 2008). As is well known, many of the dominant scientific and medical paradigms of the twentieth century followed a relatively rigid and reductionist Cartesian perspective—one that both assumed a fundamental division between the body and mind and privileged the identification of phys- ical/chemical factors as the sole model of legitimate scientific explanation. Recent scientific research, however, has increasingly demonstrated that the mind and body are not hermetically sealed and discrete units that can be ana- lyzed in isolation from one another. Instead, various fields of scientific and medical inquiry are now (re)discovering that mental practices and states can have significant, if often difficult to anticipate and understand, physiological effects (and vice versa).

New studies, for example, are showing that a variety of traditional and non- conventional practices have very specific and measurable effects on the body. In particular, studies suggest that mental practices have direct impact on physical states. For example, practices such as yoga and meditation are shown to have significant and measurable impacts on stress levels, hormone flows in the body, and a variety of other physiological indicators (Merrell 2008, especially Chap- ter 1). Other studies suggest that perceptions of "choice" can also affect physical health outcomes (Polsky et al. 2002). Still further studies have shown a variety of other effects that mental practices can have on physical states (Kihlstrom 2008; Moerman 2002; Raz et al. 2008; Wilce 2003).

Now, it is surely not the case that practices of yoga, meditation, or choice have suddenly begun having scientifically observable effects. Rather, we are only now starting to understand their physiological effects from a scientific perspec- tive both because new technologies have made available new types of evidence and because some researchers have been bold enough to develop new theories that challenge the reductionist model. One of the important lessons from this recent turn is that we often forget the degree to which the assumptions and practices of dominant knowledge paradigms and methodologies profoundly shape our (sometimes mis-) understanding of various phenomena. These new findings, for instance, were occasioned by the willingness of researchers to develop new and "fuzzier" concepts of causation, to expand the definition of what counts as "evidence," and to explore the ramifications of these new types of evidence as they became available.

These lessons are important for new understandings of the placebo effect. They suggest that the placebo effect is not a description of something that is literally inexplicable. Rather, it describes something that has an effect other than what might be predicted by "dualist" scientific knowledge paradigms. It can be reliably understood in light of new paradigms that see our mind–body relationship as a complex and inextricably linked set of reactions that respond to both "physical" and "mental" stimuli.

What are the implications of this shift in scientific understanding of the placebo effect for those of us who study politics? We believe that social scientists who are interested in the concept of a political placebo effect need also to highlight the ways in which new perspectives on the mind–body relationship can enrich our own study of the political world. It is not particularly controversial to say that for much of the twentieth century, many disciplines in the social sciences, and certainly that of political science, were heavily influenced by a Cartesian-like dualist set of assumptions that largely, if heuristically, separated mind from body and set up what some have called an "intellectualist" or rationalist foundation (see Lakoff 2008; Westen 2007). In political science, as with other disciplines, "rational actor" theories and models have been the most obvious and rigid manifestation of this basic epistemological predisposition, but many other perspectives and theories also share these assumptions, even if they differ in other ways.

This rationalist and intellectualist base, though dominant, has never been entirely uncontested, of course. Scholars from a number of disciplines, including economics, political science, and psychology, have challenged the assumptions about formal rationality that many economic-inspired models of decision making embody as being sufficient to understand the behavior of the market, the state, or the individual. Perhaps most famously, Herbert Simon (1957) introduced the notion of "bounded rationality" to account for those instances in which decision making is limited by particular contexts, where individuals must settle on less than ideal preferences. In the field of political psychology, Tversky and Kahneman have expanded on these ideas, arguing that individuals employ three heuristics when making judgements in conditions of uncertainty, even if these "shortcuts" "may lead to systematic and potentially severe errors" (Levy 2002, p. 271):

"(i) *representativeness*, which is usually employed when people are asked to judge the probability that an object or event A belongs to class or process B; (ii) *availability* of instances or scenarios, which is often employed when people are asked to assess the frequency of a class or the plausibility of a particular development; and (iii) *adjustments* from an anchor, which is usually employed in numerical prediction when a relevant value is available" (Tversky and Kahneman 1974: p. 1131 [emphases added]).

Others have generalized these concerns and, over the last fifteen years, critiques of the relevance of economic models for understanding the political world have gained in strength. In the mid 1990s, Green and Shapiro's *Pathologies of Rational Choice Theory* (1994) critiqued the ubiquity of rational choice approaches in political science, while also noting that many of these political theories had neglected to incorporate some of the important internal critiques leveled by economists and psychologists themselves. Renwick Monroe and Hill Maher (1995, p. 6) summarize the crux of the problem with applying economic ideas to the political realm:

the general assumptions underlying the economic approach to human behavior—the belief that human behavior can best be understood by assuming that people pursue individual self interest subject to information and opportunity costs—do not apply consistently enough once we enter the realm of the political. This means the market metaphor produces only limited explanations of political behavior . . . it encounters serious limitations whenever the technical foundation for the market does not exist in politics. Much political behavior falls into this category, precisely because most political acts are analogous to public goods, and all the conventional economic theories break down in the presence of public goods.

Others have shown that in the day-to-day rough and tumble of politics, large blocs of voters frequently support parties whose policies clearly work against those same voters' interests and that political rhetoric has effects that are not easy to predict using rationalist models (e.g., Fischer 2009; Marcus et al. 2000; Yanow 2000). Recent work in the field of sociology, psychology, and politics also has taken seriously the role that emotions play in structuring the terrain of collective action, and in moving beyond approaches that privilege structures of political opportunity or other "rational" features of the political environment (Flam and King 2005; Gould 2009; Jasper 1998; Lakoff 2008, Westen 2007).

Yet despite all these critiques, many influential theoretical traditions in political science have not fully incorporated these ideas and moved beyond these limitations. As Levy notes (2002, p. 271), rational economic models emerged as dominant paradigms in political science just as they came under close scrutiny from experimental economists, and they remain powerful currents even though they have been critiqued within and beyond the discipline. Recognizing the continued influence of rational actor perspectives is thus not to perpetuate an outdated bogeyman or "straw man." Rather, it is to underscore that, despite a variety of critical interventions, rational actor perspectives remain influential in political science and continue to define common interpretations and analyses of political events in ways that have limited how political science has understood and developed the concept of a placebo effect.

If we return to the question of a political placebo effect, we can see that its traditional definition reflects an assumption that political actors can be understood primarily as rational and narrowly self-interested agents. In the common journalistic usage, a political placebo is used consciously and cynically by one rational agent (the self-interested politician) to hoodwink another rational, but imperfectly informed, agent (the voting public). What is important to note is that in this usage, there is little recognition that the placebo itself has any effect other than "fooling" the electorate into forgetting about the issue and believing that it has been addressed. A political placebo, according to this view, is indistinguishable from snake oil: both are fakes that may trick the unwary consumer into parting with their hard-earned dollar or vote. Neither is viewed as having any real effect beyond that.

In contrast, we believe that political scientists should employ both the existing critiques of the rational actor model in the social sciences and the recent perspectives developed in neuroscientific and medical fields to redefine the concept of the political placebo effect. Moreover, we believe that it is useful to draw on the work of scholars who have challenged the sufficiency of rational actor models, highlighting systematic patterns of "non-rational" zones or tendencies in human decision making. For instance, Connolly (2002), Doidge (2007), Lakoff (2008), Rose (2007), and Westen (2007) have argued that we need to create a perspective that fully incorporates the fact that human decision making is, at its very core, an interaction of the mind–body complex combining emotional and "rational" calculation that cannot be heuristically separated.

What is novel about the perspective these authors bring (as compared to earlier critiques of rational actor assumptions) is not only that they suggest that political scientists expand their own theoretical toolkit to allow for the possibility that physiological phenomena can profoundly affect a wide variety of politically relevant thoughts (e.g., which ideas/concepts/language/values seem most persuasive) and actions (e.g., who we vote for, what we protest against). It is that these authors also suggest that this is true in reverse, as well: certain habitual thoughts or mental practices can stimulate and reshape physiological reactions, reshaping our preferences or actions in the process. Moreover, they argue that we need to establish new, creative sources and standards of evidence that reflect the complex nature of the mind–body interaction rather than simply reflect disciplinarily constructed (but ultimately contestable) norms of the dominant epistemological and methodological trends.

We therefore contend that the first step in a properly constituted conception of the political placebo effect is to challenge the limits of analysis prescribed by strict rational actor theories and instead embrace theoretical models that appreciate the complex interplay of mind and body. If we do not, the political placebo effect will appear as little more than the selling of snake oil, fakery, or a strategy to hoodwink the masses. We do not need more concepts or names for these types of practices, however. We should, instead, call them what they are—crude and conscious attempts to manipulate the voting public. In contrast, once we adopt a perspective that understands the mind–body interplay, we can conceptualize the political placebo effect as a situation where primarily mental stimuli (e.g., language, concepts, policy ideas) appear to have important effects *other than those that would be predicted by narrow rational actor theories.*

This, however, leads us to an important question. If a political placebo effect describes a situation that cannot be explained fully and/or clearly according to dominant dualist theories, and we do not believe that it can be dismissed as inexplicable and irrational, how do we "explain" and understand the ways in which political placebo effects function? How, in other words, does the placebo effect work? Here, a second characteristic of the most persuasive theories of the medical placebo effect is instructive.

14.3.2 **The meaning effect**

Returning to the medical context, a more nuanced understanding of the mind–body complex has led researchers to argue that scientists who want to understand the medical placebo effect need to better understand the mental context in which these phenomena are embedded. In this sense, a second characteristic of some of the most persuasive theories of the medical placebo effect in the scientific literature is the assertion that understanding the structure of meaning and expectations and "knowledge/authority" roles is crucial for understanding how, if, and when the placebo effect functions.

In this vein, we follow Dan Moerman's concept of the "meaning response" as an exemplary way to rethink the placebo effect (Moerman 2002, Chapter 7). Moerman suggests that we understand the placebo effect as being caused by the structure of meaning and expectations in which the administration of a placebo takes place. Importantly, his work implies that the structure of meaning and expectation does not necessarily even operate at the level of conscious or explicit awareness. An implicit and unquestioned faith in the goodwill, authority, and competence of a doctor, for example, is often crucial to the "success" of a placebo effect. By highlighting the fact that it is the normal case, and not the exception, in which "meaning" (e.g., conscious and unconscious psychological states of mind and thoughts) and physical responses are closely interlinked and co-constitutive, he allows us to understand the placebo effect not as something mysterious and random, but rather as something as predictable (or not) as other social phenomena whose emergence and effects are general but not universal, patterned but not uniform. Moreover, by explaining how the "reward circuitry" of the brain can help explain how expectations can have physiological effects, Enck et al. further help to demonstrate that many recent studies in neuroscience support Moerman's theory (Enck et al. 2008).

One of the implications of Moerman's theory is that researchers who are interested in understanding how the placebo effect functions will likely need to supplement their own theoretical and methodological frameworks (with their focus on direct, specific, physical, and chemical causation) with approaches that examine how conscious and unconscious structures of meaning profoundly influence the behavior of both individuals and groups of individuals. As researchers in the social sciences, this seems to open a particularly promising bridge between scientific and our own disciplines since the central focus of many scholars in the social sciences and humanities is to understand these types of questions.

In fact, many prominent theorists in the "human sciences" would be unsurprised that the so-called placebo effect is intimately connected to, and shaped by, meaning responses. Ian Hacking, the influential philosopher of science, has long argued that certain, socially recognized, roles and the types of meaning they produce, can have particularly important effects on our behavior. Scientifically and medically authorized classifications, labels, and discourses can affect the most profound levels of our self-conceptualization and behavior—as well as the ways in which others respond to us (Hacking 2000, p. 104). He calls subjects who are particularly caught up in these behavior-affecting classifications "interactive kinds" and suggests that they are "inter" actors and not just "actors" because of the complex interplay between the subject and the meanings that engender that subject. The "inter" reminds us of "the way in which the classification and the individual classified may interact, the way in which the actors may become self-aware as being of a kind, if only because of being treated or institutionalized as of that kind, and so experiences themselves in that way" (Hacking 2000, p. 104). This is what separates interactive behavior (which comprises much human behavior) from that of other phenomena studied by scientists. Interactive kinds differ from indifferent kinds such as quarks because "calling a quark a quark makes no difference to the quark" (Hacking 2000, p. 105), whereas dominant representations and discourse clearly help construct and limit public policy generally (Yanow 2000) and specifically. For instance, stereotyped representations of certain visible minorities as lazy has been shown to have demonstrable impacts on perceptions of public support for state social safety nets (Ingram and Schneider 2005, p. 8).

The impact of the embedded narratives and emotional factors can be great even in the most scientific of public policy issues—something evidenced by the controversies over the link between vaccines and autism. Despite the fact that the initial British study linking vaccines and autism has been widely refuted and retracted, many parents continue to question the safety of vaccines (Casiday 2007; Hobson-West 2003; Orsini and Smith 2010). As Hobson-West has noted (2003), the failure of public health authorities to manage vaccination fears stems from an inability to see beyond a rationalist, "information deficit" model that assumes that parents simply require reliable information (evidence) on which to base their decisions. In contrast, the vaccination case demonstrates that the meaning structure and emotional dimensions of scientific policy issues can be crucial dimensions that affect behavior.

In the context of research on the placebo effect, this perspective suggests that we need to examine more carefully the parameters of the meaning of roles, expectations, and discourses that are the meaning context in which the placebo effect occurs. Perhaps most importantly, the set of roles and expectations is characterized by a significant and explicitly accepted imbalance of power, knowledge, and authority. The person who administers the placebo is almost always a figure (whether a doctor or researcher) who is assumed to possess an expertise that is unimpeachable. Reinforced by a variety of symbolic contexts outside of the personal interaction itself (ranging from the use of medical jargon, symbols, and narratives which establish competence, specialization, and authority to the social expectations read into the architecture of a clinical space), the patient generally invests a significant amount of trust in the placebo provider and thus expects that the "treatment" will work. In this sense, it is not surprising that the areas where the placebo effect have been most consistently observed are those that are closely linked to "emotional" medical issues and situations in which self-perception is central (e.g., judgements about relative pain levels, degrees of happiness). Since these are often areas that are most closely linked to conscious conceptualization, it is reasonable that they would be most directly influenced by meaning structures. What impact any one element of the meaning context might have in any given situation—and how each is created—is an open question in placebo research, since few investigators have pursued aggressively the question of the meaning effect in this way. However, it seems clear that this should be an important avenue for future research.

What are the implications of this for our notion of a political placebo effect? Perhaps the most important point is that it highlights the need to understand the broad structures of meanings and roles—many of them implicit and taken for granted in our everyday experience—that form the crucial context for placebo-like political phenomena. Moreover, it suggests that it is unlikely that any single theory will provide a comprehensive answer to how every political placebo effect might function. While we might observe broad patterns and similarities, investigating political placebo effects will require a delicate combination of broad theoretical inspiration with careful empirical research of the specific events and their context. This suggests that researchers remain open to the diversity of social science and humanities theories and methodologies that seek to interpret and understand social structures of meaning and their impact on human behavior.

Given that many of the most pressing political issues are profoundly emotional, it also seems likely that a concept of the political placebo effect will be a valuable way of examining consistent patterns of political discourse and policy formation that, from a rationalist-tinged perspective, seem to be inexplicable and "irrational." The concept of a placebo is likely to be especially relevant to politics given the fact that scientists have observed not only placebo effects but also nocebo effects—situations in which patients demonstrate increased pain and negative pain outcomes in response to certain chemically inert, but mentally stimulating, interventions. Many of the most puzzling phenomena of contemporary politics concern the ways in which seemingly "excessive" negative emotions and attitudes are so easily, but inexplicably, intensified by political rhetoric.

Political parties wishing to elicit the support of voters feel compelled to tap into emotional landscapes of fear and anger—fear of the other as expressed in undocumented immigrants, anger over the ballooning costs of the welfare state and its "greedy" beneficiaries. Tapping into this wellspring of emotions can lead to demonstrable political gains even if the larger cause is not affected, even if the anger leads nowhere, is directionless, without purpose. In this sense, the concept of a political placebo effect might help us to better classify and understand these forms of emotional politics that can be corrosive for democracy.

14.3.3 The question of ethics

Central to most medical discussions of placebos are questions about the ethical stakes of placebos. Given the normative stakes of the study of politics, it is almost certain that the concept of a political placebo effect will inspire many questions about the ethics of political placebos, as well. While, as we have argued here, political science can learn much from the scientific and medical literature on placebos, we believe that a concept of political placebo effects will likely promote a series of very different ethical questions and analyses. Perhaps the best way to demonstrate this is to highlight some of the crucial differences in contexts between the two and then tease out some of their implications.

There is a strain of argumentation in the medical literature that suggests that placebo treatment plans are ethically defensible (Foddy 2009, Chapter 4). Taking this line of argumentation, the political analogy would be to suggest that using political placebo effects is also legitimate. It becomes apparent, however, that the types of assumptions that one can make about the clinical context are not easily transferable to the political realm. First, Foddy's argument is premised on the assumption that placebo practitioners are experts who *can* correctly diagnose and prescribe the best treatment and thus use placebos only once they have exhausted other options. This is not the case in the political realm. For example, the various selection filters and stages that characterize the path to political power do not necessarily select for and reward either expertise or competence. Rather, elected officials arrive with a wide range of relevant expertise and know-how that is appropriate to the job. Unlike scientists, they cannot claim the status of expert.

Second, Foddy's argument assumes that placebo practitioners *will* make decisions to use placebos only when they view it to be in the best interests of their patients. This is what makes most of us willing to trust doctors and accept a significant power imbalance of authority. This too differs considerably when applied to the political context. On the one hand, the relationship between public officials and citizens/voters is characterized by power asymmetries, or imbalances of power/knowledge. While this imbalance may appear to be more pronounced in the case of the doctor/patient (given the knowledge that physicians might have vis-à-vis their patients, not to mention their ability to shield themselves from patient scrutiny), in the world of politics, much of the "stuff" of decision making is also shrouded in mystery. Also in theory, elected officials have a duty to "serve" their constituents—which is why we seemingly trust our elected officials in the first place. In practice, however, citizens are increasingly realizing that this theory is far removed from reality. Elected officials do not take a Hippocratic oath when they enter office, nor is there a self-regulating and disciplinary body like the Canadian Medical Association to monitor political officials on any but the most egregious examples of ethical breaches of duty. While doctors sometimes act in their self-interest and disregard the patient's interests when diagnosing and treating a patient, these cases are largely the exception, and there are multiple levels and incentives within the medical system that are designed to guard against this. The political world stands in sharp contrast to its medical counterpart. In politics, the self-regulating institution is the political party, whose primary interest is to secure and maintain power, not protect the interests of the citizenry at large.

Another important difference between the medical and the political realm concerns the main unit of analysis. Foddy's argument is premised on the idea that a medical encounter can be reduced to the interaction between physician and patient (even if that encounter is mediated by the social context in which it takes place). Politics, in contrast, is almost never centered on the interests of a single individual. Rather, it is by nature focused on the ability of elected officials to aggregate a series of complex and diverging interests. Moreover, the success of elected officials usually depends precisely on how well they can reconcile these divergent demands—a task that usually means failing to address any single constituent's specific interests.

This context means that another assumption at the core of the ethical argument in favor of placebos is also problematic in a political context: that placebos are always safe-at worst they are merely inert, at best, they are positive. However, in the political world, they are not always safe. Since politics is about multiple interests and individuals, what might be a placebo for one person or group is a nocebo for another.

Finally, the argument in favor of placebos relies heavily on the idea that placebo-enabling deception does not vitiate the fundamental values of autonomy and truth so strongly that this would outweigh the positive clinical effects. This too is difficult to transfer into the political realm. Even if we agree with Foddy that there is no absolute duty to tell the truth and that one might be willing to accept being deceived if assured by an authority that she/he is acting in your best interests, these conditions are difficult to establish in the political environment. Even more importantly, however, the difference between a clinical context and a democratic political context is that self-governance is the first principle of democracy. As such, if deception is to be accepted as "ethical" in the political realm, it can only be in the most extreme of circumstances. In a democracy, access to the truth, and thus the ability to make autonomous decisions with reference to that information, is not a "nice to have" characteristic; it is absolutely essential.

This is not to say, however, that the opposite conclusion should be accepted— that it is clear and obvious that political placebos should never be viewed as ethical. Rather, we believe that the foregoing has demonstrated that the context (e.g., the questions posed and the stakes involved) governing the scientific administration of placebos differs radically from how we think about the notion of the placebo in the political context. At worst, this is an area where political thought will not be able to learn from the academic treatment of placebos in the scientific literature. At best, there is a need to specify some of the common theoretical assumptions underpinning our understanding of the placebo effect— in both the political and clinical environments.

14.4 The political placebo effect in practice

As previously mentioned, space does not permit a detailed exploration of the many ways in which this concept might help us to understand political phenomena. However, we think it is important to briefly illustrate its concrete relevance by using it to analyze two recent political events.

14.4.1 **Populist protest politics**

The emergence of the Tea Party movement—and its very concrete impact on electoral politics in America—has vividly demonstrated that neo-populist protest politics remains a force to be reckoned with in North American politics. It is interesting, however, that most analyses of this phenomenon often employ a series of rationalist presumptions to explain the existence and causes of these movements. Proponents of the movement attempt to explain it as rooted in deeply held logical principles and values (e.g., liberty, free enterprise, self-reliance, suspicion of government). In contrast, critics (even those as sophisticated as Thomas Frank) assume that the grassroots of this movement have been hoodwinked, fooled into privileging concerns about social issues such as abortion or same-sex marriage over what should be their defining economic self-interest. Both, however, assume that politics is best understood as "rational" (for even critiquing a movement as "irrational" presumes that there is a clear definition of political rationality that should be operative and that the cause of mass irrationality is clear, intentional manipulation).

If we employ the concept of a political placebo effect, however, other interpretations emerge. Consider, for example, the national debate in Canada in 2010 engendered by one of the doyennes of the American conservative neo-populist movement, Ann Coulter, when she visited Canada for a speaking tour. Scheduled to speak at the University of Ottawa, her organizers canceled the talk at the last minute, citing "security concerns" and claiming that the presence of more than a thousand protesters had meant that the police could not guarantee her personal safety. While these claims turned out to be false, it was the top story that night on each of the three main television networks and, in the week that followed the cancellation, no less than fifty articles, op-eds, and editorials condemning the events appeared in the largest twelve newspapers and media organizations in Canada. Articles dealing with the event were also often the most "commented upon" and "shared" articles of the online sites of those media outlets that week, indicating that the attention was not simply restricted to news editors but was also shared widely by the reading public.

Several things about this reaction were highly unusual. The breadth and duration of the media interest in this issue was notable as it embodied a level of attention that very few issues outside of highly controversial parliamentary bills or events usually inspire. It was also noteworthy that in their haste to express outrage, few media outlets bothered to question the "facts" of the case as outlined by the Coulter camp. Moreover, the emotional intensity of the condemnations was remarkable. As with the interpretations of the American Tea Party movement, Canadian supporters of Coulter tried to explain the outrage as a matter of justified, rational principle. Detractors, on the other hand, dismissed the anger as an inexplicably irrational reaction of people tricked by professional pot-stirrers looking for free publicity. Both interpretations are probably partially true.

However, are they the whole story? No. Instead, both of the dominant explanations leave us with more questions. Pure free speech, of course, is far from a universal and unconstrained right in North America, and yet one does not see nationwide editorials condemning libel laws, for example, which also censor speech. Clearly, this was not a political debate inspired purely by a rational issue of principle. Also, what of the idea that this was simply an emotional reaction of people tricked by manipulative puppet masters? Well, although it seems very clear that the persons involved consciously staged the event to garner publicity, this still fails to explain *why* people across the country became riled up about such a minor event. In other words, we are left with a puzzle. If it was not consistent principle, and it is not obvious why people could so easily be whipped up into an emotional frenzy over this, what explains the intense reaction?

Here, returning to the coverage with an eye to the concept of a political placebo effect is helpful. Recall that one of the key characteristics of the political placebo effect is the idea that there is a closer and more complex relationship between physiological and mental (especially emotional) processes than political scientists often assume. If one reads closely the media coverage, what is perhaps most surprising is the fact that almost all of it framed the issue in the same way. On one level, the vast majority discussed the issue with reference to the principle of free speech. However, the most intense anger expressed in the coverage focused on the idea that this was a selective cancellation by the administration of the university that was part of a larger bias against, and exclusion of, "conservative" ideas endemic to universities in general.

Why would this charge of bias and exclusion engender such an emotional reaction, even from media outlets that would not be easily categorized as "conservative"? One intriguing possibility comes from Geoff MacDonald's work (MacDonald 2010; MacDonald and Leary 2005; Nordgren et al. 2011). A psychologist at the University of Toronto, MacDonald suggests that a sense of social exclusion often generates intense feelings of distress. MacDonald and others hypothesize that this phenomenon has its roots in our evolutionary and developmental context—one in which social exclusion actually had a severe and negative impact on the chances of individual survival. Making this theory even more convincing is the fact that over the last decade, technological innovations have allowed neuroscience to discover that humans interpret and experience social exclusion, at least partially, using some of the same neural pathways used to experience physical pain. A sense of social exclusion—something that most political scientists would consider a purely conceptual and mental state—engenders deep feelings of distress because we actually *feel* it as pain in some sense. It is neither "rational" in the narrow sense that political scientists usually understand it (i.e., having to do with some sort of key good or value/principle), nor is it "irrational" in the narrow sense (i.e., being inexplicable or counter-productive).

If this helps to explain why the Coulter event "touched a nerve," as it were, it might also help us to understand why this distress was so strongly translated into self-righteous outrage. As Brian Massumi (1995) and others have argued, even emotions that are socially coded as negative (e.g., anger, sadness) can actually be experienced as pleasant by many people, especially if they are intense. In particular, outrage (alongside "schadenfreude") is often identified as one of those intense, "negative" emotions which nonetheless frequently makes those who experience it feel "good." If this is true, it helps to explain why the distress of social exclusion generated outraged responses. Perhaps outrage acts like a placebo by overwhelming and thus soothing the distress and pain of social exclusion. Even if it does not address the root cause or "change anything" (from the perspective of most traditional political science theories), it clearly has an impact on the emotional distress felt by those moved by the event.

If the first characteristic of a political placebo thus helps us to uncover a more complex explanation for the furore over the Coulter visit and cancellation, the second characteristic—the meaning effect—is similarly crucial. How is it that people across the country were so moved by this? Here, the idea that we always already act and feel within a web of social meaning—complete with archetypal plots, characters, moral lessons, and socialized emotional reactions—is crucial. The story that the media told about the Coulter cancellation relied on and reflected a narrative—deeply embedded in contemporary political marketing, reporting, and debate—that characterizes academics (among others) as snobby, leftist elites who are willing to use any means to silence opinions that run counter to their own. Without this widely shared and prior narrative, the specific events of that night could never have created such intense and widely shared distress and outrage. The meaning effect, in other words, is crucial for understanding why a minor scheduling change, made by the organizers themselves, and resulting from the poor logistical planning of the organizers, became a political firestorm across the country.

Finally, this case illustrates the ways in which the ethical dimensions of the political placebo effect differ substantially from the medical context. The use of outrage to salve a sense of social exclusion, while doing little to address the key issue of social exclusion itself, is significant because it feeds a larger sense of social and political alienation, cynicism and skepticism, and hyper-partisan polarization, all of which are not healthy for our democratic system. In this sense, the concept of a political placebo effect helps us to understand not only why this seemingly odd political event became such an issue but also why the ethical and political ramifications of the use of the political placebo effect are worthy of serious examination.

14.4.2 Harm reduction or immoral promotion?

A second example relates to the intensely debated Insite program, a Vancouver-based facility that allows injecting drug users to consume drugs in a safe and supportive environment where they can also access a range of healthcare services. The facility has been a lightning rod for criticism ever since it opened its doors in 2003. It has been operating under an exception to Canada's Controlled Drugs and Substances Act as the issue is, to quote one vocal critic, "punted around by the government of the day" (Montaner 2011).

Proponents of a harm reduction approach argue that safe injection sites are vital "pillars" of a comprehensive public health program to reduce the spread of HIV, hepatitis, and other infections. In addition, sites such as these help to reduce the number of deaths related to overdose. Researchers have produced numerous studies to demonstrate that investments in Insite make sound public health sense, and save taxpayers millions of dollars in healthcare costs, even if there is some disagreement about the actual estimates of those savings (see Bayoumi and Zaric 2008).

Over the last several years, however, the Conservative Party of Canada—as both a minority and majority government—has strongly opposed it. The former federal Health Minister, Tony Clement, once called Insite an "abomination" (Geddes 2010). A media investigation revealed, in fact, that the Royal Canadian Mounted Police (RCMP) had even commissioned a series of studies that were intended to attack the scientific merits of the numerous studies pointing to the positive public health effects of the safe injection site. Despite this, the RCMP had to acknowledge that the research conducted by the British Columbia Centre for Excellence in HIV/AIDS was scientifically sound (Geddes 2010)—a finding that apparently motivated Ottawa and the RCMP headquarters to cancel a joint press conference between the British Columbia Centre and the RCMP only a few days before the scheduled event. In 2011, the Supreme Court of Canada (SCC) unanimously upheld the province's right to fund and operate the facility and determined that the federal government could not prevent the facility from operating. Nevertheless, the Conservative government introduced legislation (the Respect for Communities Act) that would potentially be used to shut down safe injection sites. As such, the ultimate resolution of this issue remains unclear.

We believe that this controversy, too, might be productively understood as a political placebo effect for a variety of reasons. Here, however, we will only mention two ways. First, it helps us see that the political reaction to this public health issue is one that is deeply enmeshed in emotional, physiological responses, and that the meaning structure of already existing narratives and plots has significant effects on voters' perceptions of the issue. Particularly important here is the way in which the users of this service (so-called hard core drug users) are perceived. As Des Jarlais and his colleagues note (2008), drawing on psychological studies conducted by Harris and Fiske, deep emotional responses to particular groups help to explain the lack of support for policies that seek to reduce the harms associated with drug use. Harris and Fiske used neuroimaging to test the responses of participants to a series of images of social groups, including homeless people, drug addicts, and the elderly. They found neural evidence to suggest that some social groups are largely dehumanized in the minds of many, "at least as indicated by the absence of the typical neural signature for social cognition, as well as the exaggerated amygdala and insula reactions (consistent with disgust)" (Harris and Fiske 2006, p. 852). The ability to view drug users as less than human allows us to imagine that they make conscious choices to engage in self-destructive behaviors, and thus permits policy makers to treat them as unworthy of public sympathy or support.

Secondly, it helps us to remember that the meaning–emotion structure of the representations—in this case, moral frames—is crucial to engendering this effect. As has been shown by a variety of political theorists, most political and religious moral discourses have deep links in, and tend to evoke, disgust-based emotions (Connolly 1999, 2002; Miller 1997; Nussbaum 2004) and, as Des Jarlais and his colleagues suggest (2008, p. 1106), "within a disgust/dehumanization framework, effectiveness and cost-effectiveness are usually not important aspects of a program or policy. Rather, it is the congruency between the symbolic value of the program and the emotions of disgust, dehumanization and stigmatization that is critical." This, then, helps to explain not only why political opponents of Insite frame the issue as one of moral values rather than cost–benefit analysis, but also why that framing resonates with many voters who would likely otherwise never be so personally moved by this policy issue.

14.5 **Conclusion**

We have tried to think through how "exportable" and useful a concept such as the placebo effect is outside of the clinical realm. We have argued that drawing on recent medical, scientific, and social scientific language, it is possible to reconceptualize the political placebo effect in creative ways. Moreover, we have sought to demonstrate that such a concept allows us to interpret and understand diverse, concrete, political events in ways that depart from the explanations offered by many dominant theories in political science. As such, although only preliminary, we hope that our sketch has rendered plausible our contention that the concept of a political placebo effect is something worthy of further development.

Acknowledgement

This chapter was originally published as: Michael Orsini and Paul Saurette, "Take two and see me in the morning": reflections on the political placebo effect, *The Journal of Mind–Body Regulation*, 1 (3), pp. 125–137, © The Authors, 2011.

Notes

1 See, for example, the many studies cited and discussed in Raz et al. 2008. Some particularly relevant studies are Sherman and Hickner 2008; Nitzan and Lichtenberg 2004; Hrobjartsson and Norup 2003; Raz et al. 2009; Tilburt et al. 2008.

2 See, for example, the responses to Foddy's 2009 article in the same issue of the *American Journal of Bioethics*.

References

Bayoumi, A. M. and Zaric, G. S. (2008). The cost-effectiveness of Vancouver's supervised injection facility. *Canadian Medical Association Journal*, **179**, 1143–1151.

Brown, P., Zavestoski, S., McCormick, S., Mayer, B., Morello-Frosch, R., and Gasior Altman, R. (2004). Embodied health movements: new approaches to social movements in health. *Sociology of Health and Illness*, **26**, 50–80.

Casiday, R. E. (2007). Children's health and the social theory of risk: insights from the British measles, mumps and rubella (MMR) controversy. *Social Science and Medicine*, **65**, 1059–1070.

Connolly, W. E. (1999). *Why I'm not a secularist*. Minneapolis: University of Minnesota Press.

Connolly, W. E. (2002). *Neuropolitics: thinking, culture, speed*. Minneapolis: University of Minnesota Press.

Des Jarlais, D. C., Arasteh, K., and Hagan, H. (2008). Evaluating Vancouver's supervised injection facility: data and dollars, symbols and ethics. *Canadian Medical Association Journal*, **179**(11), 1105–1106.

Doidge, N. (2007). *The brain that changes itself: stories of personal triumph from the frontiers of brain science*. London: Penguin Books.

Dumit, J. (2006). Illnesses you have to fight to get: facts as forces in uncertain, emergent illnesses. *Social Science and Medicine*, **62**, 577–590.

Enck, P, Benedetti, F., and Schedlowski, M. (2008). New insights into the placebo and nocebo responses. *Neuron*, **59**, 195–206.

Fischer, F. (2009). *Democracy and expertise: reorienting policy inquiry*. Oxford and New York: Oxford University Press.

Flam, H. and King, D. (eds.). (2005). *Emotions and social movements*. New York: Routledge.

Foddy, B. (2009). A duty to deceive: placebos in clinical practice. *American Journal of Bioethics*, **9**(12), 4–12.

Geddes, J. (2010). RCMP and the truth about safe injection sites. *Maclean's Magazine*, August 20. Accessed at http://www.macleans.ca/news/canada/injecting-truth/.

Gould, D. (2009). *Moving politics: emotion and ACT UP's fight against AIDS*. Chicago: University of Chicago Press.

Green, D. P. and Shapiro, I. (1994). *Pathologies of rational choice theory: a critique of applications in political science*. New Haven: Yale University Press.

Hacking, I. (2000). *The social construction of what?* Cambridge and London: Harvard University Press.

Harrington, A. (2006). The many meanings of the placebo effect: where they came from, why they matter. *BioSocieties*, **1**, 181–193.

Harrington, A. (2008). *The cure within: a history of mind–body medicine*. New York and London: W.W. Norton and Company.

Harris, L. T. and Fiske, S. (2006). Dehumanizing the lowest of the low: neuroimaging responses to extreme out-groups. *Psychological Science*, **17**(10), 847–653.

Hobson-West, P. (2003). Understanding vaccination resistance: moving beyond risk. *Health, Risk and Society*, **5**(3), 273–283.

Hrobjartsson, A. and Norup, M. (2003). The use of placebo interventions in medical practice—a national questionnaire survey of Danish clinicians. *Evaluation & the Health Professions*, **26**(2), 153–165.

Ingram, H. and Schneider, A. (2005). *Deserving and entitled: social constructions and public policy*. Albany: State University of New York Press.

Jasper, J. M. (1998). The emotions of protest: affective and reactive emotions in and around social movements. *Sociological Forum*, **13**(3), 397–424.

Kihlstrom, J. (2008). Placebo: feeling better, getting better and the problems of mind and body. *McGill Medical Journal*, **11**(2), 212–214.

Lakoff, G. (2008). *The political mind*. New York: Viking.

Levy, J. (2002). Daniel Kahneman: judgment, decision, and rationality. *PS: Political Science and Politics*, **35**(2), 271–273.

MacDonald, G. (2010). *The pain of social dislocation*. Presentation at "Emotions under siege", University of Toronto, May 14, 2010. Available online at: http://www.humanities.utoronto.ca/streaming/file=media/public/serve/emotions_2.mp4&image=https:/media.library.utoronto.ca/stills/emotions_2.mp4sm.jpg.

MacDonald, G. and Leary, M. R. (2005). Why does social exclusion hurt? The relationship between social and physical pain. *Psychological Bulletin*, **130**, 202–223.

Marcus, G. E., Neuman, W. R., and Mackuen, M. (2000). *Affective intelligence and political judgment*. Chicago and London: University of Chicago Press.

Massumi, B. (1995). The autonomy of affect. *Cultural Critique*, **31**, 83–110.

Merrell, W. (2008). *The source*. New York: Random House.

Miller, W. I. (1997). *The anatomy of disgust*. Cambridge, MA: Harvard University Press.

Montaner, J. (2011). Dying for change on safe-injection site. *The Globe and Mail*, April 17.

Moerman, D. E. (2002). *Meaning, medicine, and the "placebo effect"*. Cambridge, UK: Cambridge University Press.

Nitzan U. and Lichtenberg, P. (2004). Questionnaire survey on use of placebo. *British Medical Journal*, **329**(7472), 944–946.

Nordgren, L. F., Banas, K., and MacDonald, G. (2011). Empathy gaps for social pain: why people underestimate the pain of social suffering. *Journal of Personality and Social Psychology*, **100**, 120–128.

Nussbaum, M. (2004). *Hiding from humanity: disgust, shame and the law*. Princeton, NJ: Princeton University Press.

Orsini, M. and Smith, M. (2010). Social movements, knowledge and public policy: the case of autism activism in Canada and the US. *Critical Policy Studies*, **4**(1), 38–57.

Polsky, D., Keating Weeks, J., and Schulman, K. (2002). Patient choice of breast cancer treatment: impact on health state preferences. *Medical Care*, **40**(11), 1068–1079.

Raz, A., Harris, C. S., de Jong, V., and Braude, H. (2009). Is there a place for (deceptive) placebos in clinical practice? *American Journal of Bioethics*, **9**(12), 52–54.

Raz, A., Raikhel, E., and Anbar, R. (2008). Placebos in medicine: knowledge, beliefs and patterns of use. *McGill Journal of Medicine*, **11**(2), 206–211.

Renwick Monroe, K. and Hill Maher, K. (1995). Psychology and rational actor theory. *Political Psychology*, **16**, 1–21.

Rose, N. (2007). *The politics of life itself: biomedicine: power and subjectivity in the twenty-first century*. Princeton, NJ: Princeton University Press.

Sherman, R. and Hickner, J. (2008). Academic physicians use placebos in clinical practice and believe in the mind–body connection. *Journal of General Internal Medicine*, **23**, 7–10.

Simon, H. (1957). A behavioral model of rational choice. In: *Models of man, social and rational: mathematical essays on rational human behavior in a social setting*. New York: Wiley.

Tilburt, J., Emanuel, E. J., Kaptchuk, T. J., Curlin, F. A., and Miller, F. J (2008). Prescribing "placebo treatments": results of national survey of US internists and rheumatologists. *British Medical Journal*, **337**(1938), 1–5.

Tversky, A. and Kahneman, D. (1974). Judgment under uncertainty: heuristics and biases. *Science*, New Series, **185**(4157), 1124–1131.

Westen, D. (2007). *The political brain*. New York: Public Affairs.

Wilce, J. (ed.). (2003). *Social and cultural lives of immune systems*. London: Routledge.

Yanow, D. (2000). *Conducting interpretive policy analysis*. London: Sage Publications.

Part 5

Concluding remarks

Chapter 15

Placebos as social constructs to elucidate human behavior

Amir Raz

15.1 Opening up the debate

This edited volume is a tribute to my co-author—student and colleague, Dr. Cory Harris. This writing project came about following a series of discussions with Cory in the Institute for Community and Family Psychiatry at the Jewish General Hospital in Montreal (Quebec, Canada). Once we started on the project, it was easy to facilitate this book through continuing conversations at McGill University, with national and international colleagues, and by reading and interacting with multiple experts—both scholars and practitioners. Together with Veronica de Jong, a graduate student in my lab, Cory and I were successful in getting some funding from the Social Sciences and Humanities Research Council (SSHRC) of Canada—the federal research funding agency that promotes and supports post-secondary-based research and training in the humanities and social sciences—to organize an international conference on the topic of placebos outside of medicine. Our SSHRC-sponsored conference, "Using social science to elucidate placebos: examining a powerful effect through a non-medical lens," took place in 2010 at the Jewish General Hospital and was an enormous success. By focusing on developing talent, generating insights, and forging connections across communities, SSHRC strategically supports world-leading initiatives that reflect a commitment to ensuring a better future for Canada and the world. This project was no exception.

We wanted the meeting to result in deliverables and the professionals at Oxford University Press took a quick look at our proposal and instantly recognized the value our contribution would make. Conference attendees wrote up an abridged account of their presentations and Cory gradually took charge of this production and has made the entire transition—from student to colleague—all within the process of compiling this book. He is now an independent researcher at the University of Ottawa and I am very proud of his achievements and academic prowess.

The long route this edited volume has taken over the years spanned the arrival of two children by Cory and one by me. Thus, three children and several years later, we are proud of this compilation and the contribution that it makes to the field. Cory taught me a great deal about the domain of placebo research and I am grateful to him for his dedication and persistence in connection with this writing project.

15.2 **The potential of placebos**

Placebos are undoubtedly relevant in medicine, but they are no less relevant outside of the medical sphere—as part of our social existence. Within medicine, scientific understanding of the neurobiological mechanisms of placebo effects and placebo responses is beginning to come together. However, most of our knowledge predominantly draws on findings from the field of pain and analgesia and hardly generalizes to other domains. The placebo effect represents a promising model that could potentially shed new light on mind–body interactions. Moreover, because the mental events instigated by placebo administration can trigger mechanisms similar to those activated by drugs, psychosocial and pharmacodynamic influences appear similar in their potential to impact physiology. Neurobiological insights into placebos guide our conception of clinical trials and shape our overarching views of medical practice. Outside of medicine, placebos play a role in education, parenting, social interactions, political science, food consumption, and just about any aspect of higher human behavior. This book opens an incipient lens to whet our appetite with the social aspects of placebos in our lives.

15.3 **The social role of placebos**

In the medical literature, a discussion of placebos may read something like this:

> Congruent with the working definition assumed in the high-powered world of pharmacology, most people construe placebos as the non-specific effects of medical treatment that researchers in clinical trials must control in order to assess the specific effects of new drug interventions. Placebo-like treatments, accordingly, refer to any short-term or illusory impression of improved health that some patients experience when they receive what appears to be effective and ethical treatment (but actually is not) for the condition they have.

Instead, in this book, our discussion of placebos reads something more like this:

> Congruent with common knowledge, most people construe placebos as the effects that scientists should examine in order to assess the effects of new interventions. Placebo-like interventions, accordingly, refer to any impression of improved performance that some individuals experience when they receive what appears to be appropriate help, that may actually be specious, for the situation they are in.

The difference between these two texts is hardly subtle. Moreover, in this volume, we expound on why placebos play a substantial role in our social world and interactions therein.

The placebo effect is a powerful mind–body phenomenon with a specific underlying mechanism that social scientists, beyond health professionals, should investigate and appreciate. Exemplifying the link between psychosocial factors and physiological processes, placebos are central to understanding human behavior. Furthermore, beyond the life sciences, placebos bind biology and clinical practice to the techniques and domains of social research: transcultural studies, psychology, anthropology, sociology, and phenomenology—to name a few. This placebo trip has been an exciting one, and we are just at the beginning of the ride. We hope you have enjoyed it as much as we have.

Index

Notes: *vs.* indicates a comparison or differential diagnosis, *f* indicates a Figures and *t* indicates a Table.

Notes

Notes

Notes

Notes

Notes

Notes

Notes

Notes

Notes

Notes

Notes

Notes

Notes

Notes

Notes